MASSAGE

a career ——
at your fingertips

SECOND EDITION

The Complete Guide To Becoming A Bodywork Professional

MARTIN ASHLEY

ENTERPRISE PUBLISHING

Published by Enterprise Publishing
P.O. Box 167
Mahopac Falls, NY 10542

Front Cover photograph courtesy of Le Centre D'Epanouissement Psycho-Corporel, Quebec, Qc, Canada

courtesy of Bancroft School of Massage Therapy, Worcester, MA
All other illustrations by Lorrie Klosterman
Cover design by C. Kim Design, Tucson, AZ
Typesetting by PDS Associates, Allenhurst, NJ

Library of Congress Catalog Card No. 95-090077

Library of Congress Cataloging-in-Publication Data

Ashley, Martin
   Massage: a career at your fingertips : Martin Ashley. -- 2nd
ed.
   p. cm.
   Includes index.
   ISBN 0-9644662-0-1

   1. Massage--Vocational guidance. 2. Massage--Practice.   I.
Title.

RA780.5.A75 1995   615.8'22'023
                                      QBI94-21337

Printed and bound in the United States of America

Contents

III: Sex, Gender and Touch

IV: Business, Practical and Legal Information for the Practitioner

This book is dedicated in loving memory of my father

Sam Ashley

Acknowledgements

I want to thank my friend, Doug Brodeff, who gave me the idea to write this book. I also extend my gratitude to Pete Whitridge, who took the time to read the manuscript and give me many helpful criticisms and suggestions. Thanks also to Kathleen Bennett for proofreading the text.

In addition, the following massage and bodywork practitioners all contributed to the writing of this book by allowing me to interview them, or by furnishing useful information about reference material.

Thank you all.

Paul D. Arneson
Lauren S. Bain
Kathleen Bennett
Ann W. Bertland
Wes Boyce
Gordon E. Bradford
Alberto Breccia
Iris Brown
William T. Bunting
Sharon Callahan
Robert Calvert
Norman Cohen
Karen E. Craig
Paul Davenport
Jo Anne Davies
Patrick Dempsey
Doug Deyers
Bob Fasic
Adeha Feustel
Andre Fountain
A. Ann Gill
J. Joy Gottus
Roy Gottus
Ruth R. Haefer
Susanne Setuh Hesse
Pamela Hodgson
Stuart Holland
Sita Hood
Shirley Hooker
Jeff Hopkins
Jeffrey Kates

Bob King
Apara Kohls
Shivam Kohls
Scott Lamp
Mae Leone
Glenn Lloyd
Jerrine F. Manders
Charles Mardel
Maureen A. Miller
Artie Mosgofian
Ginann Olmstead
Grieg A. Osmundson
David Palmer
Cindy Patterson
Laura Perna
Anna Pekar
Chad Porter
Cate I. Rainey
Deeta Rasmussen
Kay E. Richey
Dennis Simpson
Timothy Starbright
Christiana Stefanoff
Bruce Stephens
Kathy Tanny
Debbie Thomas
John "Shane" Watson
Dana S. Whitfield
Sherri Williamson
Carl S. Yamasaki
Etelka M. Zsiros

Introduction
Who This Book Is Written For

When I was embarking on a massage career, there was no source to turn to for information about the field, educational programs, and equipment. That was 1982, and a lot has happened since then.

My idea in creating this book was to provide you with everything you need to know to consider, plan and execute a career in massage or bodywork. This book will not only help you decide whether to get into the field, but will guide you to the best massage or bodywork school for you, and help you make the choices that bring you a rewarding career. No other source contains the information you can find in this volume.

For the novice:

For someone contemplating a massage or bodywork career, this is truly one-stop-shopping for all the essential information you will need.

For the massage student:

If you are already enrolled in a massage school, this book will expand on your school's courses in business, law, ethics and marketing. It will also provide you with information to use as you plan your career and during the first several years of your career in massage.

The practical information about professional associations, professional politics, career strategies, advanced trainings, marketing, taxes, laws, and sample forms will be useful to you for a long time to come.

For the practitioner:

If you are already a trained and practicing massage therapist or bodyworker, you may still find much of value in this book. The sections on marketing and taxes may give you much useful information. You may also be interested in advanced training programs, schools teaching different modalities, and requirements for practice in states you might move to.

You may also want to have this book in your library for the time when an aspiring massage therapist asks you how to get started in the field.

Browse the table of contents and see if you aren't interested in learning more. And whether or not you choose to enter the field, enjoy...

Introduction to the Second Edition

The First Edition of this book was a ground-breaking endeavor. No book had before been written that catalogued massage schools, bodywork trainings, equipment suppliers and laws, and also provided a career guide for massage and bodywork practitioners. The warm reception received by the First Edition has encouraged me to commit the time and energy needed to compile this Second Edition.

The information closing date for the First Edition was June, 1991. This edition's closing date was January, 1995. The growth in the massage field in just those 3½ years has been phenomenal. 190 U.S. massage schools were listed in the First Edition. This one lists 316. In 1991, the two largest massage professional associations had a combined membership of 18,500. Today these same organizations have a combined membership of over 39,000.

Curricula have expanded and schools have grown. So many more offerings are available now that it made sense to create a list for each bodywork technique of massage schools where that technique is taught. (See Bodywork Organizations and Trainings, page 173)

Over 14,000 massage practitioners have taken the National Certification Exam, which had not even been created in 1991. Six states and the District of Columbia have added massage regulation since the last edition. These new laws are summarized on page 122.

Chapter 3, which deals with current professional and political issues, has been re-written to take into account recent developments, and Chapter 11, "Working with Survivors of Childhood Sexual or Physical Abuse" is new.

The growth in the massage field shows no signs of slowing. I'm honored that, through the vehicle of this book, you and I can participate together in creating the future of the profession.

I

An Overview
of the Profession
&
What It Takes
to Succeed in It

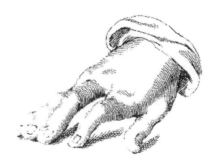

1 Is a Career in Massage for You?

Massage can be a delightful career. Your clients regard you as the person who gives them relaxation, helps relieve their pain, and assists then in improving their health. You have freedom to set your own schedule, and can earn a good living with a clear conscience.

Massage can also be a frustrating career. You have great skills and desire to help, but clients are not calling, bills are piling up, and a client has asked you for sex at the end of a massage. You may wonder whether the whole thing is worth the effort.

If you are considering pursuing a career in massage or bodywork, it is worth your while to spend a little time now examining what lies ahead and whether it is what you want. You will find information throughout this book that will help you get a fuller picture of what it is like to be a massage professional. However, certain pros and cons should be set out at the start.

First item: Money.

Many people are lured to the idea of a massage career by some simple arithmetic. The local massage therapist is charging $55 per hour. Eight hours a day times $55 per hour comes to $440 per day, or $2200 per week. Eureka! How can I get into this!?

It is true that there are *a few* massage therapists whose economic picture is like the one in the last paragraph, but they are the exception and not the rule. The vast majority of massage professionals have a very different story to tell. And it has been my experience that those who enter the field *for the purpose* of making a lot of money are not happy in the field. They either do not succeed in massage, or become so absorbed by their desire to succeed financially that they are basically unfulfilled human beings even though they earn large amounts of money.

The people in the field who are financially successful *and happy* are those who got into the field out of a sincere desire to help other people, who have good skills and who have the determination necessary to achieve success.

Second item: Drive and motivation.

What massage has in common with other professions — such as law, medicine and accounting — is that the professional has to attract a following, a clientele, in order to earn a living.

True, there are limited circumstances in which you can work for an hourly wage or on commission, but these situations are usually regarded as "entry-level" positions, or situations in which you can gain experience before you are truly established in the field. Jobs where some person or institution brings you a clientele are seldom well-paid jobs; your employer will often take up to 50% (or more) of the amount paid for your services.

Therefore, to succeed in the long run, you will need to establish yourself as an independent professional with a substantial client base. Every client is an individual who could choose any massage practitioner, but chooses you because of what you have to offer. To be worth choosing and to be well-known and respected take time, dedication, and organization. Know before you begin that this is the path you are choosing for the long run when you choose a career as a massage therapist.

Third item: Commitment.

From reading just this far, you are getting the idea that massage is not a field you just drift into and easily start making money. You can get started more easily if you have substantial experience in a related hands-on therapy field, or a solid reputation in your community. Otherwise, you can expect that during your first couple of years after massage school you will have a limited income from massage, and will be spending a fair amount of time promoting yourself in an attempt to become established.

Therefore, make a commitment to your massage career. If you approach the field in a mature way, it will be a rewarding choice for you. However, if you approach it with a half-hearted commitment, you will likely flit from place to place without staying long enough to reap the reward of the seeds you sow.

Making a commitment to your career means making some commitment to a place. That is not to say you must settle down in the first place you practice massage, but ultimately you should make a pledge to yourself to spend at least three years in a location as a massage therapist. If you don't take that step, you don't do justice to your chances to have a successful career in the field.

Still interested?

If none of this scares you off, you probably have a good chance of making it as a massage therapist. Other chapters will provide you with strategies and techniques that will enable you to minimize your frustration and maximize your success as a professional. If you are making the decision to undertake a career as a massage professional, may I extend a warm welcome to you, and a wish that you enjoy all the ups and downs and in-betweens that await you...

2 The Massage and Bodywork Field
Its Time Has Come

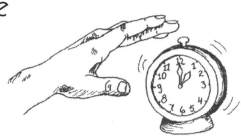

Massage is an ancient art that is having a period of tremendous new growth. Many types of massage have been developed, and many types of closely and not-so-closely related therapies have evolved in recent times. In an attempt to clarify this sometimes confusing picture, I offer the following discussion of massage and definitions of various terms.

What is massage, anyway?

In one sense, the term "massage" deserves to be many words, because one word cannot be stretched enough to include the various therapeutic techniques practiced by people who call themselves massage therapists. Consider these categories:

- **Wellness massage,** for preventative general health;
- **Sports massage,** for training, preparation and recovery from exertion during sporting events;
- **Relaxation massage,** to remove the results of stresses of daily life;
- **Pain relief,** to relieve muscle soreness, minor injury pain, headaches, or the like;
- **Personal transformation massage,** to explore emotional or psychological issues or to produce shifts in consciousness;
- **Medical massage,** as an adjunct to medical treatment for illness;
- **Rehabilitative massage,** for recovery after physical injury such as broken bones;
- **Chiropractic adjunct,** to enhance the effectiveness of chiropractic adjustments;
- **Pampering (or beautification) massage,** to provide a sensuous, pleasurable indulgence or as an adjunct to beauty services.

"Bodywork" and massage

Confusing the matter still further, many people also include "bodywork" in the term massage. Such hands-on therapies as shiatsu, Trager, Rolfing, polarity, and the dozens of other forms of bodywork now available are sometimes referred to under the umbrella term "massage," especially in the Western United States.

In order to make the information in this book easier to organize and use, I have drawn a distinction between "traditional" massage, and other newly-formed kinds of hands-on therapies. With apologies to those who prefer a definition of "massage" that includes a broad spectrum of bodywork styles, I have settled on the other, perhaps more conservative, definition.

In this book, the term "massage" is used to mean traditional "Swedish" massage, or systems very much like it. Swedish massage is characterized by the five strokes effleurage, petrissage, friction, vibration and tapotement. Other systems that work with the body are called "bodywork." The following definitions are offered for clarification.

Definitions

Please note: There are no "official" or widely accepted definitions of the terms "massage" and "bodywork." These definitions are offered to clarify the meanings of these terms as used in this book.

Massage. The application of touch by one person to another, using manual techniques of rubbing, stroking, kneading or compression (effleurage, petrissage, vibration, friction or tapotement), when done to produce relaxation, pain relief, injury rehabilitation, athletic preparedness or recovery, health improvement, increased awareness, or pleasure.

Bodywork. The application of touch by one person to another, to produce relaxation, pain relief, injury rehabilitation, health improvement, increased awareness, neuromuscular re-education, or pleasure, using any techniques other than those used in massage (see definition of massage, above). Bodywork does not include chiropractic, osteopathy, or any other system which has an organized licensing structure and grants the title "doctor" to its practitioners. (See the Bodywork Organizations and Trainings Directory starting on page 173.)

Massage Practitioner. Any person who publicly offers massage in return for money.

Massage Therapist. A massage practitioner who has received training in the theory and practice of massage, and is competent to use massage as a means of promoting pain relief, injury rehabilitation or health improvement.

Bodyworker. Any person who publicly offers bodywork in return for money.

The following definitions clarify the meaning of several words used in the above definitions:

"Compression" does not include static pressure applied to one spot (as in shiatsu and trigger point therapy), but does include pressure that increases and decreases or moves along the body, such as tapotement and friction.

"Health improvement" includes mental, psychological, emotional and spiritual health, as well as the health of the body's immune system, or any other system of the body.

"Pleasure" means the enjoyment of the sensations in the body, but does not include sexual arousal or stimulation of sexual organs.

Recent growth of massage—factors involved

In 1960, the average American had one of two associations for the word "massage." It was thought of either as a prelude to sex or a health club rub-down, heavy on the "karate chops." These images still remain for many people, especially older people whose experience of massage has been one or the other of these types. However, the last 35 years have seen tremendous growth of legitimate, therapeutic and scientific massage. Today, massage is more and more being looked to as a conventional treatment for stress and as a tool for emotional and physical health.

Several societal trends have facilitated the rediscovery of the ancient art of massage. The hippie movement in the 60's, and related consciousness-raising activities, opened doors for massage as a tool for self-exploration and personal transformation.

The explosion in fitness activities during the 70's and 80's brought acceptance for massage as both a wellness modality and a sports training aid. This acceptance of massage by the general public has allowed the development of on-site, or seated massage. Seated massage has gone into the workplace, the shopping mall, storefronts, airports, street fairs, health fairs, and many more locations. It has been a major factor in making the general public aware of the benefits of massage, and making it more available to a mass market.

Among the current factors helping the expansion in massage therapy to continue are the efforts of several companies that are doing mainstream marketing of massage therapy (see page 154), and the Touch Research Institute. The Touch Research Institute, under the guidance of Dr. Tiffany M. Field, Ph.D., has been conducting scientific experiments to demonstrate the health benefits of massage. The Institute conducts ongoing research in a number of subject areas, publishes reports in scholarly journals, and distributes a newsletter, Touchpoints, which keeps readers abreast of their work (see page 169).

As a result of all this growth, massage schools have proliferated, the membership of massage organizations has skyrocketed, and in short order massage is changing from a service for the wealthy to a service accessible to the general public.

The change is happening at a different pace in different places. In some parts of the West coast, massage has been popular for so long that there exists a surplus of massage therapists. In contrast, many remote or rural locations still have very little activity in the massage field. However, in the vast majority of places in North America, large numbers of people are just now learning the benefits of massage, and most areas are seeing a steady, even dramatic rise in the popularity and availability of massage.

What does the future hold?

People have been doing massage for thousands of years. Massage was something people were doing before surgery was ever performed, before science was even conceived. It has lasted these thousands of years because it is good. Much like gold has been the investment of choice throughout much of history because of its inherent value, massage is a part of human culture that has stood the test of time because it has real value for people.

Because massage is a service with inherent value for people, it does not need to have a market created for it in order to be in demand. Instead, massage is naturally in demand as soon as people release the artificial barriers they have against using massage services.

People's barriers to massage

These barriers are 1) anxiety about nudity and about one's own body, 2) fear of making contact with another person or oneself, and 3) a belief that spending money on oneself is indulgent or wasteful.

These are significant barriers, but they are the sort of things people tend to outgrow. The more sophisticated our society becomes, the more irrelevant these barriers will seem to the general population. The general societal and scientific acceptance of massage will help these barriers continue to come down in the years to come.

Another issue is affordability. The 1980's saw an increase in income for many, and facilitated the growth of massage in part by creating a larger group of people who could afford it. Price is a factor for many people. The economy will play a role in how widely massage is accepted, and the profession can aid the growth of massage by not pricing itself out of reach of most people.

Finally, the payment for massage services by insurance companies, if widely available, would open a whole new market for massage services. A large number of potential massage clients will receive massage only if it is covered by their medical insurance policy. Currently, insurance reimbursement plays a minor role in the overall picture of massage therapy. Whether that will change in the near future is one of the topics touched on in the next chapter.

3 Current Professional and Political Issues

This is a very lively time in the life of the massage and bodywork profession. If you liken the massage field to a growing person, it is currently an adolescent on the verge of young adulthood.

The 1960's saw the birth, or re-birth of massage as a sophisticated profession worthy of widespread acceptance in society. The 70's and 80's and early 90's were a time of phenomenal growth, and a time when the profession as a whole went in many different directions looking for a sense of identity, or for its personality. Massage expanded into many different contexts, and related forms of bodywork grew up by the dozens.

Now the profession has some sophistication, some muscle, and a lot of energy. It also has internal conflict, an evolving self-image, and an unfinished picture of its role in society. The next few years will add maturity to the field, and will continue the profession's transition to "adult" life in the next century.

The purpose of this chapter is to set out the main political and professional issues currently confronting the industry. Understanding this information may not be essential to your career as a massage or bodywork practitioner, but you might find it helpful to have a broad understanding of the political issues in your chosen field. Some of this information may help you decide which school or schools to attend, and which association or associations to join. Participating in the political process in your chosen profession may also help you avoid unpleasant surprises in the future.

What is at Stake in Political Issues?

The following scenarios are drawn from real-life experiences. Most massage practitioners will not experience the problems indicated by these examples, but some will. These scenarios are meant to alert you to a few of the real-life situations that create some of the motivation for governmental regulation of massage and bodywork:

- You have a successful private massage practice. One day, your mail carrier delivers a certified letter from the State Board of Physical Therapy, ordering you to cease and desist practicing massage unless you can prove that you have a license to practice physical therapy or chiropractic.

- You want to move to a new state, but on investigation, you learn that your educational training is considered inadequate under that state's licensing law, and you must attend school at a massage school in that state and then take that state's licensing exam.

- You are working with a car-crash victim who could benefit from massage therapy. She asks you "are your services covered by my medical insurance?"

This chapter will give you an overview of the current political situation and some of the conflicting views that are being advanced, and will suggest some directions for progress in the future.

Governmental Regulation of Massage

Massage is the newest member of the group of regulated professions. Dentists, doctors, psychologists, nurses, lawyers, physical therapists, and chiropractors, among many others, have all gone through the process of establishing procedures to regulate who can and can't practice the profession. That regulation process has begun in the massage and bodywork field, but is far from over.

At present, 19 states have laws regulating massage. The requirements in those 19 states are different from state to state. Texas, for example, requires 300 hours of educational training. Oregon requires 330 hours. Several states require 500 hours. Ohio requires 600, New York 605, New Mexico 650, New Hampshire 750 and Nebraska 1000. Some of these states have licensing, two have certification and two have registration. Some use the National Certification Exam as their written test, others do not.

The 31 states without regulatory laws require *zero* hours, and do not restrict the practice of massage. Although some municipalities and counties in those states regulate massage, most practitioners in those 31 states do not have to answer to anyone.

Why regulate the practice of massage and bodywork?

Why not just let people do what they want, and let the free marketplace take care of who succeeds and who fails? Some believe that's the best approach and for that reason oppose governmental regulation of massage.

Proponents of governmental regulation put forth several arguments in favor of governmental regulation of massage:

First, the public deserves protection.

When a state agency regulates the practice of massage, they maintain a hearings board or grievance board to consider complaints by members of the public about how they were treated by a practitioner. In this way, the profession gives the public a quick and easy remedy against a practitioner who is incompetent or unethical. This inspires trust and confidence on the part of the public and enhances the respect of the entire profession.

If there is no agency regulating massage in a state, it is much harder for an injured party to get satisfaction from the practitioner who injured her. The only remedy available is to hire a lawyer and pursue a lawsuit, which is usually a very lengthy, traumatic and expensive undertaking.

Second, state licensing protects the massage profession from other professions that claim *they* are the only ones with the right to do massage. Physical therapists in Maryland are trying hard to restrict the practice of all massage therapists in that state. They have instituted legal proceedings against massage therapists, charging them with practicing physical therapy without a license. Similar challenges have taken place in Oregon and the District of Columbia. State regulation of massage prevents this kind of headache — the state, by regulating the field, ensures the right of massage practitioners to practice.

Third, governmental regulation of massage helps greatly in getting rid of those who offer sexual gratification as part of a massage. Where massage is regulated by the government, there is a quick and easy process for suspending the license or registration of one who is unethical. However, where massage is not governmentally regulated, the only remedy against unethical practitioners is the criminal justice system, which is notoriously slow and inefficient. Therefore, in areas where massage is not regulated by the government, it is much harder to stop those who offer sexual massage.

Finally, some believe that state regulation of massage encourages mainstream society and the medical profession to take massage practitioners seriously. The desire for acceptance as a mainstream health care provider has been an undercurrent in the licensing and certification debate for a number of years. The effect of governmental regulation on this issue is unclear, however, since there are places where unlicensed practitioners receive insurance reimbursement, and there are places where licensed practitioners do not.

Why Some Oppose Attempts to Create State Regulation

A few people are against governmental regulation on principle — some people are suspicious of government and don't want any outside authority taking control over their lives.

Others oppose regulation because the situation in the practice in their location does not need improvement. Perhaps the profession is well-established, unlicensed practitioners are able to receive insurance reimbursement, and there is no lack of respect and acceptance for massage and massage practitioners. Governmental regulation adds expense, burdens and restrictions. If there is no problem to be solved by regulation, then regulation is unnecessary.

However, most of the attention that is paid to the issue of governmental regulation of massage does not concern whether or not licensing is a good idea in principle. The major controversies arise because of *the way* in which the attempts to enact licensing laws are sometimes made.

Specifically, some groups within the massage profession keep legislative proposals secret, propose legislation without consulting the majority of practitioners in the state where the law would be in force, and propose legislation that favors the members of the group sponsoring the legislation, as opposed to considering the interests of all practitioners in the state.

Many groups are interested in the outcome of legislative efforts. However, the two largest national professional organizations have some of the strongest interests concerning these issues. These organizations, the AMTA and the ABMP, sometimes have different ideas about how the licensing process should proceed. From published articles and editorials about licensing issues, the following seems true of the current situation regarding attempts to create governmental regulation for massage:

The AMTA (American Massage Therapy Association) often initiates attempts to create new state licensing, but does not necessarily advocate licensure for every state.

The ABMP (Associated Bodywork and Massage Professionals) is not against licensing, nor is it against the AMTA, but it opposes unilateral attempts to impose massage licensing without input from the majority of practitioners who will be affected by the law.

Both organizations have programs whereby they accredit or approve the curriculum of massage schools. The AMTA's approval/accreditation program is based on a prescribed 500-hour educational standard, and has been in operation for a number of years. The ABMP's approval/accreditation program was created in 1995, and as of press time, the ABMP's standards for program approval/accreditation had not been finalized.

Membership in AMTA requires 500 hours of educational training, with a prescribed curriculum. Many members of ABMP, IMA, and other professional organizations have education of 500 hours or more, as do many massage and bodywork professionals who are not members of any professional organization. Others, however, have less than 500 hours of education, or have education from schools with curricula different from AMTA's established educational standards.

For example, the great majority of California's massage schools offer less than 500 hours of training. Therefore, many individuals in that state practice massage professionally with educational training of 100 hours or 200 hours. These people are concerned that they would be forced out of their chosen profession if the state were to adopt licensure based on a 500-hour standard.

Currently, the ABMP is maintaining a network to alert practitioners about attempts to enact laws regulating massage. The ABMP's goal is to be included in the process of formulating the law, so the law will be responsive to all groups within the profession. In some states, AMTA representatives have invited the members of other groups to join in a coalition to formulate legislative proposals acceptable to all.

Licensing, Certification and Registration

These terms can be confusing. They do not mean the same thing. In order to properly understand the political issues in the massage and bodywork field, you must understand the differences between these three terms. Once you read the following, their meanings will come clear to you.

First, ask yourself this question: Does the term apply to what a government is doing or what a private group is doing?

Governments can create any of the three kinds of regulations mentioned — licensing, certification or regulation.

When a government requires a *license* to practice massage, then practicing without a license is a criminal act. The license law sets out the requirements for obtaining a license and establishes a procedure by which qualified individuals can apply for a license.

When a government *certifies* practitioners, that is usually a voluntary procedure that carries some benefit. For example, in Maine, certified practitioners may use the title "Massage Therapist" and non-certified practitioner may not. In Delaware, certified practitioners are exempt from the "Adult Entertainment Law" but non-certified practitioners fall under its authority.

When a government *registers* practitioners, they generally do not restrict the practice, but keep track of practitioners by requiring them to submit certain information to the government. However, Texas requires registration as a mandatory condition to practice massage, so registration operates much the same as a license in that state.

Private groups can give *certification*. They cannot give a license or registration. Private groups that give certification are giving an individual their official approval, or are certifying that the person has completed specified requirements for certification.

While certification of a private group is never a legal requirement to practice massage, some forms of bodywork are protected by trade-name or service-mark protection. As to those forms of bodywork, permission from the owner of the name is required to use that name in connection with your work.

Now that you know this much, you are able to understand how the National Certification Exam fits into the picture.

This is a standardized written test that is created by a private group (not by a government). However, it has been adopted as the *written exam* by governments in ten states that regulate massage: Connecticut, Florida, Iowa, Louisiana, Maine, Nebraska, New Mexico, Rhode Island, Washington, Utah.

These states have other requirements, such as educational requirements, licensing fees, and sometimes character references. However, in these states the government has chosen to adopt the National Certification Exam as the written exam for state regulation of massage.

Those states that require the National Certification Exam as their written test do not require individuals to comply with other aspects of National Certification, such as continuing education. Once an individual passes the test and obtains a state license, the individual's subsequent activities regarding National Certification are not of interest to state licensing authorities.

Therefore, the National Certification Exam is kind of a hybrid — part private certification, part governmentally-required exam. The history of the creation of this exam is the subject of the next section.

A Brief History of the National Certification Exam

During the late 1980's, the AMTA announced its plan to create a voluntary, nationwide certification exam for massage. It was initially to be an AMTA project, and was to be a Swedish massage certification exam. Although the exam was to be voluntary, many therapists became concerned that it would nonetheless become a practical requirement, since the goal of the exam is to standardize the qualifications of professional massage therapists.

Some non-AMTA massage therapists became resentful that a standard was being created without their input, which could damage their ability to earn a living. Some were angered that this action was being taken without consultation with any industry leaders outside the AMTA.

In the wake of this initial controversy, some organized attempts at reconciliation took place. A series of "Head, Heart and Hand" conferences, or "summit meetings" took place in an attempt to secure some unity among the different groups on the scene in the massage profession.

In the course of these meetings, the AMTA explained that it planned to make the certification project separate from the AMTA. The newly formed certification project had been funded by a loan from the AMTA, and seven of the nine original members of the steering committee were AMTA members. These connections to the AMTA caused some non-AMTA members to believe that the project was still an arm of the AMTA.

After the exam had been created, the steering committee was dissolved and replaced by the National Certification Board, which now administers the test. The National Certification Board is incorporated as a separate entity in the state of Virginia, and Board members are elected by mail ballot from all nationally certified practitioners. The Board has a stated commitment to cooperate with the AMTA toward mutual goals, although it is administratively independent from AMTA.

The National Certification Exam certifies basic competence in massage, and does not test for competence in any specific area of practice, such as sports massage, medical massage, shiatsu or the like.

The exam is administered twice per year. It was first administered in June 1992, and as of January 1995, over 14,000 practitioners had taken and passed the exam. To date, the overall pass rate is approximately 94%, with a pass rate of 90% on the most recent administration of the exam in November 1994.

To be eligible for the exam, a practitioner must have completed 500 hours of education in massage or bodywork. Professional experience can substitute for a portion of the educational requirement. The exam covers anatomy and physiology, clinical pathology, massage assessment and technique, business practices and ethics. Continuing education is required to maintain certified status, but not to maintain state licensure in states that use the test as their written exam.

Suggestions for the future

For the immediate future, it seems that individuals and organizations that are concerned about licensing will continue to work out their process state by state. I would like to offer a slightly broader perspective that could be a goal for the industry to aim toward.

That is the idea of *specialized credentials* for massage therapists and bodyworkers.

The idea of a basic, or entry-level credential for massage and bodywork is receiving a lot of attention. State licensing and the National Certification Exam both aim to assure basic professional competence and to confer professional status to the practitioner.

In the years to come, additional states may adopt the National Certification Exam, and other states may create licensing that uses a different written exam. In either case, the trend in licensing laws seems aimed at a 500-hour standard. This amount of training is enough to provide entry-level competency in massage. However, 500 hours is probably not enough to provide training both as a massage practitioner and also as a specialist in a particular branch of massage, such as medical massage.

The next issue for the profession to address is the creation of unified *specialty* certifications. Medical massage seems to be an ideal candidate for unified specialty certification.

With forms of bodywork that are protected by trade-name or service-mark protection, the owner of the name performs this function by requiring that certain standards are met before an individual is allowed to use the name, such as "Rolfer" or "Trager Practitioner."

Providing a specialty certification for massage specializations will let the public know who is properly trained, and will give mainstream society some way to judge the qualifications of a practitioner who claims to be an expert in a particular field. If there were a unified medical massage credential, it would be much easier to convince hospital administrators and physicians to use massage as a healing modality for medical patients.

The great challenge, as with national certification, is to foster dialogue among all the practitioners and educators so that a unified credential is created that appropriately represents the specialty.

Massage in the United States has come a very long way in the last thirty years. The profession is on the verge of stepping into a mainstream role in American life. You, as a practitioner, will have the power to help shape how that takes place, and unless you participate in the process, you will give others the voice to speak for your future on these important career issues.

II

Career Options,
Strategies
and Tactics

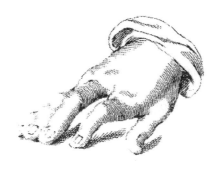

4 Your Career in Massage or Bodywork
Let's Get Organized

A surprising fact is that most massage school graduates never create a massage practice that supports them financially. They either never make an organized effort to practice massage professionally, or they give it a try but abandon their efforts before they achieve a successful practice.

The purposes of the chapters in this section are:

1. To help you gain clarity about what it is you want from your professional life in massage or bodywork.

2. To help you make a sensible plan for achieving your goals.

3. To help you follow through on that plan with a minimum of wasted effort and a maximum of success.

Common misconceptions

Many would-be massage therapists have certain wrong assumptions about the paths their careers will take. One very common expectation about a massage career goes like this:

> I will attend massage school, where I will learn everything I need to know to be a successful massage therapist. When I finish school, I will set up a practice. Clients will come to me and I will be busy and happy.

Several misconceptions are evident in this scenario. First, massage school will not teach you everything you need to know, either about giving a good massage or about operating in the business world. In fact, you should look at your first 1,000 professional massages as completion of your education as a massage therapist. Your skill level and confidence level will grow for years to come.

Second, you probably will not be in a position to set up a practice right out of school. Unless you have a very good reputation in the community, it will take time and effort to build your reputation sufficiently to establish a clientele.

Third, clients will not come to you just because you make yourself available. If you get yourself an office and say "Here I am, world!" the world will respond with a deafening silence. In order to be a busy massage therapist or bodyworker, you will need to take organized, affirmative steps to let people know you are there and make them want to take advantage of your services.

Finally, being busy and being happy are not necessarily the same thing. You want to attract those clients that most suit you. Even when you do not have enough work, there are still clients out there whom you do not want to have. Your clients will be a significant part of your life when your practice is going, so take the time to attract a clientele you will enjoy serving.

Typical career paths

In imagining what your career will be like, and taking logical steps to reach your goals, it will help you to have the benefit of the experiences of those who have walked the path before you. Numerous interviews with successful massage therapists and bodyworkers have disclosed many common elements in their career paths.

Below are capsule versions of the careers of some actual massage therapists and bodyworkers. Some are more successful than others. All are earning their sole livelihood at massage or bodywork.

"A" started his career in massage when he had a wife and a baby and was very poor. His wife was very supportive. During the early years, he did very little else to earn money, except some painting work for Christmas money. He chose this approach so that he would be fully immersed in the profession and would be forced to overcome any obstacles. It took two years to achieve a steady client load. After four years, he was so busy he was turning away clients, and now travels with world-class athletes to international sporting events.

"B" went to massage school, then went traveling in Asia for 15 months. On his return to California, he found he was seriously depressed. After three months of depression, he pulled himself out of it and began working at a health spa and promoting himself locally, working out of his home and doing house calls. Newspaper coverage of him and his Asian trip helped his practice grow, and within eight months, he was doing upwards of 20 massages per week. His business is growing, yet he plans to spend only one or two more years in the area before moving on to some other location.

"C" had a marketing background, and when she graduated from massage school, used newspaper ads, coupons and flyers to gather a practice quickly. She worked out of her home in San Diego, and had 10 to 15 clients per week within a month of starting her marketing program. After two years, she got out of massage completely, finding she was "fed up" with dealing with men who were asking her for sexual favors. She currently works as a receptionist in a wholistic health center.

"D" opened a store-front massage office in Chicago right out of massage school. She did a great deal of personal promotion in the neighborhood. Almost all of her clients in the early days were men, many of whom presented her with requests for sex. Her husband supported her financially for the first few years, and despite aggressive promotion, it took about three years for her practice to reach a profitable level, especially in light of the very high rent she had to pay for a corner store-front business location. After four years in practice, she is seeing 20 to 30 clients per week.

"E" did massage for about five years as a hobby, accepting donations, before ever attending massage school. He has been out of massage school eight years, and does 6 to 15 massages per week. The slow growth of his practice and his current pace of activity are exactly to his liking.

"F" spent quite a few years not succeeding in the massage field. He worked as a physical therapy assistant for three years, and also tried to establish a massage practice in a hair salon. Then he "took some time off" from the profession. He returned to the profession and became involved in his state massage associations. He became active in the AMTA and went into practice with a prominent sports massage teacher and practitioner. His massage practice reached full capacity within three months of starting in this office, and he has since taken on a significant leadership role in the AMTA.

"G" had 10 years experience as a swimming trainer and worked as a case manager in a chiropractor's office while she attended massage school. She did some massage in the chiropractor's office for a few months after graduation. A cardiologist who had heard of her invited her to rent an office in his tasteful, downtown practice building at a very reasonable rent. She accepted, and once there, she was able to work on some very influential community members who spread the word about her skills. Within three months of moving to the cardiologist's office, she had a thriving practice.

"H" started out in the field as a new mother, and very poor. She was always moving from one home to another in search of cheaper rent. Her main priority was to be very good at her work, and it took her several years to begin to earn a living at massage. She has now been in practice 10 years, specializes in pregnancy massage, and works at a birthing center. She sees 15 to 20 clients per week, most of whom are regulars. She would welcome having more clients.

"I" made a point of having non-massage work that supported her when she began her massage career. She was concerned that if she were financially needy, clients would sense that neediness and be put off. Instead, having her financial needs met, she could approach her clients with warmth and openness. Within one and a half years, she was seeing 20 clients per week, and only then did she quit her other job. She has kept her practice at that level ever since.

"J" did house cleaning at the beginning of her massage career to meet expenses. The first year brought only enough massage income to pay expenses such as office rent and supplies. After fifteen months, she was earning enough from massage to stop doing cleaning work. After 18 months, her client load was 10 to 15 per week.

"K" was a public school teacher. She started gathering a practice during after-school hours, and as the practice grew, she switched to substitute teaching, and eventually was able to let go of substitute teaching, and be a full-time massage therapist. The entire process took four years, which was longer than she thought it would take. She currently sees 15 to 20 clients per week.

"L" has a practice as a polarity therapist, which she took six years to build. For the first year, she kept her job as a university teacher, and saw one to three clients per week to decide if she wanted to pursue polarity more seriously. For the next three years, she held a consulting job two days per week, and built her polarity practice up to about six clients per week. She currently sees 12 to 15 polarity clients per week, teaches four yoga classes per week, and markets her own yoga instructional tapes.

"M" opened a practice in the town she grew up in immediately after finishing massage school. During the next two and a half years, she worked in at least six different locations in and around the area, gaining experience and slowly gaining a client base. She then opened an office in a charming, wealthy seaside resort town a few miles away. She coordinated this new office with a direct mail promotion and a public speaking engagement. Within weeks of moving, her practice doubled, and within two months she was seeing 30 or more clients per week.

"N" worked for four years as a physical therapy assistant and sports therapist before going to massage school. She has been supporting herself with massage work during the first year after massage school, doing house calls and working in a chiropractor's office doing massage for $14 per hour. Her goal is to be a physical therapist.

"O" worked full-time for AT&T, and practiced massage in her off-hours, doing house calls in an affluent community. After about one and a half years, she left her job and went into massage full-time. She went to work in a hotel health spa to supplement her practice, and has a busy practice.

"P" went to massage school after several years in practice as a lawyer. After graduating from massage school, he took a job teaching law, and did one to three massages per week on the side. He did this for three years, and then set out to establish a massage practice in a new location where he knew very few people. It took two years for the practice to produce enough income to meet his living expenses. He used some of his spare time to work on a book about the massage profession. After three and a half years of practice, he is seeing between 12 and 20 clients per week.

Elements these career paths have in common

The experiences summarized above display several elements that are repeated in more than one story. Consider the following:

- Those who had substantial experience in a hands-on field before going to massage school became established massage therapists much more quickly than those who had no such experience.

- For those without such prior experience, the average time needed to establish an income-producing practice varied quite a bit, but two years was about average. Some made it in a year, some took three or four years. Those taking longer than four years probably were not making an organized attempt to become established.

- Attempts at rapid growth through advertising tend to bring sexually-oriented male clients.

- It appears to take longer for most men to become established massage therapists than it does for women.

Main causes of career failures

The two main ways in which would-be massage therapists sabotage their careers are moving too often, and being reluctant to promote themselves.

As you can understand from reading the career capsules above, success as a massage therapist comes only after a period of building a reputation in the community. The two essential elements in this process are 1) doing things to become known and 2) giving the process some time.

Recent massage school graduates are often very unsettled. Perhaps you are "in transition", having moved away from home to attend massage school, and not knowing where you want to settle to start a new life. Perhaps you are living in your home town, and you are apprehensive about becoming established, for fear that if you acquire a successful practice, you will never leave your home town and see the world. Perhaps you do not have confidence in your ability to give a professional massage.

If you are in such a situation, or in a similar situation that makes you unsure or reluctant about becoming established, you have at least three logical approaches you can take:

1.   **The side-step.** Do some other kind of work to earn a living, and do massage on the side. This will give you the opportunity to see if you really enjoy massage work, and will give your skills a chance to slowly improve. It also will give you time to become better known in the community. If and when you decide to move to full-time massage work, you will have a stronger local reputation.

2.   **The trial balloon.** Take any job you can get doing massage, such as working in a health club, resort, spa or chiropractor's office. These jobs will give you substantial experience doing massage, will give your skills a chance to grow, and may yield some contacts that can lead to a different job opportunity. While the pay usually will not be high, you retain the opportunity to leave town without sacrificing any time and energy spent in reputation-building.

3.   **The leap of faith.** Act as if you have decided to stay in town for awhile. Commit yourself to staying for two or three years and take some steps to build a clientele.

If you don't know where you'd rather live, and you can't figure your life out, there is a good chance that three years from now you will either be right where you are now, or will move to a new place and still not be sure what you want to do. If you decide to take a stand wherever you are now, you may find that any major issues in your life are just as easy to wrangle with while you build a massage career as they would if you moved somewhere else or did something different.

The golden keys to career success

Having discussed what holds some people back from succeeding in the field, what is it that generates success for those who succeed? There are four keys to success in this field, and all four are indispensable. Imagine them like the four legs of a table. If any of the legs is short or missing, the table is not of much use.

The four golden keys to success in this field are:

Location   Personality   Skills   Desire

Location. You might be the greatest massage therapist on earth, but if you are in a town filled with people who cannot afford your services, or who have overwhelming resistance to trying massage, you will not do well.

Location refers also to the part of town your office is in. Neighborhoods have characters, as do streets, as do individual buildings. The character of the surroundings seeps into people's attitudes about you and your office.

Personality. Your clients are not simply coming to you for a physical treatment. They are coming to you for your presence as well as your skills. They may come in for work on the body, but it is the whole person who decides whether to come back for another massage.

Not only should your clients feel completely comfortable in your presence, they should look forward to coming to see you as a chance to be with you for an hour. Successful massage therapists develop personal, often warm relationships with their clients.

Skills. You need to have the ability to do a good treatment. The client must feel better leaving than coming in. The client must also feel there is some good reason for choosing your therapy over the competition.

In short, whatever type of massage or bodywork you practice, you need to know what you are doing and do it well. This can mean not just education, but experience. Your skills as a massage therapist will improve throughout the first few years of your massage career.

Desire. Consider whether you whole-heartedly want to succeed in your practice. If not, what is it that is holding you back? Your deepest and most honest desires deserve expression. If you honestly want to be a professional massage therapist, you will focus your efforts efficiently and effectively.

Do your best to look inside and discover what you really want from your massage career. If you have reluctance to really put yourself in the public eye and build a clientele, ask yourself why, or talk it over with a trusted friend. Understanding yourself is a valuable asset in making choices that will bring you a career you can really enjoy.

How do you rate yourself on the Four Golden Keys?

Re-read the four golden keys to success. This is the most important information in this book. If you embark on a massage career with a significant weakness in any of these four areas, you should understand that you need to work on this area in order to become successful. Before you put yourself through any needless hardship, consider very carefully your assessment of yourself and your career.

Make a commitment to strengthen your weaknesses

If any of these four keys is missing or deficient in your assessment of yourself, make a commitment to yourself that you will work on this area. Here are some suggestions for how to improve.

Location. Do some research about the town, neighborhood and building you are planing to be in. Find out about the residents' income and standard of living. Find out how well any massage therapists in that area are doing.

Generally speaking, it is more difficult to be the only massage therapist in town, because that indicates there is no established massage clientele in that area. On the other hand, if you are the first and only practitioner in an area, you will have a secure professional foundation once you do become established.

Imagine the best neighborhood, street and block for your massage office. What other businesses are on the street? What is the look of the neighborhood? Imagine yourself as a client coming to this office. Is it difficult to get to? Is it on the way to other places you may want to go? As you come onto the block and into the building, what thoughts do you have? How do you feel?

Coming to your office is what every client will do at the start of your sessions. Evaluate the experience of coming to your office, and make sure you choose a location that makes coming to see you a pleasant and comfortable experience.

Personality. If you have an abrasive personality, make a commitment to yourself to soften it. If you are shy, make a commitment to yourself to be a little more outgoing so you can put your clients at ease.

You yourself enjoy being around people who are caring, accepting, warm and easy-going. These traits are important for the massage therapist. If you are too talkative, judgmental, sarcastic, crude or angry, these traits will tend to discourage your clientele and make it difficult for you to become established.

Of course, you cannot become someone you are not. However, you can choose to suppress the aspects of your character that would interfere with your career. Remember that the tongue often acts as a sword, so when in doubt, say less rather than more.

Skills. Understand that your skills will continue to grow for years to come. Take continuing education workshops, and professional trainings. Get massage often, not only to feel good but to learn from the skill of others. Continue to grow psychologically as well, as growth and maturity will lend their own added value to your manual skills.

Look for opportunities that match your skill level, and understand that your fees will rise with your skills and reputation.

Desire. Take steps that are consonant with your true desires for success — don't reach for the stars if you heart is not in it. You may not be ready for success today. If you are not ready, don't struggle — do something else for awhile and do massage on the side. When you have the desire that fosters organization and commitment, it will be much easier for you to get started in this profession. Be honest with yourself about what you want.

Weaknesses can be worked into strengths if you have the commitment to do so. These are the keys to success in your career. Use them well.

5 Career Options in Massage

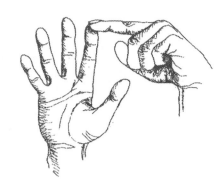

This chapter's purpose is to expose you to the broad range of options for the kinds of massage work you can do, the types of clients you can work with, opportunities for self-employment, and what you can expect in various employment situations.

Kinds of massage, types of clients

The six categories described below pretty much cover the field of massage at the present moment. Each of these types of massage attracts its own type of client, and requires its own set of skills on the part of the practitioner. You might practice several of these types of massage, but in most cases you will not practice more than one or two types in any one location.

1. Relaxation/stress reduction. The most common kind of massage, relaxation or stress reduction massage includes the types of treatments common in resorts, spas, private offices and clients' homes. This category would also include wellness massage, or preventative health massage.

2. Sports massage. This rapidly growing field encompasses athletic training massage, and massage designed to help an athlete prepare for competition and recover from competing.

3. Medical massage. Working by prescription, or in a hospital, or in a physical therapist's office, the medical massage therapist works with pathologies, pain or recovery from injury. Medical massage can also be adapted to a non-medical clientele, and practiced in a home or office setting.

4. Chiropractic adjunct. Working in chiropractors' offices is becoming more and more common, especially on the West coast. Some practitioners operate relatively independently from the chiropractor, with a cross-referral agreement. Others work by prescription of the chiropractor, working on specific parts of the body that the chiropractor designates.

5. Psychotherapeutic massage. Some massage therapists focus on shifts in awareness and psychological insight that can be brought about with massage. These therapists often work by referral from

psychotherapists, and usually work out of a private massage office. They often combine another form of bodywork with massage.

6. Pampering. Probably a branch of relaxation massage, pampering refers to the type of treatment that might be found in some spas and hair salons. This treatment is usually thought of as more of a beautification treatment than a health treatment, and might include salt glows, loofa rubs, and light Swedish massage.

Settings for the practice of massage

The following are locations where massage is currently practiced. Some of these locations are traditional locations for massage, and the arrangements establishments make with massage therapists are fairly uniform. Others are not so well established, and the arrangements may vary from place to place.

In general, the more the owner of the location provides in terms of linens, booking service and client base, the less she or he will expect to pay the massage therapist. If the location has a built-in clientele, such as a resort, the owner will usually take at least half of the fee.

At the other end of the spectrum, if the massage therapist brings additional business to the location, or adds a sense of uniqueness to what the location has to offer, the owner may make a very favorable deal with the massage therapist, on occasion even allowing the therapist to retain 100% of the fee.

Health clubs. Home of the "rub down" in the old days, health clubs are increasingly being staffed by well-trained massage therapists, who may practice relaxation massage or sports massage.

Some clubs will hire a therapist for an hourly wage, usually between $6 and $10 per hour. Some give an hourly wage plus a small percentage of the price of the massage, and some offer the therapist anywhere from 45% to 100% of the price of the massage.

Generally, clubs where the massage therapist has to cultivate the clientele will offer the therapist a larger percentage of the proceeds. Clubs where massage is an established part of the routine, especially where there are two or more treatment rooms, will usually pay less to the therapist, since they are supplying the clients.

Common disadvantages of health clubs are relatively low pay, noisy environments, and clients who may not have a sophisticated understanding of the value of massage.

A major advantage of health clubs, especially for newly trained massage therapists, is the chance to get lots of experience in a short period of time. If your health club will allow you to bring outside clients in, it can also serve as an office location for you while you develop a private practice, and this can be a substantial advantage.

Spas and resorts. Many of the same comments that apply to health clubs apply to spas and resort facilities. The pay tends to be low. La Costa, an internationally-known spa near San Diego, pays massage therapists around $7 per hour. The

Hilton hotel in Long Branch, New Jersey has a beautifully equipped spa, and pays its massage therapists 45% of the price paid by clients. However, the more elegant the location, the more likely the massage therapist is to make good tips.

The therapist in a spa or resort usually does not need to supply anything. The massage room will be equipped, and the spa or resort will do the bookings. The clients are supplied for you, but since they are vacationers, they seldom will become repeat clients for you in your local practice. They will be repeat clients only if they come back to the spa or resort again.

Spas usually have clean, comfortable and quiet massage rooms, and the clients are there for vacation or healthful relaxation, so their mood is usually conducive to enjoying a pleasant massage experience.

Hair salons. There are no reliable generalizations to make about the practice of massage in hair salons. Sometimes the service offered is a pampering-style light Swedish massage, and sometimes it is expert massage therapy.

Some salon owners expect a large percentage of the proceeds or a fixed monthly rental from the massage therapist, and some offer more reasonable arrangements to the therapist. It may depend in part on whether the salon owner sees the massage therapist as bringing new business or prestige to the salon, or simply relying on the salon's established clientele.

The salon owner will often offer a "day of beauty" or "day spa" experience which includes a massage, usually a half-hour full-body massage. The price of the package will be discounted, and the salon owner will usually expect the massage therapist to offer her services at a discount for the day of beauty clients.

Common disadvantages of practicing in hair salons are noise, noxious odors, and an approach to massage as a "pampering" or beautification service. Advantages include a strong clientele for referrals (in an appropriate salon) and an atmosphere in which massage stands out as a unique service.

Cruise ships. Again, few generalizations are possible. Working conditions and pay can vary a great deal from ship to ship. Cruise ship massage jobs are very difficult to get unless you have a contact in the cruise ship industry. Once you are known to those who do the hiring, however, it may be easy for you to find work on a ship, as schedules are often changing, and companies are often looking for experienced massage therapists to fill in on relatively short notice.

In looking for massage employment on cruise ships, writing to the cruise line generally does not produce any positive results. The hiring may be done through a separate company, or through a franchised health spa. Even the published guides for cruise ship employment do not provide much help with massage jobs for cruise lines. Here, more than anywhere else, it is necessary to "know someone" who has contacts within the cruise industry.

On-site or chair massage. On-site, also called seated massage, or chair massage, is a fast-growing part of the massage industry. October 17, 1989 was the date the Wall Street Journal ran a front-page story about on-site massage, and its growth has accelerated ever since. On August 15, 1990, the Associated Press carried a photograph of an on-site massage session being given to a customer waiting in line at the new McDonald's in Moscow.

When practiced in the workplace, the practitioner usually offers a ten to fifteen minute massage to the employees. Sometimes the company hires the practitioner and provides the service as a fringe benefit, and sometimes the employees pay individually for their massages. Currently, other locations for seated massage are gaining in popularity, such as shopping centers, airports and store-fronts. Seated massage can be used as a marketing device when done at fitness fairs and craft shows.

The type of treatment done is often a shiatsu-like treatment, done in a specially designed chair that supports the client's chest and face, exposing the back and shoulders.

There are two ways to approach on-site — as a practitioner, or as an entrepreneur. As with other forms of massage practice, the hardest part of the job is acquiring a clientele. In this case, that means convincing a corporate executive that your services would be beneficial to his or her workers, or arranging some other setting for a practice.

Once you have a contact to perform services in a workplace or other location, you can perform them yourself, or hire others to do so. If you establish a large number of clients, you can keep yourself and others busy, often making a percentage profit on the work done by those you hire.

Chiropractic offices. Especially in California, business relationships between chiropractors and massage therapists have become quite common. Chiropractors typically employ massage therapists to work in the chiropractor's office. The chiropractor most often prescribes massage for his or her patients, handles the insurance billing procedure, and pays the therapist either a commission or an hourly wage.

Some chiropractors pay the therapist 50% of the amount charged for massage. Some pay 50% but require the massage therapist to pay a monthly rental out of the therapist's 50%. Those who employ therapists at an hourly rate often pay in the neighborhood of $15 to $20 per hour.

Chiropractors have traditionally had great reluctance about prescribing massage for their patients. Some clients enjoy massage much more than chiropractic, or believe they benefit more from massage, and choose to stop going to the chiropractor and go to the massage therapist instead.

Chiropractors combat this by having the massage therapist in their office, and prescribing massage so that insurance reimbursement will cover the cost. The client sees massage as a no-cost added benefit of chiropractic care, and therefore has an added incentive to keep coming to the chiropractor.

The chiropractor not only gains a unique service to offer, but makes a large profit, since chiropractors can bill massage services to insurance companies at far more than they pay the massage therapist (in the neighborhood of $80 per hour). The massage therapist, usually a recent massage school graduate, has a way to make a living wage and to gain a great deal of professional experience quickly.

The massage/chiropractic relationship varies greatly from state to state. In some states, like California, New York and Virginia, no restrictions exist on practice relationships massage therapists and chiropractors may enter into. In other states, some barriers do exist. Maryland and New Jersey chiropractors have all received a letter from their state boards advising them that only chiropractors can perform massage services in a chiropractic office, disrupting established relationships between chiropractors and massage therapists.

Hospitals. Hospitals equipped with massage therapists are rare today, although some pioneering hospitals are incorporating massage therapy as part of their healing approach. One writer estimated in 1993 that 50 U.S. hospitals had one or more massage therapists working in some capacity with patients. (*Massage* Magazine, March/April 1993)

The acceptance of massage in these hospitals is usually the result of a good working relationship between doctors or administrators at the hospital and educators or practitioners in the massage community. The exchange of information and ideas in personal and professional relationships brings about the possibility of establishing a program by which the hospital offers massage to its patients.

Making massage more available to hospital patients would be a morale booster, would be a great public relations advantage, and could even result in shorter hospital stays by helping strengthen patients' immune systems. However, this may be an area of practice that will remain undeveloped until enough standardization takes place in the massage profession to make the medical profession comfortable with massage as a credible therapy.

Those who wish to work in hospital settings or who want additional information about this area of practice may want to contact the Healing Healthcare Network, or subscribe to their newsletter. Healing Healthcare Network is an association of organizations committed to developing healthcare that heals as well as cures. Contact the Healing Healthcare Network at P.O. Box 339, Brighton, CO 80601, (303) 659-2446.

House Calls. If you talk to massage therapists about house calls, you will find that most therapists either love them or hate them. The majority seem to hate them. I personally love them.

All of the massage therapists I have talked to who hate house calls charge only a few dollars more than they charge for studio massage. Those who love house calls generally charge 40% to 50% more for a house call than for a studio massage.

Clients expect house calls to cost more. If your price is $50 for a studio massage, consider charging $75 for a house call. Another method of pricing is to start with your basic fee for massage; add $5 for carrying and setting up your table, and add 50 cents per mile for your commuting fee.

House calls have several advantages. First, there is no office rental to pay. Second, the higher fee includes compensation for your time in driving to and from the client's home. It's nice to be paid for driving time, especially if your body is feeling the effects of a busy massage schedule. Third, the client usually finds it easier to fit a house call into their schedule, and may have an easier time relaxing at home than she or he would in an unfamiliar environment. Finally, you get to visit lots of people's homes, many of which are quite interesting.

Certain disadvantages exist as well. First, you have little control over the environment. You can turn off the phone ringer, but the kids might cry, the dog might bark, the room might be cramped and it might be too hot or too cold.

Second, people dawdle more at home than they would if they came to your office. They will take a phone call, or someone will come to the door, or they will be late getting home. It is not uncommon for a one-hour massage to extend to an hour and twenty minutes. Add commuting time, and you might spend well over two hours doing a one-hour massage.

Third, carrying the massage table in and out of the car, in and out of the house, and up and down stairs can be tiring. It helps tremendously to purchase a carrying case with side handle and shoulder strap.

The real beauty of house calls comes when you can establish yourself in a community, so that you have enough business to go from one house call to another, thereby reducing your commuting time. Another advantageous situation is the couple, each of whom wants a massage. Some therapists do house calls exclusively, and when they become established can make a very good living.

Suggestion: Keep your oil bottle in a zip-lock plastic bag when traveling to avoid messy leaks and spills.

Office in your home. Home massage office practice has major advantages and major disadvantages. The advantages are fairly obvious—no commute and complete control over your massage environment. One disadvantage is the increased vulnerability of your home because of contact with the public. Another is that some zoning boards prohibit massage as a home occupation, fearing either that you will conduct a prostitution service in you home or that your business traffic will disturb the neighborhood.

A practitioner operating in a home office must have all the permits and licenses that would be necessary for any massage office. However, some communities will not issue a permit for a home massage practice, even though they would issue a permit to a dentist or psychotherapist in the same location.

In communities that refuse to permit massage practices in the home, some practitioners simply keep a low profile and hope they do not get caught violating the law. It is a shame that professionals are required to do this, but it results from local government officials who believe that massage equals prostitution. Consider organizing the home practitioner massage therapists in your town and trying to work through the governmental process to get the zoning restrictions changed. If you choose this option, consult your professional association for guidance and support.

The challenge in a home office is to create a professional massage environment. This means no dogs barking, no music or television sounds wafting into the room. It also means keeping your massage environment separate from your living environment, and if possible, having a separate entrance so that clients do not have to walk through your living space to get to the massage room. If there is no separate entrance, the massage room should be the first or second room one comes to on entering the house.

If you are going to base your business in your home office, treat it as professionally as you would any other office space. Charge the going rate, have a separate phone line, and create the ideal massage room. Your efforts to create a professional atmosphere are just as important in a home office as in any other office you practice in.

Group Practice. Joining in practice with other massage therapists or other health practitioners can be a great way to share expenses, generate cross-referrals, and create a sense of community in which each member draws support from belonging to the group.

The disadvantage that is most often reported by members of group practices is that everyone shares the responsibility for making decisions that affect the group, so there is a need for regularly scheduled meetings in which everyone must participate. This can be time-consuming, and can take lots of energy, especially when it comes in the middle of a busy week.

Some group practices hire a receptionist, and others use the group members to answer the phone on a rotating basis. A receptionist is a substantial expense that has to be split among the practice members, so sharing phone duties substantially lowers the overhead. However, if the practice is well-established, having a receptionist can be a luxury for the practitioners who would rather not deal with telephones and scheduling. The presence of a receptionist also designates the office off as a successful and professional operation.

Entrepreneur with associates. Similar to a group practice, several massage therapists or other kinds of therapists practice in a single location. Instead of being a group venture, however, it is the business venture of one or two who lease or own the establishment. The other practitioners either rent space or pay a percentage of the fees they charge. Payment of rent is much more common than fee-splitting.

The entrepreneur can often arrange things so that the rents paid by the other therapists cover the entire expense of the building, giving the entrepreneur a rent-free office. Generally, the entrepreneur is someone with a strong reputation in the community and good business skills.

Individual massage office. In an individual office, you have complete control over your environment and your schedule. You also have complete responsibility for getting done everything that needs to be done, including paying the rent and all other expenses. You have the most freedom and the most responsibility; the most potential for debt and the most potential for large income.

Legal relationships

Any two people who have a business relationship also have a legal relationship. These relationships can apply to people in all of the categories discussed above.

Sole proprietor. When you are the only one in charge of your business, you are the sole proprietor. In the eyes of the law, you and the business are one. Business income and personal income are pooled together for income tax purposes, as are business deductions and personal deductions.

If you work in another person's office, you will need to understand whether you are working as an employee or as an independent contractor.

Independent contractor/employee. This refers to the two different legal relationships you can have when you make an agreement to work in another person or organization's location.

The main difference to you lies in how your income taxes are handled. If you are an *employee,* your employer is responsible for paying social security tax on your earnings, and must withhold money from your pay for this purpose.

However, if you are an *independent contractor,* you are responsible for paying your own contribution to the social security system, called a self-employment tax, and nothing is withheld from your pay. This can make a significant difference to you and to the person who may have to pay social security tax on your wages.

Another difference between employees and independent contractors relates to insurance. The person you are working for will normally have business insurance that covers employees but *not* independent contractors. For this reason, some massage employers will hire only employees, so that they will be covered under the business insurance policy.

The key fact that distinguishes between your status as an independent contractor or employee is who has *control* over the way in which you perform your services. If you are in charge of setting your hours and your fees, and choosing the specifics of the treatments you give, then you are an independent contractor. If the person or organization you work for controls your hours, your prices, and your therapeutic services, then you are an employee.

If your situation has elements of both, then you have to examine it to see whether it more closely fits the description of an independent contractor or an employee. If you are really an employee but your employer treats you as an independent contractor, the IRS can charge substantial penalties to your employer for failing to withhold the appropriate social security tax.

6 Career Strategies

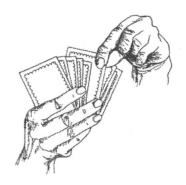

The purpose of this chapter is to help you acquire a "big picture" of your possibilities for a massage career. This chapter will examine the ways you can organize your career, from the investigation phase through the building of a practice.

The following four steps form a framework for your massage career:

1. Investigate the field—explore the field to see if you are interested in pursuing a career.

2. Go to massage school—make a choice based on geography, educational standards, or specialization.

3. Choose one of three approaches for professional growth: cautious exploration, planned transition or total immersion.

4. Create a business plan and follow it through.

1. Investigate the field

This book contains some of the flavor of a career in massage, but your own experience is the most reliable guide you can consult. Use the resources and ideas you pick up from this book to find people who can complete your picture of the field. Get a professional massage. Talk to professionals about their careers. Listen to what people say about massage.

Imagine yourself in the profession. Can you? Is it easy, enjoyable and exciting, or awkward and unnatural? Ask yourself why you want to go into the field. Are your motives based in service and a desire to connect with other people, or are you thinking more about what you can get from the profession?

This is the time to be as honest with yourself as you can. Choosing massage as a career can be very rewarding for the person who wants to grow and serve. It can be frustrating for the person who does not have the determination to make a commitment and follow it through.

2. Going to massage school

Some massage schools offer evening programs so that you can go to school without changing your life. Others require full-time attendance.

If you are unsure about pursuing massage as a career, you might consider taking some adult education massage classes, or classes for the general public offered by the massage school in your area. This can be an excellent way to "get your feet wet" without risking your whole lifestyle. It may also have the advantage of making the rest of your professional education tax-deductible (See Chapter 18).

Your choice of a massage school will set the tone for your career. The items to look at in selecting a school are:

A) Consider the licensing requirements of the states you are interested in living in.

If your chosen state has a licensing requirement, you will probably find it easiest to attend a massage school in that state. The school will be aware of the licensing requirement in its home state, and will tailor its curriculum to those requirements.

If you go to an out-of-state school, be sure their training is acceptable to the authorities in your state. The specific requirements for licensing in each state are unique. Even states with the same number of required hours of education may require study of different subjects.

Some states have "reciprocity" with certain other states. This means that they recognize a license from another state as equal to their own and will admit a licensee from that state without further examination. The state Licensing Chart notes reciprocity in the states in which it exists.

B) Give yourself a strong educational foundation to support your career in the years ahead.

You might choose a 100-hour massage program, learn all you need to establish a career, and enjoy tremendous success in the field for years to come.

You might choose a 100-hour massage program, and on graduating find out that the state you want to practice in has adopted a 500-hour educational requirement.

This is an unsettled time in the massage profession, and no one can tell you what the future will bring. The trend seems to be for the profession to settle on 500 hours as a "normal" amount of professional training. All things being equal, it would be prudent to obtain 500 hours or more.

Of course, all things are not equal, and more training costs more time and money. You will have to gather all the information you can, and use your own judgment and intuition to make the best choice for yourself.

C) Choose a school that offers the approach to massage and the specializations that most interest you.

The State-by-State directory contains enough information to understand the emphasis, or general orientation of all the massage schools described. Almost all schools will send a brochure or catalogue upon request, which will give a more complete picture. You may find it useful to compare several schools' catalogues before making your decision.

Some schools require a personal interview, and even for those that do not, it is a good idea to visit the school before making a commitment to attend. Get the flavor of the place. See how you feel there. See if you would expect to fit in comfortably with the students currently there, and with the overall atmosphere. Get the details of the financial arrangements, including the school's refund policy for those who leave early.

Massage school is very often a "different" sort of school than the ones you are used to. Since students practice on each other, a large part of your curriculum will consist of giving and receiving practice massages. Receiving massage can bring about emotional awarenesses and unexpected changes. Receiving massage several times a week during your massage school program can accelerate the process of change.

Many massage schools recognize this and integrate this aspect of learning into the program. In fact, many schools consider a student's personal growth an essential component of the curriculum. These schools will recognize the psychologically transforming effect massage can have for clients.

Other schools emphasize "medical massage" or the "medical model." Schools with this emphasis present Swedish massage with an emphasis on medical massage. These schools tend to minimize the focus on consciousness and personal growth.

Still other schools present a focused approach to career growth, emphasizing a strong work ethic. These schools will place a greater value on building technical skills, business skills and practical experience. Their programs will be more directed toward the goal of achieving professional competence and career placement in the most efficient way.

Think about these issues, but also let your intuition guide you to the best school for your needs. Going to massage school can be a very special and life-changing experience. Choose with your mind and your heart, and have a great time.

3. Choose your approach:

cautious exploration, planned transition or total immersion

Your massage career will take some time to grow. Your skills as a therapist will mature for years after you finish massage school. Your reputation in the community will likewise take time to build. It is best to have a plan that will allow you to integrate that period of career growth into the context of your life.

Plan A: Cautious Exploration

This is a low-risk alternative. The idea is to make no significant changes in your current lifestyle, but integrate massage education and exploration of massage practice into your life.

You can do this by going to a massage school that has evening or weekend classes, and using your after-hours time to experiment with doing massage professionally. You can charge for your services or not, as you see fit. (In states that require a license, you can charge only after licensure) The idea is to gain experience, and to learn whether massage is a field you want to put some real energy into.

After exploring the field in this way, you will be in a position to know whether it is something you enjoy and can commit to pursuing for a living. At this point, you can move to Plan B or Plan C.

You can also keep massage as a part-time activity in your life. Many massage therapists have other professions or occupations, and have no desire to make the practice of massage their sole livelihood.

Plan B: Planned Transition

This is for those who are committed to pursuing a career in massage, yet want to do it in a way that creates a minimum of disruption in their lives. It is a plan that is particularly well suited to teachers, part-time and flex-time workers, and others with substantial free time to pursue a massage career.

A teacher might build her massage practice after working hours. When it reaches a good level, she can switch to substitute teaching. When the practice will support her fully, she can quit teaching and rely fully on massage. Similarly, a waiter or waitress can cut back on hours as the massage practice grows, eventually giving up waiting tables completely.

In order to make this option work, you will need to be committed. Making a living at your "day job" can take a lot out of you, yet you need to have the energy and drive to become established in your new field during your after-hours time. In the next chapter, you will read about the many marketing techniques available to you. Make sure you will have the energy to keep your current job and also apply yourself to building a massage practice. The transition may take several years, so be sure you are prepared.

Plan C: Total Immersion

This is a sink-or-swim approach in which you quit your job, rely on whatever financial support you have, and focus 100 per cent on establishing yourself as a professional massage therapist. This option requires some means of financial independence — either a bankroll, a generous spouse or benefactor, or a talent at living without much money.

Most marketing techniques require you to have an office setting for the practice of massage. To pursue Total Immersion, you should have an office. This will of course add a significant expense for which you must be prepared. Give some thought to the economics of the situation, and decide whether you could essentially go without any income for a year. There is a good chance that your first year will be a very lean one, and that your second may not be a great deal better.

Some prefer this approach because it forces the person to do everything possible to make a success of their massage career. To pursue this option requires a clear sense of commitment, and also an understanding of the balance between self-promotion and patience. You should also be prepared for some long, lonely days.

This option will be easier for the individual who has lots of contacts and a strong local reputation. Such a person will have the best chance of establishing a practice relatively quickly. It is not advisable for someone who is new in the community.

4. Create a Business Plan and Follow it Through

A business plan is like a blueprint. You can build without one, but having one is likely to make your task easier and your result better.

The specifics for creating a business plan, and a form you can use to create your own, are provided in the next chapter.

7 Marketing Yourself as a Massage Therapist

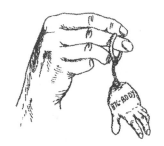

This topic mystifies more massage therapists and bodyworkers than any other. Books, marketing kits, seminars, instructional videos, and other items are on the market to teach you how to acquire a following in your chosen profession.

This guide will give you the benefit of my experiences, as well as those of many other therapists I have interviewed, as to principles and techniques you can use to market your professional services. Before examining the specific techniques you can use, however, there are a few questions you should ask yourself.

1. Preliminary questions

Are You Ready?

Do you feel your massage is worth $55 per hour (or whatever is the going rate in your area)?

How would you feel about having a strong clientele in the town you are now living in? Are you prepared to call this place home?

Imagine introducing yourself to a variety of people in your town. You tell them you are a massage therapist. How does that feel to you?

The above questions touch on the chief reasons that massage practitioners, even after they have gone to massage school, are reluctant to make a commitment to building a massage practice. If you are not ready to present yourself to the public as a professional deserving their time and money, take the time to grow before making a sincere effort at professional marketing.

That growth may mean gaining new professional skills. It may mean confronting issues of self-image or self-esteem. It may mean learning to be comfortable relating to a broad variety of people. Your growth on all these levels will continue for a long time, well into your professional career. You do not need to be perfect to succeed as a massage therapist—just ready.

How Long Do You Expect This To Take?

How much of a hurry are you in? Are you expecting to throw yourself into a marketing campaign for six months and then have a thriving practice? Are you willing to spend two years or longer creating a practice for yourself? If you are looking for the six-month version, you will probably be disappointed in the results. These things take time.

Consider advertising, for example. One study has shown that the average consumer will notice your ad only one out of three times you run it, and that the same consumer has to *see* your ad nine times before she is ready to purchase the advertised goods or services. Therefore, you may need to run an ad 27 times to have your client actually come in for a massage.

Word of mouth can be similarly time-consuming. A new client recently told me that his friend had been urging him to try my massage for two years. Two years is an exceptionally long delay in accepting a referral, but I include this example to give you the idea that some aspects of marketing simply cannot be rushed. Successful marketing involves a blend of *commitment* and *patience*.

What's your plan?

Make a plan for your career—what your practice will be like in six months, one year, two years, three years, five years. Use the form below or create your own planning form.

All sources of professional business guidance will tell you, as a business person, that a business plan is an essential part of your growth process. Advantages of a business plan are:

- It helps you know where you want your career to go;
- It helps you keep track of your progress toward your goals;
- It helps you organize your efforts toward meeting your goals;
- It gives you the clarity to express your goals to others so that they will help you find opportunities.

At the same time, it is important to stay flexible and be quite willing to depart from the plan. In fact, every few months or so, you may want to completely rewrite your plan to reflect what you have learned or how your goals have changed.

For example, let's say you make a business plan that emphasizes house calls in an affluent suburb. It includes working at a health spa in that area part-time and using advertising in a community newspaper to try to break into the house call market. Midway through this project, you meet a cardiologist who offers you an office in his group practice. This is a terrific opportunity that you had not even realized was possible.

Do you pass up the cardiologist because you are in the middle of a different plan? Of course not. You change your business plan. At the same time, it was important to have the business plan even though you changed it; you might never have met the cardiologist.

When you make your plans for six months, one year, two years, three years and five years from now, be as detailed and specific as you can. Include your best predictions about all of the following:

- Location for doing massage
- Target clients
- Type of work you want to be doing
- How clients will learn about you
- Number of clients you want or expect to have
- Workshops, professional trainings and meetings to attend
- Advertising and other promotional plans
- Expenses you are likely to incur

Mark on the top of each plan the date you write it, and the target date for the goals you create. Take your group of plans out every few months and see how things are going. Revise the entire group of plans at least once a year.

Sample Business Plan

On page 41 is a sample business plan for Mary Jones. Mary has been out of massage school one year, and is seeing 8 to 12 clients per week. Some of these are house calls, and some are in a resort 15 miles from her home. She has a part-time job doing cleaning work to supplement her income.

Create Your Business Plan

Use the form on page 42 as a sample to create your business plan. If you feel the form does not suit your particular needs, by all means modify it to take into account the planning you need to do.

You will be creating more business plans as time goes by, so you may want to create a form that suits you and make a few copies of it. Keep your business plans in a folder and keep the folder with your other business materials, such as business receipts, client records, and professional books.

2. Nuts and Bolts of Marketing for Massage and Bodywork

You have examined your readiness for success, your expectations about your career path, and your plans for making your goals take shape. You now have an understanding of the larger picture that your marketing efforts will fit into.

Before discussing the specific marketing techniques you might use, there is one broad principle to consider:

Person-to-person contact is the most effective.

Because massage is a personal service, and because it is relatively expensive, people want to have a good idea that they are going to like both the person and the person's treatment before they come in for a massage. It is much harder to convey this level of confidence with impersonal contact, such as advertising, than it is with person-to-person contact.

To overcome people's natural shyness and resistance to the idea of nudity and being touched, you need to let people know enough about you to trust you, and enough about your work to have confidence in it.

Keeping this in mind, consider the following techniques you can use to promote your professional services.

A. Person-to-person marketing techniques

All professions depend chiefly on referrals, or word-of-mouth, and massage is no exception. A certain amount of word-of-mouth marketing happens naturally. If you give one client a great massage, she naturally wants to tell her friends, and some of them may be curious enough to try you out sooner or later.

MARY JONES' BUSINESS PLAN   May 7, 1997

Goals:
   To increase clientele to 25 per week
   To keep commuting distances to a minimum
   To emphasize sports massage in my practice

Target clientele:
   Amateur and professional athletes
   Local residents
   Professionals and their spouses

Possible new locations to work in:

...try club newsletter
...th physicians and attorneys in the area
...ss trainers and athletic trainers in the area
...circulation newspaper

...nonth goals:
...st where I can see clients; meet at least
...letic trainers and give them complimen-
...t at least four doctors or lawyers in the
...and my work.

...year goals:
...ascular therapy and sports massage tech-
...nal fitness trainers and athletic trainers;
...12 per week; obtain a quality office en-
...deal setting for sports and rehabilitative
...massage.

...ear goals:
...litative massage office, seeing 20 clients
...occasional house calls for professional
...hletes in preparation for competitive

...ear goals:
...ts, hire other sports massage therapists
...work in my clinic when I am away.

Five year goals:
Offer sports massage trainings; employ at least one full-time massage therapist in my clinic; work exclusively with competitive athletes.

SAMPLE BUSINESS PLAN   date _____

Items to consider:
        Location for doing massage
        Target clients
        Type of work I want to be doing
        How clients will learn about me
        Number of clients I will have
        Workshops, professional trainings and meetings
        Advertising and other promotional plans
        Expenses I am likely to incur

Goals:

Target clientele:

Possible locations to work in:

Means of reaching target clientele:

Six month goals:

One year goals:

Two year goals:

Three year goals:

Five year goals:

The art of marketing yourself, however, lies in accelerating this process as much as possible. The main task to accomplish in that regard is to become widely known and accepted within as many groups as possible in your community.

The following are some proven methods for making people familiar with you and comfortable with you, and interested in trying your therapy:

1. Demonstration/lecture at health clubs, professional groups and social groups

These can be a very effective way to become known and accepted, and to increase your clientele. The idea is to present a short speech on the nature of massage, the benefits it can have, and what is to be expected during a session. This is followed up by a brief demonstration on a volunteer.

If you are doing it in a place where a massage room is available, such as a health club, you might consider following it up with an offer to do a ten-minute foot massage on anyone who is curious.

A presentation of this sort accomplishes many marketing goals all at once. As you establish rapport with the group, you become known, familiar and accepted. They learn the theory of massage and how it can help them, and they gain an understanding of the process and what to expect. Then, after your demonstration, they see and hear from your client how wonderful a person feels after one of your treatments.

For someone who is curious about massage but fearful about nudity or about being touched by a stranger, the lecture/demonstration is perhaps the only marketing tool that will give that person the confidence to try a massage. By creating confidence in yourself, taking the mystery out of the massage process, and giving the person a clear idea of what she has to gain by having a massage, you can effectively break down some strong barriers to using your services.

One therapist gave several lecture/demonstrations at her health club, a women-only club. She made such an impression that practically each time she went into the club for a workout after that, one or more members came up to her asking to schedule a massage appointment.

Other locations for this type of presentation are civic, professional and social groups. Ask your friends and clients about any groups they are members of, such as the Rotary, local women's club, yoga group, exercise class, or toastmasters. These groups are often glad to have outside speakers, and the fact that one of their members recommends you will be an advantage.

Many people have a great fear of public speaking, and will feel it is impossible to do a lecture/demonstration in front of a group. If you can't, you can't. However, if you can't you are missing out on one of the most effective and successful marketing opportunities you can use. Remember that the group you speak to will be there because they are interested in you and in massage. They are on your side and they want to like you. Prepare in advance what you are going to say and do, and just be yourself.

2. Free introductory massages for selected individuals

Anyone who is likely to be the source of repeated referrals should be cultivated as a contact. Such people are psychotherapists, medical doctors, chiropractors,

acupuncturists, wholistic practitioners of all sorts, team coaches and sports trainers, dancing teachers, other massage therapists and bodyworkers, and people who
are well-known and well-respected members of the community.

Any of these people, who are in a position of trust with their friends, neighbors, clients, and patients, will generally be listened to by those they know.
Therefore, once they believe in you and your work, they can be a good source of
referrals.

You may wish to seek out these people and try to introduce yourself, or you
may wait until you meet someone in the natural course of events. Either way,
offering a complimentary massage can be an excellent way of introducing that
person to you and your work. Once they know you and have confidence in you
they will be more willing to refer clients to you.

3. Discounts to clients for referrals

One therapist gives a ten-dollar discount on the next massage to any client who
refers another client. She believes this fosters referrals, as it gives clients a motivation to spread the word about massage.

In a similar vein, one therapist offers a "buy two gift certificates, get your
massage free" promotion. I have not tried either approach. My hunch is that clients have a natural desire to tell their friends and neighbors when they like you
and your service. However, it is possible that a financial incentive would give
them more of a reason to do so. Those of you who do try it, let me know your
experiences.

4. Join the local Chamber of Commerce

Consider joining the Chamber of Commerce in your community. These are local
business people who are getting together to share matters of common concern. You
are such a person, and there is no reason you should not be involved in such a
group.

The contacts you make in a group like this will be valuable for your career, in
that these are people who know many members of the community. The more
you become known and accepted as a "normal" business person, the less resistance people will have to the idea of coming to you for a massage.

5. Do on-site promotional massages

This means going where the people are and working either for free or for a small
amount, doing brief treatments. You can rent a booth at a health fair, craft fair,
workshop center or convention and offer five or ten minute massages. You can
arrange in advance to set up at the end of a sporting event, or at a shopping center during busy times. The exposure you get from such activities may bring you
clients immediately, and also may have a long-term benefit in getting you known
in the local community.

6. Join as many organizations as you comfortably can

The goal is to meet large numbers of people and to become known. Don't join
organizations just to accomplish a marketing goal. You won't have fun, and you

may seem pushy. Join organizations you are interested in, but don't be shy about telling people what you do, and never get caught without your business card handy to give out to an interested person.

B. Person-To-Paper Contact

There are some people who are your potential clients, whom you cannot reach in person or through a personal recommendation. Reaching them through the printed word may be your only means of making contact.

Advertising is a quick way to reach large numbers of people. The difficult aspects of using advertising effectively are *avoiding* the people you do *not* want to find you, and making a persuasive impression on the people you do want to find you.

Advertising has the disadvantage of being impersonal contact. It will let people know who you are and where you are and perhaps what you offer. However, it will not tell them that they will like you, that they can trust you, that you have a great touch and tremendous skills, or that they will feel much better after one of your treatments.

Therefore, advertising will most effectively reach those clients who are already familiar with massage but do not currently have a massage therapist whom they go to. This is a relatively small percentage of the general population. However, it takes only one new regular client to make any advertisement worth its cost.

The biggest disadvantage of advertising is that it opens you to sexually-oriented massage clients. A great many men have had sexual experiences that were billed as "massage." In many areas of the United States today, it is easier to find sexual massage than it is to find legitimate massage. Though great progress has been made in legitimizing the profession in recent years, confusion persists.

Doing any general advertising virtually guarantees that you will be confronted by at least some men calling to find out if they can get sexual services from you. Every massage therapist I know finds this to be draining, degrading and infuriating. However, at this point in the history of massage, it is an unavoidable side-effect of using advertising as a tool to build your practice.

Suggestion: In any person-to-paper advertising you do, consider including a photo of yourself. This will do several things. First, it will help dispel any idea that you are offering sexual massage. Second, it will convey some information about you — it is the best substitute available for personal contact. Finally, it is an eye-catcher. In a print medium, a photo tends to draw attention, and it can help clients see an ad they might otherwise miss.

1. Flyers and Business cards

Flyers and business cards are best used after you have made person-to-person contact, to further explain your work or to serve as a reminder about you and your services.

Most therapists who have tried leaving flyers for the general public and posting business cards in places like health food stores and supermarkets find that the results are poor. The main people you are likely to reach by posting your business card are the other therapists who see your card when they post theirs.

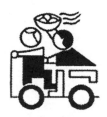

One flyer that worked was the one used by Wes Boyce in southern California. That is reproduced on the preceding page. Wes used this flyer as part of his plan to become established quickly from the ground up. This flyer brought him 100 clients within seven months, and at that point he canceled the promotion. His promotion had raised $1,000 for Meals On Wheels.

He did not make much money directly from these massages, although some clients tipped him, and a few became paying customers. However, he was able to get a lot of practical experience in a short time, and also generated a great deal of public awareness about himself and his work.

2. Direct mail

This refers to those packets of ads and coupons we all get in the mail from time to time. Some massage therapists have used these very effectively to build their practices.

These direct mailings generally go to 10,000 homes at a time. The cost to have your ad or coupon included will usually be a few hundred dollars. This may sound like a lot of money, but consider that one weekly client will repay the entire cost of the promotion in two to three months.

Two useful approaches to direct mail are to use it when you open a new office, and to use it at holiday times to advertise gift certificates. It can also be used as a major promotion to boost an existing practice.

To get in touch with direct mail companies, look in the mailers for their phone number and address, or get the Business-to-Business Yellow Pages if there is one for your area. (available free from your local phone company's business office) Look in the listing for "Marketing Programs and Services."

The direct mail sales person will help you design your promotion. Most such promotions include a special offer, such as an introductory massage for new clients at a reduced price.

3. Yellow Pages

All of the massage therapists I interviewed who have yellow pages listings agreed that the listing more than paid for itself with the business it generated. However, they also agreed that the quality of calls that came from the listing was poor. A large percentage of these calls are from men seeking sex, and a significant amount of time and energy is taken in screening these calls.

Some localities have two listings in the yellow pages — one for massage, and one for massage therapists. The idea behind the distinction is to tip off the sex-seekers that those listed as massage therapists are legitimate. Unfortunately, the sex clients either don't see the distinction, or figure that you're really offering sex massage and you put the listing under "massage therapist" to fool the police. If your listing has the word "massage" in it, you can count on sex calls.

You can help create the image you want by carefully selecting the name and information you present in the yellow pages. One practical option is to choose a business name at the beginning of the alphabet, since you will get more calls if you are listed first.

Another practical option is to choose a name like "wholistic health center" to generate a minimum of sex calls. The business name you choose for your yellow pages listing need not be the same as the one on your business cards or bank account. The people who publish the yellow pages will accept most any business name you supply.

Yellow pages ads are expensive. A basic listing with no more than name and phone number will cost around $15 per month, or $180 per year. A small block ad with some basic information can cost around $50 per month, or $600 per year. Larger ads can cost a great deal more. This will be more economical for a group practice than for an individual.

Getting into the yellow pages requires some planning in advance. In my area, the deadline for new orders is in March, and new books are distributed in July. If you are opening a new office, or changing locations, you may want to coordinate your move with the schedule of the yellow pages publisher to minimize the disruption in your practice.

4. Newspaper coverage of you and your practice

One way to become better known is to have a local newspaper reporter write an article about you, about massage, and about any particular aspect of you or your work that is unique or interesting.

Make contact with a reporter for your local newspaper, and give her or him a massage. Discuss anything about yourself or your work or training that may be of interest, and let the reporter decide what angle might serve as the basis for a story.

After the story appears in the paper, frame it and put it on your office wall. Your clients will be gently reminded that you are a special person worthy of respect.

5. Placing ads in newspapers

Many successful massage therapists have never advertised in newspapers and never will. Others have found newspaper advertising to be a way to shorten the time needed to build a practice to a self-supporting level. Others have advertised and been so frustrated by the clients who responded that they have burned out on massage as a profession. The following information about newspaper advertising should help you make the most of newspaper advertising.

Two types of newspaper ads—classifieds, display ads

Two types of massage ads are available in newspapers—display ads and business classified ads. Display ads (also called block ads) appear in the body of the paper, with the news and features articles, and therefore are seen by more readers than business classifieds. Display ads are larger and substantially more expensive than business classifieds. Display ads make sense in small-circulation newspapers, when you are trying to break into a new market. In larger newspapers, massage ads almost always run in the business classifieds.

Business classifieds

Business classifieds is a separate section of the classifieds, devoted to business services such as painting, carpentry, cleaning and hauling. While these ads are much cheaper than display ads, they cost a great deal more than a normal classified ad.

The response to advertising in the business classifieds tends to be immediate. If the response to your classified ad is going to be good, you will know within the first few days. Start with a short run for your ad, so that if the response is not good, you have the opportunity to try a different newspaper.

Generally speaking, business classified advertising is cost-effective for massage therapists. In other words, you will generally make more money as a result of placing the ad than you spend on the ad. The other question, however, is how much grief you will have to put up with in the process.

Display advertising

Display advertising is quite different from business classified advertising. Someone looking up massage in a business classified is ready for a massage — today, if possible. Someone just reading the news or features, who sees your display ad in the newspaper, was not thinking about massage until she saw your ad. She may not be ready for massage for quite a while.

In fact, it may take many exposures to your ad before this person feels you are sufficiently "familiar" to give you a try. After seeing your ad a few times, she will begin to get the idea that you are not just a passing fad, but a true fixture in the community.

The more times a person sees your ad, the more familiar and accepted your name will be to that person. After five to ten exposures to your ad, the person may be sufficiently comfortable with your print image that she would consider trying a massage. The more nervous the person is about massage, the longer it may take for her to begin to feel comfortable about you by repeatedly seeing you ad.

Therefore, display advertising is generally best used in small circulation newspapers, where you have a particular desire to break into a new market that you feel has a good potential for your practice. Choose your newspaper and plan to place your ad many times. Keep your ad the same each time you run it, so that the "familiarity" factor works best. Use a picture of yourself in the ad — this will be an eye-catcher, will help the person feel she knows you and will give more of a sense that you can be trusted.

Types of Newspapers

Many types of newspapers exist, and you can use each differently in aid of your marketing goals. The different types of newspapers are general circulation dailies, special interest newspapers (usually weekly or monthly), and local or regional papers (usually weekly).

General circulation newspapers

These are the daily newspapers read by the general population. The general circulation newspaper I advertised in is the Asbury Park Press, which serves a region within about a 25-mile radius of Asbury Park, New Jersey. Their business classified directory includes a listing for massage, and at the top of the massage listing each day is the following notice:

> ATTENTION ADVERTISERS: The only copy permitted in a massage ad is: name, address, phone number, rates & hours. The only exception is a licensed spa listing their facilities (sauna, steam room, etc.)
>
> The terminology 'Professional or Licensed' can be used if customer sends copy of certificate from a school of massage prior to ad running.
>
> Ads must be paid in advance.

This notice appeared for the first time shortly after the same newspaper ran a story about a prostitution ring that had operated through the massage classifieds. The management placed the notice at the top of the massage listing in an attempt to prevent the use of its massage ads for prostitution.

I advertised in this listing immediately before and immediately after the story about the prostitution ring operating through the massage classifieds. Despite the notice at the top of the listing, and despite the story in the same newspaper about prostitution arrests, roughly ninety percent of the calls I received from this ad were men looking for sexual massage. This percentage did not seem to change as a result of the prostitution story or as a result of putting the notice at the top of the massage listing.

Phone calls at 7:00 a.m. and 11:45 p.m. in response to my ad were not uncommon. I chose to answer my own phone, although some therapists who advertise leave the answering machine on and selectively return calls. I found that, in general, people calling at unusual times were looking for unusual massage services. My first name (Martin) indicated I was a man, and my ad apparently attracted a great many gay or bisexual callers. Calls for sexual massage dropped off dramatically after the first week.

Most of the clients looking for sex had the sense to stop trying when I explained in no uncertain terms that my massage was completely legitimate and did not include any sexual contact. A few, however, apparently regarded that as a challenge and made appointments anyway.

These men would wait until the end of their massage, or in some cases until their second or third massage, to verbally or non-verbally make their wishes known. This was quite a growth experience for me, as I had to learn how to deal with my own feelings of anger and resentment in such a situation.

My growth brought me to a point where I could comfortably take charge of the situation. I learned to discuss any suspect signs of arousal immediately, carefully watch the client's attitude about the subject, and terminate the massage immediately if the client was being inappropriate. Once I realized that I had control of the situation, my emotional response lessened dramatically.

The several regular clients I acquired through this advertising exposure are lovely people whom I appreciate very much as clients, and who never would have found me without the ad. The total expense for the ads I ran was about $250 over a period of several weeks. Despite the irritation factor, on the whole it was well worth doing.

Special interest newspapers

There may be newspapers for special interest groups in your area that can be good sources of massage clients. Such papers include:

- New age or wholistically oriented newspapers

- Religious or community-oriented newspapers

- In-house newspapers for institutions such as retirement communities and hospitals

Two such newspapers I have advertised in are written for the Jewish community.

The cost involved is usually low, and the response level probably will also be low. However, such exposure can be useful in gaining entry into a new market. In my case, my small ads in two Jewish newspapers generated enough new business to at least pay for the ads, and also served to gain some name recognition.

Local and regional newspapers

Many communities have small local papers, which are published once or twice a week. These are sometimes mailed to all households in the community at no charge. These papers often have a "business classified" section similar to the one in general circulation newspapers.

Before advertising in one of these, get the flavor of the other ads in the paper. If a massage ad would seem distinctly out of place in comparison to the other types of ads that are currently running, it may not be a good idea to place your ad in that paper.

As with special interest newspapers, the circulation of local papers will be small, as will the cost to advertise. One advantage is that you can be sure that any potential clients who see this ad will be close to you and able to conveniently come to see you.

C. Broadcast Media

Radio, broadcast television, and direct access cable television are also possibilities for massage marketing. Generally speaking, the cost of commercial advertisements on radio and television is too great for a massage practice.

Direct access cable, however, can provide opportunities for exposure. A pair of chiropractors in my area produced a multi-part feature on wholistic health modalities for showing on direct access cable. One segment was on massage, and the therapist they chose for that segment received significant exposure at no expense to her.

D. Ethereal marketing techniques

"There is more to the world" says Shakespeare, "than is dreamt of in your philosophy." Many successful practitioners believe there is more to making contact with another person than operating in the world of the physical senses.

These are some of the unorthodox marketing tips used by some successful massage practitioners:

- Visualize an open field, and see clients coming across that field to you.

- Meditate, tell the universe you are ready for people to come into your life.

- Imagine that you have a dial you can turn to control the flow of your practice. Turn it up to become busier, turn it down when you need freedom from your practice.

If this sounds like so much hocus-pocus to you, don't bother with it. You may find, at some point, that it has meaning for you. For example, several therapists have said that when they find themselves feeling frantic and wishing they had spare time instead of appointments, their clients often call in and cancel.

A skeptical person can always see something like this as coincidence. It is not scientific and cannot be proven. If it intrigues you, simply suspend disbelief. Allow the possibility that it is hogwash and allow the opposite possibility that it is a real phenomenon. Then stay with your experience, see how things go and form opinions later.

E. Fostering Repeat Business

The first goal of your marketing efforts is to get potential clients to try you out. The next goal is making them realize they should come back and make massage a regular part of their lives.

The two main ways you can foster repeat business are to create an understanding of the benefits of massage, and to stay in touch with your clients.

Create an understanding of the benefits of massage

After receiving a massage, the client's body will understand how healthful it is, but the person's mind may not. Many people guide themselves primarily by their mental processes, and unless these people have an understanding of the value of massage, they may not become repeat clients.

You can help them understand the process by honestly explaining how massage benefits people in general, and how they specifically could benefit from a regular program of treatment. There is no need to be a salesman, or to be pushy. If you are honest and forthright, people will respect your professionalism and appreciate the information—they want to take care of themselves once they understand how.

Stay in touch with your clients

Some therapists call their clients a day or two after their first massage to ask how they are feeling. This is especially appropriate with clients who have come in for relief from a specific condition.

Other ways to stay in touch with clients are:

- Send birthday cards

- Photocopy an article of interest about massage and send it to all your clients with a short note

- Send holiday greeting cards at Christmas or Rosh Hashanah

- Send a flyer or post card reminding clients that you offer gift certificates at holiday time

- Send flyers or post cards advertising any special offers you are making on your services

- Send announcements to your clients when you begin working in a new location or take on an associate in your office

- If you have a seasonal clientele, send thank-you letters to your clients at the end of the season for their patronage.

If initiating contact of this type feels unnatural to you, do not bother with it. If it is a genuine expression of your interest in your clients, they will take it as such and respond positively.

For further information about marketing

A book that will expand on several of the concepts in this chapter is *Guerilla Marketing* by Jay Conrad Levinson, published by Houghton Mifflin (The sequel, *Guerilla Marketing Attack*, is not as useful). This book emphasizes the creative, low-budget techniques and principles you can use in marketing. Much of the information is inapplicable to marketing professional services such as massage, but it is worth looking through if you are seriously interested in marketing yourself. It is widely available at libraries and bookstores.

Other marketing aids tend to be expensive, and you should be cautious about using them. The best marketing devices you can obtain are education and motivation—these turn you into your own best resource. I have included reference to *Guerilla Marketing* because, as I have tried to do in this chapter, it educates you so that you can understand and use effective marketing techniques. It is more worthwhile to invest in training yourself about marketing than it is to buy the expensive videos and packets you may see advertised.

8 Opening a Massage Office

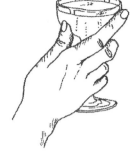

Opening an office is a big step. It is the mark of maturity of a massage career. It requires confidence in your professional skills, your business ability, and your commitment to your practice.

When the time comes in your career to open your own office, it should be a joyous venture. It will bring you the chance to make a better living and have a clear professional identity. This chapter will help you be fully prepared and ready to take this step, and will give you the basic information you will need to make the best choices in bringing your office to life.

The topics covered in this chapter are Governmental requirements, practical requirements, and business decisions. Business decisions include subjects like measuring your readiness to open an office, choosing a location, and negotiating a lease. In addition, you will find a checklist for office opening, and discussions of opening a group practice and buying an existing practice.

Governmental Requirements

You are becoming a local business owner, and as such you are taking on a new identity in the eyes of your local government. One of the main functions of local government is to regulate the operations of businesses. By the same token, one of the chief sources of revenue for local government are the license fees and taxes paid by local business owners.

So you are in a two-way relationship with your local government. On one hand, the government wants to exert its authority over you to make sure you do things to their liking. On the other hand, the government wants to see you succeed, so that you will make money and share it with the government.

Your first step is to visit your local government, whether it is a town hall, city hall, municipal complex, or village governmental center. Bring a note pad and pen. Ask for assistance about the following items:

1. Massage licensing law

Most towns and cities do not have laws regulating the practice of massage, but many do. These laws often were written more to guard against prostitution than to realistically regulate massage practice. You may find that the local law regulates massage quite heavily. Some local laws prohibit massaging members of the opposite sex. A few towns prohibit the practice of massage completely.

If your town has a restrictive law, you will have to choose 1. meeting all of the restrictions, 2. giving up the idea of practicing there, 3. fighting to have the law changed, or 4. practicing there and risking being penalized for violating the law. If you think you may choose number 4, it is probably not a good idea to march into city hall and identify yourself as a way of getting information.

2. Practitioner license, establishment license

If the town has a licensing law, it will probably have two parts to it. One will give the requirements for a massage practitioner license, and the other will give the requirements for a massage establishment license.

The practitioner license applies to your right to practice massage within the town, and the establishment license applies to the office in which you will practice massage. Each will have a separate procedure and a separate fee. A sample zoning map appears on page 56.

3. Zoning requirements

Almost all towns have zoning laws, which regulate the types of "uses" that may take place in different "zones." In other words, zoning laws restrict the kinds of businesses you can operate in different neighborhoods. Certain neighborhoods are set aside for residences only. Others may be zoned for industrial uses, such as factories and warehouses. Others will be for stores or professional practices.

Before committing to a particular location for a massage office, you should be sure that the location has the proper zoning for use as a massage business.

Different communities will use different zoning classifications for massage. Some will call it a personal service. Others will call it a profession. Others will call it a health service. Still others refer to it as "adult entertainment." What they call it will have an effect on which zones you will be allowed to locate in.

The town clerk can direct you to the zoning map for the city. If the zoning board can tell you exactly which category massage is considered to be for zoning purposes, you can check the map to see which neighborhoods are open to you for an office location. If there is doubt about which category they consider massage, you may need to go before the zoning board to get a definitive ruling before choosing your office location.

If you are opening a home office, the zoning board may require a hearing before deciding whether to allow you to operate a massage practice in your home. They may consider factors such as the burden placed on neighborhood parking, the percentage of space in the home devoted to your business, and whether you will be the only one who performs massage services in your home. If you need to appear before the zoning board, consider consulting an attorney beforehand for advice about how to proceed.

4. Health, police and fire department inspections

Inquire of the health department, police department and fire department what their policies are about inspecting a massage office before it opens. Ask about any requirements you will need to meet. Write down the answers you receive, the name of the person who gives you the information, and the date.

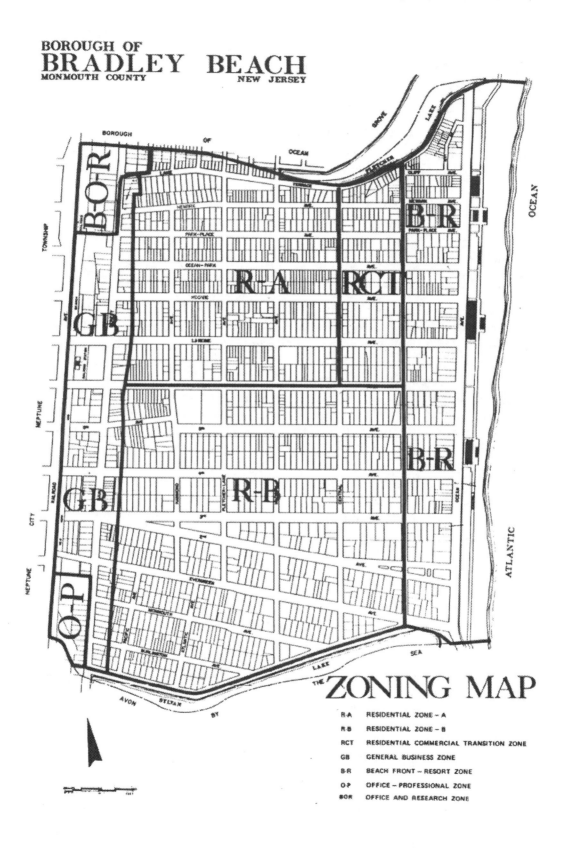

BOROUGH OF BRADLEY BEACH
MONMOUTH COUNTY — NEW JERSEY

THE **ZONING MAP**

R-A	RESIDENTIAL ZONE — A
R-B	RESIDENTIAL ZONE — B
RCT	RESIDENTIAL COMMERCIAL TRANSITION ZONE
GB	GENERAL BUSINESS ZONE
B-R	BEACH FRONT — RESORT ZONE
O-P	OFFICE — PROFESSIONAL ZONE
ROR	OFFICE AND RESEARCH ZONE

5. Local business taxes

Ask the clerk about any local taxes, such as sewer tax, business property tax, or other local business taxes. Make a note of this information, as you will want to know what your expenses will be in operating your business.

Practical Requirements

1. Fictitious name statement (also called "assumed name" or "doing business as")

If you will give your business a name other than your own name (such as "Wholistic Massage Center" or "Beams of Light Massage") you will need to register your fictitious name with the county government. This allows the public to know who owns a business when the owner's name is not included in the business name. This certificate does not give you exclusive rights to the name. For that you must seek trade-name or service-mark protection.

To register your fictitious name, you must go to the county seat, the town in your county that houses the county government offices. If you do not know where that is, someone in your bank or city government office can tell you. Contact the county clerk, and find out the cost for registering a fictitious or assumed name, the hours you can go and do so, and the procedure for doing so. In some places, the procedure includes advertising your fictitious name in local newspapers.

In most cases, you will be required to do your own checking through the county's records of business names to make sure that no one has already chosen that business name. This can take awhile, so give yourself enough time to take care of this. After you have checked the records, you pay your fee (bring cash and keep your receipt) and you will receive a "fictitious name certificate" (or "assumed name certificate").

2. Business bank account

Your bank will require a fictitious name certificate in order to open an account in the name of your business. It is a good idea to have a business checking account, and to pay for all business expenses with your business checks (or business credit card). Your business will appear more credible and established than it would if you pay for business purchases with your personal checks or credit cards. Having a separate account will also make your task easier when it is time to prepare your year-end income taxes.

3. Business stationery, cards, gift certificates, flyers

Choose a print shop that you can be comfortable with. You will probably be a repeat customer for your printer. You should have a printer that you have confidence in, as to quality, prompt completion of orders, and competitive price. Consider recommendations of others and your own observations when in the shop.

The bare minimum you will need to open your office is business cards. Consider whether to also invest in customized gift certificates and business stationary.

Also consider: A rubber stamp with your business name and address, a rubber stamp with your bank account number to endorse the back of checks, flyers that describe you and your business, a printed coupon for purchasers of pre-paid series of massage, and promotional items to publicize your office.

Business Decisions

1. Financial and Professional Readiness

Start-up costs

First consider that you will need some money up front in order to open an office. You will need money for office furnishings, first month's rent, security deposit, telephone and utility deposit, printing needs and advertising or other promotional costs. If you have established credit, you may be able to get a loan. Otherwise you will need to use your savings to meet these start-up costs.

As a guideline for planning purposes, the following figures probably come close to the amounts you will need to spend on start-up costs:

Massage table	$400
Desk	175
Table or shelf	40
Hamper	35
Phone/ans. mach.	75
Music system	150
Sheets/towels	200
First month rent	400
Security deposit	400
Phone deposit	150
Utility deposit	75
Printing	100
Ads/promotion	300
Miscellaneous	100

Any of these items can be more or less than the amounts shown, depending on your particular circumstances. The start-up costs in the sample above total $2600.

Monthly expenses vs. income

Next examine your ability to meet the continuing financial obligations of operating a professional office.

Perhaps you work in a health club, hair salon, or doctor's office. Would most of your clients stay with the new massage therapist who replaces you or would they follow you to your office?

Estimated Monthly Business Income

Take an honest look at your client list, and imagine the first month in your new office. Examine your records to see what your business income has been for the last few months, and any upward or downward trends you notice.

Consider, also, that once you have an office of your own, it may be easier for you to create new growth. First, you will have strong motivation to do so. Second, you will have a location that is conducive to the kind of work you want to do. Third, you will have an established office that will serve as the focus of your marketing efforts — promotional ideas such as direct mail, lecture/demonstration and advertising will be more open to you than they would be if your were working in an employer's space.

Make an estimate of your first month's income. If in doubt, choose a lower figure for planning purposes. For purposes of making a sample financial projection, we will assume you can start in your new office with an income of $1,200 per month. This is your "estimated monthly business income."

Other Monthly Income

Calculate your other sources of income, apart from your business. Include any sources of income you know you can count on, such as interest, alimony, dividends, pension, or the like. Total all this income, and figure how much you receive in an average month. For purposes of this example, we will use the figure $150 per month for your "Other Monthly Income."

Total Estimated Income

Add your "estimated monthly business income" to your "other monthly income." In this example, the total is $1,350.

Estimated Monthly Business Expenses

Calculate the amount you must spend each month for your office rent, telephone, and yellow pages. Also include a twelfth of your annual business expenses, such as advertising, oils and linens, business taxes, professional association dues, accountant fees, insurance costs, and the like.

The total of your monthly business expenses is likely to be between $300 and $1,200. This is the amount you need each month to support your business. We will use the figure of $600 per month as an example of "estimated monthly business expenses."

Estimated Monthly Personal Expenses

This is the amount you need to live on each month, for such essentials as home rental, food, automobile, health insurance and taxes. One way to calculate this is to look through your checkbook for last year. Add up all the money you spent on personal expenses, plus your best guess for how much cash you spent, and divide by 12. Another way is to add up your fixed expenses and then add an estimate for your spending money.

Let's say you come up with a total of $1,000 per month for your "estimated monthly personal expenses."

Estimated Total Monthly Expenses

Add the "estimated monthly business expenses" of $600 per month to "estimated monthly personal expenses" of $1,000 per month to find your "estimated total monthly expenses." This is the amount you will need to earn each month in order to support your new office and your current lifestyle. In our example, this is $1,600.

These estimated figures are summarized in the chart below.

New Office Financial Projections

INCOME
Estimated monthly business income $1,200
Other monthly income   150
Total estimated income   1,350

EXPENSES
Estimated monthly business expenses
   in new office location   600
Estimated monthly personal expenses   1,000
Estimated total monthly expenses   1,600

NET DEFICIT $250 per month

This projection shows expenses will be higher than income. Subtracting income ($1,350) from expenses ($1,600) shows an estimated deficit of $250 per month for this person's overall lifestyle after opening the new massage office.

If your financial planning estimate shows a net deficit per month, you should plan to have a reserve of at least one year's worth of deficits before you decide to open your office. It may take a year for you to see any significant increase in your business, so plan to start with the ability to sustain your practice at its current level for at least a year.

In this example, that would mean you should have a capital reserve of $3,000 to supplement your income for the first year.

Consider choosing a larger figure for your capital reserve, since it is possible your second year may also produce a net deficit.

Additional Reserves For Business and Personal Expenses

In addition to the predictable expenses, you should ideally be prepared for the unforseen ones as well. For example, your car's transmission falls out. You need $600 to fix it. You decide it would help business to do a direct mail promotion. You need $400 for the cost of the mailing.

This kind of expense can come up without warning, so you should plan on at least another $1,000 to draw on for such emergencies.

Total Needs for Financial Readiness

Add your Start-up Costs, your first year's Net Deficit, and Additional Reserves. This is the amount you can expect to need in the first year to start your business and supplement your income. In the example above, this total would be $6,600.

If your skills, personality and location are good, and you approach your marketing with commitment and organization, you should find that after the first year you begin to see some increase in your practice. You may still have a net deficit each month in the second year. If you proceed with organization and commitment, you should have a net profit after the second year, and have a net operating profit for the rest of your massage career.

2. Location

There is an old joke in the real estate business:

> *Question:* What are the three most important factors in the value of real estate?
>
> *Answer:* Location, location and location

This expresses a basic truth about the business world. Location counts for a great deal in business. Choose a location that is central, easy to get to, enjoyable to go to, and that conveys a positive image for your practice.

WIZARD OF ID

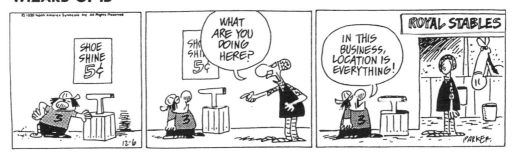

Take your time finding a location. Consider a broad range of questions.

Consider the town:

- Is the town one that can support a massage therapist?

- Are any massage therapists currently earning a living in this town?

- Will I be in direct competition with them or will we draw on different client bases?

- Is there another town in the area that would afford a better image or a more receptive client population?

Consider the neighborhood and building:

- What is the ideal location within my town for my particular practice?

- Will this location be one my clients are comfortable coming to? One they will look forward to coming to?

- Is the building attractive and well-maintained?
- Is the building visible to large numbers of people on a daily basis?
- Are the other offices in the building ones whose images fit comfortably with the image I want for my practice?
- Is the neighborhood safe and pleasant?
- Is parking convenient?
- What other businesses are nearby?
- Will this location support my plans for future growth?
- Do I feel comfortable thinking of this as "my" office?

Your choice of an office location can make your whole professional life easier or more difficult. Do yourself a favor, and make the selection of an office your highest priority. Investigate, think, feel and take some time with this decision. Your efforts will pay great dividends for years to come.

3. Negotiating a Lease

Look for items in a lease which give you flexibility and control and avoid items which give power to the landlord and obligate you excessively.

For example, your lease should include a statement that the office provided will be suitable for use as a professional massage office—as to noise level, temperature control and good repair of all fixtures. This gives you a legal right to complain if the landlord fails to provide you with a quiet and warm massage environment.

If you have any doubts about the zoning for the location, put in the lease that it becomes void if the city refuses to approve zoning for a massage business at that location. Otherwise, you could be stuck with a lease on an office in which you cannot open your business. Also consider making the lease conditional upon being granted a local massage practitioner license and a massage establishment license.

You also may want to negotiate for a lease that is renewable at your option. After all, you do not know for sure that you will succeed in your business, or that you will like the location. Give yourself the option to leave after a year. At the same time, give yourself the option to renew for a second and third year at the same rental (or a small increase) so that you know you will be able to enjoy the reward for your efforts if your practice is very successful.

Spell out in the lease any other items that you consider of special importance to you, and make sure you understand all of the provisions of the lease you sign. As a precaution, it is good practice to show the lease to a lawyer or experienced business person to get an informed opinion before signing.

One further thing to keep in mind is that, while your lease gives you legal rights, these may not amount to anything in practical terms if you wind up having a conflict with your landlord. If you need to hire a lawyer and file a lawsuit, your expenses in suing will almost certainly be more than you would recover even if you win. You can sue in small claims court if you meet the local requirements.

LEASE CONTRACT

This contract is entered into this 15th day of January, 1988, between Martin Ashley (Martin) and Anthony Marzarella, doing business as Anthony Louis (Anthony). The parties agree as follows:

1. Anthony will furnish a massage room in Le Club salon on Route 88, Brick, New Jersey. He will also furnish a receptionist to take appointments for massage and to collect clients' payments for massage. The receptionist selected shall be a courteous individual who presents a positive image of massage and of the massage therapists employed to work at Le Club.

2. Martin will pay a monthly rental to Anthony of $400.00 per month, payable on the 1st day of each month. Martin will also pay Anthony 17% of the cost of advertising which advertises massage at Le Club.

3. This contract shall be for a period of three months, and shall be renewable at Martin's option for additional periods of three months, up to a total of one year. In addition, after the first year, the contract shall be renewable for an additional year at a monthly rent not to exceed $500 per month.

4. Anthony shall obtain a Brick massage establishment license, and Martin shall obtain a Brick massage practitioner license. All massage therapists employed by Martin at Le Club shall have Brick massage practitioner licenses. Martin shall have the right to transfer or sell his rights under this contract to any other individual who has a Brick massage practitioner license.

5. Permanent improvements to the premises made by Anthony shall be the property of Anthony, and furnishings placed in the massage room by Martin shall remain the property of Martin.

6. Collection of the amount due to be paid for massage shall be the responsibility of Anthony. The receptionist shall collect payment from massage clients.

7. Liability to clients and customers for any accidents or injuries shall be Martin's if the accident or injury occurs within the massage room, and Anthony's if the accident or injury occurs elsewhere on Le Club premises.

_____	_____
date	Anthony Marzarella
_____	_____
date	Martin Ashley

However, even that takes preparation, time, energy and expense. While your lease should afford you legal protection, steering free of conflict is worth much more than having right on your side.

The lease on page 63 is the one I signed when I moved into a massage office in a beauty salon. It's not perfect, and the rent was too high, but it will serve as an example of the kinds of items you might want to include in a business lease.

4. Taking Credit Cards

Consider taking Visa and Mastercard in payment for your services. The disadvantage is that the card company will take a percentage of the amount you charge for your services, usually 3 to 4% for Visa and Mastercard (sometimes higher for new accounts), and around 6% for American Express. (Members of the International Massage Association can take advantage of reduced-rate credit card accounts — see page 105.)

The advantage to taking credit cards is that you present a very established and professional image. This can be a good asset to a massage office, which is susceptible to being thought of as outside the mainstream of the business world.

Practically all clients find it convenient to write a check or pay cash, but you may find that there is a small amount of business you will do that you would not do without taking credit cards. Credit cards make it very easy for clients to buy gift certificates — they can order them much as they do flowers from a florist.

To investigate taking credit cards in your business, go to the bank where you have your business checking account, and ask for assistance. You can also do some comparison shopping — call other local banks and ask them about their arrangements for credit cards. Also, check the Yellow Pages and the Business-to-Business Yellow Pages under "Credit Card Equipment and Supplies" for other companies that issue merchant numbers and credit card plates. The initial fee for the imprinter will be in the neighborhood of $50.

5. Furnishing Your Office

The furnishings you choose for your office will reflect your personality and your preferences for a setting in which to practice your particular type of work. You might choose pastels and crystals if you lean toward the ethereal, and whites and stainless steel if you lean toward the clinical. Only you know the atmosphere you want for yourself and your clients.

Certain basics, however, apply to most or all massage rooms:

- In general, you should keep your office spacious and uncluttered, as this generally promotes a more comfortable and relaxed feeling.

- Arrange for lighting that is not harsh. Avoid ceiling lights, as these will be too bright for clients when face up. Dimming switches are inexpensive and easily available. One type installs in the wall switch and another screws directly into the bulb socket. Also consider stained glass lamps designed to hold low-watt bulbs and night lights that plug into wall sockets.

- Your diplomas will add an air of professionalism to the walls. Consider also some artwork to create an appropriate atmosphere.

- Keep a desk in your office. The desk is the place for your telephone and answering machine, phone books, schedule book, client files, and business card collection.

- Linens can be kept on a shelf, in a cabinet, or under the massage table. Choose your linens after you decide on a color scheme for the office, or use white linens, which can go with any office colors.

- Have a mirror available to your clients.

- Give your clients ample hooks for their clothing. Create a private space for dressing and undressing or leave the room while clients are dressing and undressing. Have a table or counter where clients can put their jewelry and personal belongings.

- Have a computer, word processor or typewriter in the office so you can do paperwork between appointments if necessary.

- Have your business cards out in a spot where clients will see them and can take one.

- Consider having bottled water available for you and your clients in your office.

Checklist for office furnishings

massage table	mirror
linens	desk
hamper	table or counter space for client's use
oil	telephone and answering machine
chair	
clothing hooks for clients	typewriter
business card holder	lighting system
bottled water cooler or other dispenser	artwork, diplomas or other decorations for walls

6. Telephone Reception

One advantage of a group practice is that the group can pool resources to either hire a receptionist or rotate duties on phone reception. This assures that callers will reach a person who can answer their questions about massage and schedule an appointment.

If you are practicing alone, it is much more difficult to answer your own phone. Hopefully, you will be too busy doing massage to be serving as your own receptionist. The choices available to you are hiring an answering service or using an answering machine.

Practically all therapists, faced with this choice, choose an answering machine over an answering service. The service may seem to have the advantage of presenting the caller with a live human to talk to, but the person who works for the answering service is not likely to be familiar with massage. Therefore, she or he cannot answer the potential client's questions about your services. The answering service can take messages for you, but that is about all.

Answering machines have one major drawback—a great many people simply hang up when an answering machine answers a call. A person who has a strong desire to reach you will leave a message. However, someone who has been given your card, or who has seen an ad, may not go to the trouble to leave a message. For this reason, having a live human being answer the telephone is a significant advantage.

Caller I.D.

In most areas, phone companies now offer a feature that lets you know the phone number of the person calling you. The service costs a few dollars per month, and requires a separate caller ID device costing around $60. Consider ordering caller ID on your business phone, or your home phone if you use that for business calls.

After two rings, the caller ID device displays the phone number of the person who is calling you. The machine also stores the numbers of the last twenty or so people who have called your number. When making an appointment for someone for the first time, you can say to the person "Can I call you at 555-3456 to confirm?" The fact that you know their phone number will be a strong deterrent for any sex clients who may be calling you.

Checklist for office opening

The items in this checklist are arranged in chronological order—in other words, do number one first, number two second, etc. Begin this process three to six months before your target date for opening your new office.

Three to six months before opening:
1. Contact local government for information about zoning, and any regulations of health, fire and police departments
2. Contact direct mail company to learn the date of their next mailing; contact phone company to learn deadline for next yellow pages listing
3. Consider possible locations and look at offices for rent
4. Negotiate a lease for your office location, select starting date with enough lead time to make all preparations
5. Obtain all necessary governmental approvals, licenses and permits

Two to four weeks before opening:
6. Register fictitious name with county

7. Establish business checking account

8. Contact telephone company to connect new service

9. Order stationery, business cards and any promotional items you plan to use to publicize your office's opening

10. If appropriate, plan an advertising push when you open to create an increased clientele for your new venture

11. Shop for office furnishings

12. Notify all your clients of your new office opening and any introductory promotions you may be having

13. Get to know the neighbors in your new location and use any opportunities to gain clientele through your neighbors

Opening a group practice

Group practice refers to several massage therapists or related professionals sharing a suite of offices. Group practices have some significant advantages over individual practices, as well as some disadvantages.

The two main advantages of group practices are shared expenses and cross-referrals. The main disadvantage is the group decision process.

Renting an office suite and sharing the cost usually results in a lower price to each member than she would have to pay for a similar office space rented individually.

A group practice has the potential to become well-known as a center, thereby attracting a larger clientele through the reputation of the group practice. Once such a reputation is established for a group practice, it will generate a significant walk-in trade, and all the group members will benefit by having additional clients.

The disadvantage of a group practice is that decisions must be made by the group as a whole. This usually means devoting one evening per week to the process of group decision-making. After a busy week of massage, an evening of group process can seem like a burden. However, if you choose carefully which other practitioners you associate with, these group meetings can be an opportunity for learning and socializing.

Buying an Existing Massage Practice

Occasionally, practitioners sell their practice. You may have an opportunity to purchase an existing practice. This may seem like an appealing way to have a ready-made practice. However, buying an existing practice is very risky, and you should be extremely careful if you choose to do so.

Ask yourself several questions:

1. Why is this person selling her practice? She may not be giving you the real reason. Ask to see her appointment book, and take a minute to look at it. See how busy the office really is.

2. Will she take any of her clients with her? This can be a problem if the selling therapist plans to stay in massage and to stay in the area. You may find you have paid for a practice that evaporates as soon as you arrive.

3. Will her clients like you? It was the selling therapist's style of massage and personality that attracted her current clientele. If your massage and your personality are different from hers, her clients may be dissatisfied with you and may leave to try other therapists.

If I were buying an existing practice, I would want to first become an associate, and work in the office on a part-time basis. By so doing, I would get the feel of the clientele, and know whether they would accept me, and whether I would feel comfortable working with them. I would also have the opportunity to see first-hand how busy the practice is.

Ask the seller if such an arrangement is possible.

You could try it for a couple of months, at which time you would decide whether to buy the practice for a pre-set amount of money.

The real value of an established practice is the client base, the group of people who are in the habit of coming to this practice for massage on a regular basis. The client base can be a valuable asset if you are new to a community and want to become established quickly. I suggest you base a selling price on the number of clients you believe will stay with you after you take the practice over. You will need to make your best estimate of this.

If the client base will give you only enough income to meet the office rent, it is not worth much to you. On the other hand, if you will be able to step in and immediately earn enough to meet expenses and take home an income of $500 per week, that is worth a great deal.

Figuring the value of an existing practice is tricky, but consider this formula. Project the income you expect to earn immediately after taking over the office. To do this, you must have some basis for knowing how many clients will stay with you after the selling therapist leaves.

Assume your projected income for the first month is $1300. Next, total the expenses you will have for rent, phone, yellow pages, insurance, taxes and supplies. Assume this is $750 per month. Subtract the expenses from your expected income. You can project your estimated profit to be $550 for the first month.

Offer the seller three to five times the amount you expect to take home as profit for the first month. If your assessment is correct, you will be able to recover your investment within a year or so, and you will then have a successful practice with a minimum of marketing effort on your part.

The figure you offer will probably be less than the seller was hoping for. The seller may hope for a figure that represents a year's profit. If the business is very attractive and you can afford it, you may want to agree to such a price. However, you should only offer what the business will be worth *to you*. If you were buying a store that sold brand-name goods, the established trade would be reliable. In your case, the value of this business depends very much on how much it will change after you take it over.

III

Sex, Gender
and Touch

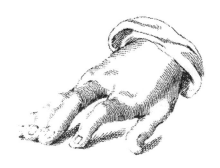

9 Sex and Massage

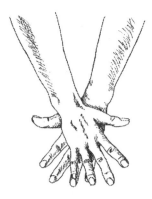

About half-way through my massage school course, I began to wonder when we would have the class about sexuality and massage, to help us understand and deal with sexual feelings that may arise for the client or the therapist during a session. I kept waiting for such a class, but it never arrived.

When I set up a practice in the "real world," I encountered sexual issues that deserved to be discussed in schools. While some schools now include a discussion of sexuality and massage in their programs, it is still relatively rare for a school to give its students any meaningful preparation for what they can expect in the "real world."

Differences in approach

The approach I suggest for a professional massage therapist or bodyworker is to set up clear boundaries for the therapeutic session. Any sexual intention by the client or the therapist is outside those boundaries. A client who presents sexual intentions should be confronted, and if the client acknowledges sexual intentions, the treatment should be ended.

Some authors and some educators differ with that approach, and regard a client's sexual desires not so much as a problem, but as an opportunity to foster the client's growth by exploring the psychological issues he has concerning sexuality. Be aware that if you choose such an approach, you are crossing the line between massage and counseling. If you have psychological training and the therapeutic skills needed to work in that way, there is nothing wrong with doing so. I don't, and most massage therapists don't. Therefore, my advice is to simply terminate a massage when a client presents the wish for sexual gratification.

Clients who want sexual massage

Occasionally, a woman massage client attempts to initiate sexual contact, either with a male or female massage therapist, during a massage session.

Instances in which men attempt to initiate sexual contact, either with a male or female massage therapist are, unfortunately, much more common.

Since you should expect to deal with clients who attempt to initiate sexual contact, the following are offered as guidelines for what to expect and how to deal with what takes place. Since the great majority of sexually oriented clients are men, the male pronoun is used throughout this chapter.

Arousal need not be considered a problem

A few men experience a partial erection at some point during a massage. These men are not necessarily after sex, and may actually be somewhat embarrassed by their arousal. The simple fact of a male client having an erection should not be seen as a problem, as long as the man's attitude is appropriate and he presents no verbal or non-verbal sexual expressions.

Arousal plus inappropriate action is a problem

Signs to watch for if a male client has an erection are: touching the genitals; grinding the hips into the massage table; moving the hips in any way; using muscular contraction to flex the penis.

These activities should alert you that this client will probably present a request for sex. You should confront him immediately about his arousal. Unless he can explain his actions to your satisfaction, terminate the massage immediately.

Other, subtler signs to look for are very shallow breathing or sighs of appreciation or pleasure. If you have some experience with clients who want sex, you will learn to "feel" that desire coming from them. It may be a subtle change in the mood in the room, or a change in *your* breathing or thinking that you cannot explain.

If in doubt, confront

If a client has an erection and you perceive signs that lead you to believe this client wants sex, ask your client questions to find out if you are right. Mention that he seems to be aroused and ask his feeling about that.

If the client's response tells you his attitude about the arousal is one of enjoyment, terminate the massage immediately. If the client continues to make any voluntary movements of a sexual nature, such as grinding the hips or touching the genitals, terminate the massage.

Your massage room is your environment, and you are in control of what does and does not happen there. Do not allow a client to threaten that control. Do not be afraid of losing business — any client who is sexually oriented is a client you want very much to lose anyway.

If you are alone in your office, you may want to have a phone number handy for someone you know you can reach in an emergency. I have never heard of a massage client actually becoming aggressive, but it may help you to feel more at ease to know someone is available to help you just in case.

Understanding the big picture

Sex and massage have undoubtedly been linked for thousands of years. One explanation for the persistent connection between the two has been offered by

David Lauterstein, co-director of the Lauterstein-Conway School of Massage in Austin, Texas:

> … we rather awkwardly encounter the one good reason massage and prostitution were ever associated. Both address people's need for love. However, prostitutes simply don't deliver—selling sex as love is robbery. That's a good reason why it's illegal. Massage therapy recognizes that underneath each person's tension, stress, even illness and injury, is an unmet need for energetic nourishment, i.e., love.

Unfortunately, many men are not aware of the distinction Mr. Lauterstein refers to. They *think* that what they need to be happy is sex, and there are plenty of "practitioners" who are willing to indulge them in their illusion.

In some parts of the world, a manually-stimulated orgasm is the normal and accepted conclusion of a professional massage. In many parts of the United States, a sexual massage is more common and easier to find than a legitimate massage. In some areas (San Diego, for example) the sexual massage ads in the yellow pages completely overwhelm the few listings for massage therapists.

In recent years, newspapers have carried stories of "acupressure" parlors fronting for prostitution in Los Angeles County, California, and massage parlors fronting for prostitution in the Oyster Bay area of Long Island, New York. The New York parlors were closed only after a march by licensed massage therapists, who announced plans to hold a press conference in front of their local senator's office unless action was taken.

Millions of men have had sexual massage experiences, and continue to have them today. As such, it is understandable that they would have some confusion about what it is you do. That is why you should be 1) non-judgmental and 2) completely clear in your communications before beginning a massage.

Screening new clients

It is a good practice to ask anyone who calls you how they heard about you. First, you want to be able to thank clients for referrals, and keep track of how successful your various promotional activities have been. Second, if the person does not come as a referral from a trusted client, you want to be able to make sure the person does not have the wrong idea.

Most sex clients will find you either through the yellow pages or through a newspaper ad. With male callers who have located me through advertising, I make a point of stating at the beginning that my massage is strictly non-sexual. I may use terms like "legitimate" or "therapeutic" to reinforce the message. I then ask them if this is the type of massage they are looking for, and pause to give them an opportunity to answer.

Massage clients understand the need for such an explanation, and are not put off. Most of the sex callers will hang up at that point, but some persist. During the conversation that follows, I have learned to watch my breathing. If my own breathing becomes shallow, and my heart starts beating fast, I have learned that this means my unconscious is getting the message that there is something dishonest about the caller.

Clients looking for sexual massage will try to find out what they can get without saying anything incriminating. Typical questions the sex caller may ask, in an attempt to find out if he can get a sexual massage, are these:

> Is this a nude massage?
>
> Is this a "complete"?
>
> What will you be wearing during the massage?
>
> Is tipping allowed?
>
> Are there extras?
>
> Can I get a release?
>
> What else is included?
>
> Does a girl give the massage?

If you hear any of these questions, politely tell him he has the wrong office, and hang up.

To minimize sex clients, get a first *and last* name for any first-time clients, and a phone number you can call to confirm the appointment. Try to avoid same-day appointments with first-time clients, and phone to confirm the appointment the day it is to take place. If any difficulty or confusion results from your attempt to confirm the appointment, be prepared for a no-show or a client who may be using a wrong name.

One Massage Therapist's Story

The following essay is one of four essays in a work called Massage Portraits, originally published in 1984 in CoEvolution Quarterly/Whole Earth Review, issue No. 43. It is written by Anneke Campbell and is reprinted with her permission. I include it here because it captures well many of the aspects of dealing with a client seeking sex.

CHIP

It was nine in the evening when the phone rang, and a male voice asked if he could come for a massage. "How did you find out about me?" I asked, always cautious. "Connie usually works on me when I'm in town, but she's out for the evening."

I knew Connie did good work, so I relaxed. "My old football injury is acting up," the man continued, "Could you see me tonight?" "Well …" I didn't much feel like it, but my rent was due at the end of the week. "Alright then." "I sure do appreciate it."

The fellow who walked in my door was a massive six-foot-four, dark-haired, jowly. I was going to have to work for my money. Chip had played football at college in the sixties, and nearly gone pro. Partly due to his back problem, he had opted for business, and was doing quite well, if he did say so himself. He also told me he was divorced. He took off all his clothes with bravura, as if to let me know he had no hang-ups about his body, not him.

His back was a sheet of lumpy, tight muscle. I stood close to the massage table and leaned all my weight into my hands. I began by pushing on the bunched-up erector spinae, and to my surprise, they softened up right away. Chip was responsive. I concentrated with my fingers on the vertebrae, which were buried in fibroid connective tissue. While I worked, Chip told me about the injury which had left him with some weakness in the sacral area. He had experienced both numbness and aching in his legs for years.

"There's nothing I can do about nerve impairment, if that's what the problem is," I explained, "but your entire back is a mess, probably due to compensating for the injury. And I can do something about all these tense, bunched-up muscles." I used long, firm strokes down the erector spinae and up the latissimus dorsi. I kneaded the well-padded abdominal obliques and trapezius. I worked so hard that the muscles in my own arms started aching, and drops of sweat ticked at the small of my back.

After about forty minutes, he began to moan. I was feeling pleased with the results of my work; his back was definitely less rigid than when I started. "Doesn't it feel better?" I asked. "It does, oh yes, but you're not getting to where most of the pain is." "Which is?" "Lower down."

I chased an uncomfortable thought from my mind, and moved my hands down to his sacrum and pelvic brim. I focused on the tiny muscles that lie over the sacrum; they were mushy in texture, a mushiness I associate with damage, and I could see that these could well be the source of his "weakness." Underneath, my fingers discovered some cyst-like formations. Here I worked carefully, but thoroughly. "Lower," he said.

I ignored the request. Chip's heavy body seemed suddenly disgusting to me. "Massage my thighs, that's where the problem is, on the inside of my thighs." "I've only a few minutes left." "How about another hour?" "I don't work two hours in a row," I lied.

I did some long, firm strokes down the length of his legs, trying to ignore the slight grinding of his pelvis into the massage table. I moved up, and took his bullish neck into my hands. Muscle like rock. He needed another hour, that was clear, but he wasn't going to get it from me.

"My masseuse in Florida, she does a full-body massage." I felt a sudden stab of hatred for the masseuse in Florida. "Yep, but she's a strong lady," Chip continued, "bigger than you are. You're just a little thing, aren't you. Well, what this lady does, it doesn't take much strength really."

I remained silent, kneading away at his sterno-cleido-mastoids. "She massages me down there, you know ..." "I don't do that kind of massage." "I'll give you fifty dollars." "Thank you, but no," I say, clear I would never do such a thing. "One hundred dollars then." "I don't do that kind of massage," I repeated, thinking, good Lord, one hundred dollars for a hand-job, he must be filthy rich.

"Please," he said, "One hundred and twenty?" Half a month's rent, I thought. Is it really that different, rubbing his penis or rubbing his trapezius? What's a little come on my hands? And what difference would it make to anyone but me?

"No," I said, and left the room. As I washed my hands, I noticed they were shaking. I felt a little sick to my stomach, and worried about being alone in the house with this huge man. I sat down in an easy chair in the living room. After a while, Chip appeared, fully dressed. He handed me a twenty-dollar bill. "Thanks," he said, "my back feels a hell of a lot better."

For the first time in that hour, I looked him fully in the eye. The cringing I saw there took away my fear. He was obviously embarrassed, but more to the point, terribly lonely. I knew what he needed was not sex, but warmth, contact, friendship. I nearly wished I could help him, but I had no desire to be his friend. "I'm glad your back feels better." I said, getting up. I opened the door, and extended my hand. Chip held it between his for a moment. "Good hands," he said.

Therapists who have sexual feelings toward clients

Very likely, at some point in your career, you will feel sexually attracted to a client on your table. It is your responsibility to your client and to your practice to work with your own feelings and control your thoughts and actions.

Your touch transmits your thoughts

Your touch communicates an unbelievable amount of information to the person you are touching. If you are viewing them with sexual intention, they will feel that in your touch. They may not be consciously aware of what they are feeling, but the communication will take place nonetheless.

If you have ever had the experience of receiving a massage from someone who had sex on their mind, you know what I mean. You can feel it in their touch. It is a totally different experience than being treated by a therapist.

Transmitting sexual feelings in your massage can sabotage your practice. The client whom you approach sexually will feel uncomfortable, and is not likely to become a repeat client. He or she is also likely to communicate to others a feeling of discomfort, uneasiness, or general dissatisfaction with your massage.

Monitor your own thoughts and feelings. If you start to slip into sexual thoughts about a client, try to determine whether these are originating with you or the client. If you find that you are responsible for originating these feelings, simply choose to stop. Remind yourself of your therapeutic intention, and focus your thoughts on your techniques and therapeutic goals for this client.

Never initiate sexual contact with a client

Occasionally, stories are reported about professionals, including massage therapists, who sexually accost their clients. This is damaging to the profession as a whole, and disastrous to the lives of the therapists involved.

It is one thing to decide to date a client, to become friends, and then to have whatever personal relationship you both decide to have. That presents no particular moral or ethical problem.

It is another thing to attempt to initiate sexual activity with a client *during* a professional massage. This is immoral, unethical, and illegal. The massage relationship involves trust on the part of the client, who becomes vulnerable to the therapist. In this sense, the relationship resembles that of a doctor and patient, or priest and penitent. The trust placed in you by your client gives you a greater responsibility to be honest and above board in your dealings.

If you feel a desire to initiate sexual activity with your clients, seek professional help. You may be able to learn something about yourself in the course of working with this desire. If you are unable to control this desire, your best course of action may be to stop practicing massage, or to limit your practice to men only or women only.

10 For Men Only

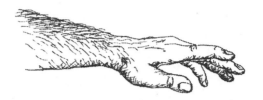

The challenge for a male massage therapist

In the massage field in general, attracting clients and becoming established is more difficult for a man than for a woman. This is not true in certain specialties, like sports massage, on-site massage, Rolfing, Trager, polarity, and other forms of bodywork that do not involve nudity and stroking. It is also not true in some other countries, such as Germany, where men tend to be accepted as massage therapists more easily than women.

However, in the field of Swedish massage in the United States, experience shows that most clients prefer having a woman give them a massage. Most women are shy about becoming undressed and being touched by a man they are not intimate with. Many also have self-image issues and are embarrassed to have a man see their bodies. Many men feel uncomfortable being touched by another man, and prefer the nurturance they receive from a woman's touch.

Some groups of clients that prefer male therapists

Some men prefer a male therapist because they want to avoid any possibility of arousal. Such groups include Catholic priests, orthodox Jewish men, and men with strong moral principles.

Many gay men prefer a male therapist, apparently because they are more comfortable in the company of men.

Many athletes and very muscular men prefer a male therapist, having learned by experience that women usually lack the strength to give a satisfyingly deep massage.

Some clients are gender-neutral

A certain number of clients do not care whether their massage therapist is male or female, but choose a therapist on personality and skill level. Such clients are a small minority. Generally speaking, such clients are probably more common in cosmopolitan areas and in the Western U.S..

The task for a male massage therapist

Because the available client pool for men is smaller, men have to try harder, be better, and have more patience than women when establishing a massage practice.

Men can and do succeed in the field, and some men become tremendously successful. Do not allow the challenge to discourage you. Knowing the situation in advance will allow you to better plan your career and focus on target groups which are likely to produce clients for you.

The male as pursuer

Societal conditioning, and perhaps instinctual patterns, result in men generally pursuing women sexually and initiating sexual contact in relationships. As a result, men tend to be in the habit of seeking sexual encounters.

One very successful male therapist told me that he considers it a great advantage to him that he is married. His desire to couple is focused on his wife, and he feels much more relaxed than he otherwise would about working with his women clients.

If this issue is a problem for you, there is no magic solution. Simply be honest with yourself, and exercise your will and creativity to avoid confronting your clients with sexual energy that will create problems in your professional life.

11 Working with Survivors of Childhood Sexual or Physical Abuse

Recent years have seen a dramatic increase in society's awareness of childhood abuse as a prevalent social problem. Those who have been abused as children may or may not remember being abused, may have been abused sexually or non-sexually, and may or may not have begun the journey of healing the effects of that abuse.

As a massage practitioner, chances are you will come in contact with a number of clients who experienced childhood abuse. Some of these clients will have normal reactions to massage — they will appreciate your services, and will pose no difficulty to work with. Others may have extreme reactions that include terror, convulsions and withdrawal. It is these other clients, who may have dramatic reactions, that are the subject of the cautionary advice in this chapter.

Because your touch may re-activate childhood trauma, there are certain fundamental things you should understand in order to work with these clients without doing additional harm to them. This chapter seeks to give you the basics you need to know to avoid doing harm and to serve these clients to the best of your ability.

Most massage clients are women, so the female pronoun is used throughout this chapter. Be aware, however, that many men have also experienced childhood abuse, both sexual and non-sexual.

I wish to thank Mary Ann DiRoberts, who provided substantial assistance in the preparation of this chapter, and also Diana Lonsdale and Anya Seerveld, both of whom provided information for use in this chapter.

Childhood abuse and the damage that results

Children have natural mechanisms to deal with stress, but extremely strong experiences can overwhelm these mechanisms. Sexual or physical abuse is too much for the child to deal with, and it can prevent the normal integration of the psyche as the child matures.

One aspect of this process is numbness, or dissociation. Minor dissociation is a natural part of life for most people, taking the form of spacing out, daydreaming, or similar behaviors. However, more significant dissociation can result in a state in which the person is not aware of the physical sensations of the body, or is not consciously present in the experience of the body. In extreme cases, multiple personalities are created and the person lives a life as different personalities who may not even know each other.

Psychologically, childhood abuse destroys the child's sense of safety and trust, and drastically violates the child's boundaries. The child may grow into an adult who has difficulty trusting and is confused about boundaries. One who experienced childhood sexual abuse may have guilt about the sensations she had during the abuse, feel shame or responsibility for the abuse, and have terror buried in her body from these childhood experiences. As an adult, she may feel like "damaged goods" and may believe that sex is all she is good for, or that she is not even good for that.

While you should not attempt to diagnose someone psychologically, certain traits can clue you in that childhood abuse *may* be an issue in someone's life. Signs to look for include depression, lack of emotion, extreme changes in emotion, feelings of being different or defective, dysfunctional relationships, irresponsible sexuality, anorexia, bulimia, obesity, childishness or excessive vulnerability, inability to take care of one's self, workaholism, compulsive rituals or other compulsive behaviors, and anxiety attacks.

It is important to remember that unless you are trained as a mental health professional, you should not attempt to be a psychotherapist for a person who experienced childhood abuse. In fact, unless you have specialized training in practicing massage with abuse survivors, you should consider declining to practice massage with such a client. Without the understanding and skills necessary to work with such clients, you may do more harm than good by giving a massage.

The intake interview

When initially interviewing a client, do *not* directly ask if she experienced childhood abuse. Asking this question violates the client's boundary; it requires her to either lie or disclose something she may not wish to share with a person she does not yet trust.

It is better to ask generally whether bodywork brings up feelings for her. You may tell her orally or in your printed information that you invite her to let you know if she is in psychotherapy. However, avoid probing too deeply, as this violates a client's boundary. It is better to carefully listen and watch for signs that may alert you to a history of abuse.

During the massage

The abused child has been dis-empowered, has had trust violated, and has not had boundaries honored. When massaging this adult client, be careful to empower her and to operate with clear boundaries. Be scrupulous about giving control of the session to the client. Be clear about your permission to touch in specific places or in specific ways. Check in often with your client to be sure she is comfortable with the session and is present in her body.

Even a client who is not an abuse survivor will appreciate being empowered, respected, and given control. Since you likely will not know that a particular client is a survivor, consider these guidelines with all clients.

It is especially important to check in often during the massage with a client who has a history of abuse. When your touch triggers an emotional response or a memory of abuse, this client may be unable to tell you what is happening. The abusive experience often includes training in "not telling," and when a memory of that experience is triggered, the training to be silent may prevent the client from letting you know what is happening.

If a client recalls a portion of the abusive treatment during a massage session, it can be extremely upsetting for the client and a difficult situation for the massage therapist. A "flashback" can feel to the client like a flood of terrifying feelings. She may dissociate from current time and reality and be completely immersed in an experience of the childhood events. She may shake with terror, convulse, go into tetany, curl up in a ball, or shout at the perpetrator.

If you as a therapist find yourself with a client having such an experience, remember that this person is re-experiencing a terrible event from her past. If you can, talk to her in simple language, telling her where she is and what is happening in the present moment. Suggest that she open her eyes and describe the room you are in, or make eye contact with you, or change her position to sitting or lying on her side.

If she tells you about her experience, let her know you understand what she tells you by rephrasing it in your own words. Maintain boundaries and give her control over what happens, and assure her that you will stay with her and keep her safe as long as she needs you. After the experience has passed, she may still need your support and attention. Help her make specific plans for the rest of the day, and encourage her to use whatever support is available in her life. If the client is not in psychotherapy, this would be a good time to make a referral to a qualified practitioner.

Because flashback experiences can be so very unsettling, it is advisable to assure that a client with a history of childhood abuse has a psychotherapist if she is going to work with you doing massage. Because of the likelihood that your work will bring up such an intense experience, the client should have the services of a professional who can help process such an event if it occurs. If you intend to specialize in working with clients with histories of childhood abuse, you should have additional training in this area, be in supervision, and have done your own psychotherapy.

One survivor's experiences with massage

The following is excerpted from an article that appeared in The Journal of Soft Tissue Manipulation. Written under the pseudonym of Tess Edwards, it describes the experiences of a woman who experienced ritual satanic abuse as a child, and became a massage therapy client as an adult.

Her descriptions of various massage experiences and suggestions for therapists have great value. As you will see from reading the following, Tess is a client who dissociates during massage. Her massage therapist practices safe touch work, which requires specific training to do.

I wish to express my gratitude to "Tess" and to the Journal of Soft Tissue Manipulation for permission to reproduce this essay.

One trauma survivor's experience of massage
by Tess Edwards

I believe strongly in the importance of massage for survivors of child abuse. I feel very lucky that I am one of the few survivors I know who can both afford and tolerate a weekly massage.

In my search for healing, I saw an applied kinesiologist who told me that my trauma has settled mostly in the muscle and skeletal systems instead of the organs, as is more common. So for me, I believe that massage is crucial to the healing process because the toxic effect of the trauma is lodged in my muscles. Even when the toxic effect of abuse is primarily in the organs, I believe that massage is essential to the healing process—not only because safe touch is an important and unusual experience for most survivors, but also because trauma is held in the body.

Dancers talk about muscle memory—that is how they learn the intricate moves they must make on stage. We all have muscle memory. I have never been comfortable placing my arms above my head—I have never been able to paint a ceiling or hang curtains without going into a state of panic. Similarly, I usually postpone washing my hair for as long as possible. I always called myself lazy, stupid or other nasty names because I could not do these tasks. And I never understood that this had any meaning.

I now understand that many of my worst life experiences took place while my hands were tied above my head for long periods of time. I still have trouble with this. In fact, as the memories surface, difficulty with these tasks has increased. Now even in aquabics class I have tears rolling down my face when I try to do the above-the-head arm exercises. This is typical. As the memory surfaces, the symptoms intensify.

I've always thought that massage would help me, but it has been a long battle to allow myself to afford it and to learn how to tolerate it.

For three or four years, I got massage treatments about three times a year. For the most part, I don't think they helped me at all because I simply left my body during them. Touch of this type is really a re-enactment of the original abuse and in fact gives me even further to go in my healing journey. In one case, the massage I received was truly a re-enactment of the abuse and for months undermined the healing work I was doing.

One massage therapist really upset me when she was giving me her new-age philosophy about how we all choose our lives—have choice even about abuse in childhood. One of the hardest things to recover from is the guilt and shame that every survivor I've met feels about the abuse. Hearing their stories, I have noted that in most cases, the abuser blames the victim: "You're too sexy." "You make me do it." "You love it." "You know you want it."

"You're making me evil" was what my father used to say to me and he even taught one of my personalities to beg him for intercourse at an early age. So for my massage therapist to tell me that I chose either to come back in this life as a victim of child abuse, or that I as a child had some choice in the matter, pushes all my shame and guilt buttons. If I'm lucky, this makes me very angry. If I'm not, I feel despair.

My biggest difficulty with massage, although it took me a long time to realize it, was that any touch was triggering. Two years ago, a group of four survivors of sexual abuse started a self-facilitated group based on giving and receiving safe touch. In our weekly five-hour sessions, we would ask for what we wanted that night—anything from getting a back rub, to being rocked while we sang lullabies, to massaging just a hand, to building a protective igloo with pillows, to brushing hair. Any activity involving touch that the survivor could accept that evening.

During these sessions two of us began retrieving new memories of abuse while in the group. Instead of being a group for safe touch, the group became, temporarily, a group for memory retrieval. The memory work triggered by the touch was so intense for the other two members of the group that they asked us to stop. We then formed a group specifically for memory retrieval, which has been going on for over a year now and from which I have benefitted enormously.

Another survivor I know began the process of retrieving memory when she began to receive massage. This is why I feel that massage is so very important and so very tricky for survivors.

Currently, I see a massage therapist once a week, and it is helping enormously. Three nights ago, I had a dream that my body turned from metal into flesh. Last Sunday in my memory retrieval group, I was able to feel and express many more of the feelings that I felt as a child than I have before.

The massage is still hard sometimes. We're still trying to develop a system so that I can ask her to stop. We haven't found a good way yet because when I need her to stop, I'm in a child part who was trained not to speak; stopping wasn't an option, no matter how desperately she wanted to. It's hard for my massage therapist to help when I go there because the signs are subtle to non-existent. This is partly because I received tons of training on how to pretend everything was alright.

I think my massage therapist is learning my body enough to notice when I hold my breath or, more often, when my flesh just feels dead or uninhabited. I don't know how she does it. She checks with me a lot, which for me is great because it can sometimes give me permission to say that I am in trouble.

I have learned to set some boundaries. We do not work on my bum. I allowed her to work on my upper legs once and got so badly triggered that I was unable to say so until a week later. During that week, I wandered around in flashbacks. My inner thighs are now off limits.

My massage therapist tells me a lot of things about my body which are very useful to me because I've spent most of my life outside of it. She is helping me to learn about my body, making it easier to reside there.

There are a number of things I feel that a massage therapist should do when working with me. I am sharing these ideas so that other massage therapists might learn about how to help someone who has been abused.

- First and foremost, I am more important than your technique. If I can't lie face down, I need you to accommodate me. Maybe massage me while I'm on my side, even if it means you can't give me what you feel is your best work. Give me what is best for me, not your best work.

  If I leave my body, you can make my circulation shoot around better, but that's it. For me, the purpose of massage is to get more into my body, not leave it more. If I'm not present, I'm not getting what I need. I need to learn to feel pleasure in my body. Pleasure is something that has never been safe for me.

- Be creative. If I can't tolerate lying down, you could have me sit on a chair with my arms on the table and do just my head and neck. If I need to keep my clothes on, figure out how you can help me with my clothes on. Encourage me to bring my teddy bear if I am terrified.

- Help me to feel safe and comfortable. I love to be rocked and so do my inner kids. I love to be warm and adore my massage therapist's heating pad and the warm blankets she covers me with.

- Find out what you need from me in order to help me. Find out my other support systems. You can't be all things for me. You're not my therapist and you're not responsible for my healing or the bad things that happened to me. If you sense that my support structure is weak, be careful if you trigger memories that you can't take me through.

- Respect me and my process. I know best about me, just as you know best about you.

- One of the skills I value the most in my massage therapist is her understanding of emotional release. It is wonderful to know that she can handle anger, grief or terror as they come up and work with them, instead of being terrified by them. She has a big bucket with a pillow on it for resting my hands on when I am on my front or hitting if I need to release some anger.

- Learn to detect the difference between re-enactment and release. Re-enactment and release can look the same but have an opposite impact on the survivor. Both re-enactment and release can cause the survivor to show physical symptoms of grief, fear or anger. However, in re-enactment, the survivor is lengthening the work she has to do. She has yet one more incident of feeling powerless and victimized to recover from. In release, she is letting go of some of the abuse and actively reclaiming her life.

Being placed in a re-enactment can help enormously if I am ready for it and I choose it. I went to my massage therapist once after a particularly nasty memory where my hands were tied. I specifically asked her if she could work on my wrists and as she did, it felt as though hundreds of wrist restraints fell off as I cried. The relief was wonderful.

- Learn about triggers: what they are, how they work and how to cope with them.

- Please refer me if you are uncomfortable working with me. Don't sabotage my courageous act of attempting to find safe touch and learning to re-inhabit my body.

To me, my healing process involves recalling my life and integrating the sensory information that I blocked or dissociated from my awareness. This includes my emotions, my spirituality and the events, sights, sounds, smells, tastes, textures that I have been unable to allow into conscious awareness. I want to experience my life as a whole.

One of the most useful parts of healing is massage. To be touched without sex, without violence, is a first for me and a great gift. To learn that it is safe to allow someone into my space is incredible. To begin to release the trauma is a relief.

IV

Business, Practical and Legal Information for the Practitioner

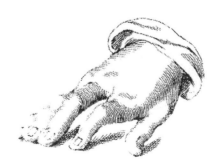

12 Business Basics and Practice Pointers

Practicing massage means operating in the business world. If you have no significant experience doing business, certain expectations of the business world may not be familiar to you. The purpose of this chapter is to give you enough information to avoid pitfalls and facilitate your success.

The subjects covered in this chapter are Steps You Can Take Toward Professionalism, What to Expect From Clients, and Pricing Your Services.

A. Steps You Can Take Toward Professionalism

1. Communicate Clearly and Keep Agreements

The business world operates by mutual agreement. In order to run smoothly, agreements must be unambiguous, and both parties must be able to rely on the other to keep the agreement.

In practice, this means you and your client should have no confusion about where or when appointments are to take place, how long they are for, how much they cost, and what sort of therapy the client is expecting you to provide. Keeping your agreement means arriving on time to all appointments with all the equipment you will need.

If an appointment is tentative, make sure both of you know when you will speak again to make it definite. If there are any questions in your mind about an agreement, speak to the client about them. The chances are that your client also has questions.

2. Present a Well-Groomed Image at Work and After Work

Most massage therapists understand the need to present a professional image at work. Your physical appearance announces who you are, and if you are proud of your work the image you present should convey that pride.

As a community member, you will see and be seen by your clients after working hours at unexpected times. Your appearance and your actions at these times will also have an effect on your clients' perceptions of you. While you need not constantly look over your shoulder, keep in mind that anything you do in public reflects on your professional character. If you have a wild side, you might want to keep it indoors.

3. Answer Your Phone in a Business-like Manner

Even if you have separate office and home phone numbers, you should answer both your home and office phones in a polite way. You never know who is calling with what opportunity, and it is a shame to spoil an opportunity by creating a poor first impression.

4. Return phone calls promptly

Make a point of returning your phone calls as soon as you can. Keeping people waiting for a return call will train them to expect you to be hard to reach; they may think twice about calling you next time. You also run the risk that the person who is trying to reach you will find someone else to meet her needs, and you will have missed an opportunity.

5. Make Cleanliness a Priority

Massage clients are very sensitive to the issue of cleanliness. If they find you or your office unclean, they will not tell *you*, but they will tell others.

Since massage is such a personal service, clients will want to be sure the linens are fresh, the carpet is clean, and your clothing and body are clean. If in doubt, go overboard, as some clients have a very critical eye when it comes to hygiene.

6. Avoid Talking Too Much During a Massage

If your client wants to talk, let her talk. It's her massage and her hour. However, do not use the massage as a time to talk about yourself, your problems and your opinions. If your client is being quiet, then you should be quiet as well, unless your conversation concerns an issue related to the massage session.

Several of my clients have told me they left their previous massage therapist because he or she would not keep quiet during a massage. Notice that they did not tell the talkative therapist — they told their new therapist.

7. Watch the details of client comfort

Show concern for your clients' experience. Their perception of their entire experience with you is important, not just the result of your hands working their muscles.

On a physical level, make sure your clients are warm enough. Be aware of any modesty issues. Avoid getting oil in their hair, and offer to towel off excess oil. Avoid causing any pain during the massage, unless you and your client both agree that aggressively working a body part is the best thing to do.

On the level of emotions and boundary issues, make sure you honor the right of your clients to reveal or not reveal facts about themselves, to have portions of their body worked or not worked, and in general to be in charge of their session.

For example, ask permission to work the abdomen unless you know your client will not mind. You do not know much about your client — he or she may have experienced sexual or physical abuse, and your careless touch may trigger a very painful experience. Don't let your desire to give override the client's wishes about what to receive.

8. Finish on time

Clients are often on a busy schedule. You may want to do that extra five or ten minutes, but your client may feel it's more important to be on time for her next meeting. If you need to go over the agreed time, get the client's permission beforehand.

9. Get to know the other therapists in your area

Become acquainted with as many massage therapists, fitness trainers, physical therapists, bodyworkers, chiropractors, acupuncturists, psychotherapists and medical doctors as you can. The more people who know you, the more opportunity there is for them to assist you in your professional growth.

Remember that you are becoming a service professional. Allow yourself to assume membership in the community of those who are serving others' health needs. Knowing a large number of health professionals gives you a broad perspective on the field, and on the level of activity in your community. Be as involved in the total picture as you can.

10. Foster Your Own Personal and Professional Growth

As one therapist told me "There are massage therapists, and there are massage therapists, but the ones who make it are the ones who are working on themselves."

Examine what it is you offer your clients — what benefits your work gives them, and what kinds of difficulties your work helps them get through. Chances are, you are offering your clients help with the kinds of issues you also face in your life.

Acknowledge that you are also a client. Practice what you preach. Nurture your own growth through finding therapists and healers and teachers who help you grow. In the process, you will also learn new techniques that you can incorporate in your bodywork. The process of growth has no end.

B. What To Expect From Clients

1. Cancellations

Clients will cancel; plans change. It is an unavoidable fact of life. You can create a cancellation policy to protect yourself, so long as you communicate it to your clients. One fair cancellation policy is to require 24 hours advance notice, and to charge a penalty (such as $20) for canceling on shorter notice. A notice on your desk or office wall, where it can be seen by your clients, is adequate to commu nicate your policy.

2. Great expectations

One lesson I have learned over and over is not to place any importance on statements by clients like "I'm going to get a massage every week" or "I've got half a dozen friends who have been looking for someone like you." If I had the fee I would have charged all the people who told me they were coming in for a massage, I'd be considering retirement by now...

I'm sure they mean it when they say it, but the fact is people talk about getting massage much more than they actually follow through. Once you are an established therapist, these "great expectations" are not of great importance. However, if you are seeing four clients a week and needing the rent money, it can be harder to keep this sort of thing in perspective.

3. No-shows

Some clients make an appointment, do not cancel, and do not show up. This is about as frustrating a situation as you can get practicing massage, and there is very little you can do about it.

The great majority of no-shows are clients who have never been to see you before, and who learned about you either through the yellow pages or a newspaper ad. One way to control the problem is to require that all people making appointments give you first and last name, and a phone number where they can be reached to confirm the appointment.

If you call the number and they never heard of the person, don't be surprised if he does not show up. If you call the number, and they sound shocked that the person is getting a massage, don't be surprised if he never arrives. With experience, you will learn to evaluate the likelihood of the person showing up for the appointment based on your experience in calling to confirm.

When a first-time client fails to cancel or to show up, let that person go. This is a person you will not hear from again, and it will not do you any good to try to track him down. Put your energy into those who want and need your services.

The decision what to do when a regular client fails to cancel or to show up for an appointment is more difficult. It helps to have an announced cancellation policy, but if you do not you will need to decide whether to charge your client for the missed appointment or simply reschedule.

4. Angels

Once in a blue moon, you will get a client who takes it upon herself to be your fan club, publicity agent, networker and marketing strategist. Say a prayer of thanks.

An angel is someone who thinks so much of you and your work that she is inspired to do anything she can to help you succeed. This person will be thinking about you and talking about your work many times a day. Some are able to do more than others, but all act out of a feeling of love and caring.

My angel is one of my less affluent clients, and as a gesture of my appreciation, I have never raised his rate from the low introductory rate I was offering when he first became my client several years ago.

5. Constructive Critics

Most clients will not let you know that you caused them pain, or that they were too cold or too hot, or annoyed about something in your massage room.

Although they will not tell you, such unspoken dissatisfactions cause many clients not to return for another massage.

That is why you should be grateful for the very few clients who ask you not to do a certain stroke, or complain about the temperature, or ask you to change this or that about your massage or the surroundings. In all likelihood, these clients speak for many others as well.

One such client of mine is a chef with a very acute sense of smell. One day while I was seated and working on his face and head, he asked me to please breathe to the side. Apparently, he was able to identify just what I had eaten several hours ago.

Until this time, I had not realized that I have a tendency to breathe through my mouth, and to exhale onto my clients' faces. Most clients probably did not notice any breath odor, but they probably did feel my breath on their faces. Either way, I no longer breathe on people's faces. Unless my constructive critic had spoken up, I would never have realized what I was doing.

C. Pricing Your Services

Pricing your services can be a difficult issue. This discussion is meant to give you guidance in what to consider in order to find the most appropriate price for your services.

Several factors enter into a decision about pricing. The factors to consider are the "going rate" in your community, your expenses involved in providing the treatment, the price you feel comfortable charging, and the effect your price will have on your clients' ability to come to you.

1. The "going rate"

This refers to the customary charge for your kind of services in your area. The "going rate" for a one hour massage may be as low as $25 or $30 in some areas, and as high as $80 in other areas. Usually, there is a variation of $5 or $10 between the low and high ends of the "going rate." In my area, for example, the price for a one-hour massage ranges from $45 to $55.

Consider that the "going rate" is the rate charged by established professionals who have a clientele. A time-honored custom among newly-trained professionals is to slightly undercut the going rate when they are first attracting a clientele. To the cost-conscious consumer, the lower fee is an incentive to try this therapist. In addition, the lower fee is an acknowledgement that a newly-trained professional is still learning, and has not yet acquired fully mature skills.

If you choose a rate *far* below the going rate, for example $15 per hour, people will become suspicious that you are not really a trained therapist, and it may actually be harder for you to attract clients than if you charged a fee nearer the going rate.

As your skills and reputation grow, you will naturally raise your rates to a level that reflects your growth. Your clients will adjust to your new rates without much difficulty, especially since your new rates will be in line with the rates established therapists are charging. While some clients may find it hard to accept a rate increase after becoming accustomed to a lower price, most clients who know and like you will not leave you when your rates rise to the "going rate."

2. A price you are comfortable with

For you to be comfortable with the fee you charge for your services means at least two different things. It means, first, that you are comfortable asking your client to pay your fee — you believe your service is as valuable as the money you receive for it. This touches on issues of self-worth. Your fee should be one that you can ask for and receive without mixed feelings.

Second, being comfortable with your fee means that it creates an income for you that meets your needs. You should feel that it compensates you for what you have given in your therapy session, and that it provides you with the means to have the material things you need to keep your life and practice going. If you feel you are not being nourished in your professional life, you may find yourself resentful and unenthusiastic about your work.

3. Effect of pricing decisions on clients

One massage client told me "If massage costs $40, I'll come in twice a month. If it costs $55, I'll come in once in six months." I suspect this client speaks for many others.

Massage clients are generally quite cost-conscious. Many people would like to have massage on a regular basis, but feel they cannot afford it. Compared to items like a bag of groceries, a movie ticket or a tank of gasoline, massage is an expensive item to fit into a budget.

Even the wealthy are often quite cost-conscious. Many wealthy individuals either do not believe they have enough money, or resent people trying to charge them a premium because they are wealthy. They will shop for the best price, and reject a therapist who charges what they consider too high a price. This may not apply to a celebrity clientele, or the enormously wealthy, but the run-of-the-mill millionaire often watches prices very closely.

Therefore, your pricing decision may well affect the amount of business you get, the ease with which you generate new business, and the frequency of your repeat business.

4. Working on a "sliding scale"

Sometimes meeting all the goals mentioned above with one set fee is not possible. In some cases, you may need to make exceptions to your price or work on a "sliding scale." This means that you charge some clients a lower fee because that is all they can afford.

Some clients refuse to pay a reduced fee, as a matter of pride. Others may ask you directly for a reduced fee. If you are comfortable working at a reduced fee for those with a financial need, there is nothing wrong with doing so. Charge a fee they can afford and you can comfortably accept. Do not price your work so low that the client no longer places a value on it, or that you become resentful of the imbalance in the relationship.

My normal fee is $45. For clients with financial hardship, I will reduce my fee as low as $30. If I worked for less than $30 I would feel taken advantage of. However, for someone who cannot afford $30, whom I feel really needs my services, I will work without charge.

5. Discounts for series purchase

A common device therapists use is to offer a discount to clients who purchase several massages in advance. For example, if the cost of one massage is $45, a therapist may sell a series of five massages for $200 ($40 per massage).

This benefits both parties. The client saves $25, and the therapist has the use of the money in advance for any necessary expenditures. The client has the option of giving one of the series massages to a friend, which brings a potential new client to the office.

To offer a series, you can have a coupon printed up and sell the coupon. It may have five places to punch holes, or five numbers to cross off, or any system you prefer for keeping track of when the massages are used up. You can also create a system without coupons, by keeping track in your record book, or in a separate ledger.

6. Other discount arrangements

Create any discount arrangement that serves a business purpose. This can include discounts for those who refer new clients, or promotions in which you give a free massage to someone who buys two gift certificates, or any other such idea that makes sense to you. One discount I offer is $10 off the second massage in one week for any client.

Sometimes it is appropriate to offer a discount to a client for becoming a "regular." Take the example of Ray, one of my clients. Ray came for massage an average of once a month. Sometimes he would come more often, sometimes less often.

At the end of a massage, I asked Ray if he would come in regularly if the price were lower. He said he would, and we discussed possible agreements.

We decided that he would like to come twice a month, and could afford to do so if he paid $30 per visit instead of the $40 I was then charging. This seemed advantageous to both of us, and we agreed to adopt this plan. Now Ray comes in twice a month. He enjoys receiving more massages and I appreciate the added business and income.

I would not make this offer to most of my clients. It felt right to do so with Ray, in part because Ray does not know any of my other clients, so I knew I would not be presented with multiple requests for the same arrangement. I offer this as an example of the creative marketing you can come up with to fit a particular situation.

13 Staying Healthy in a Demanding Field

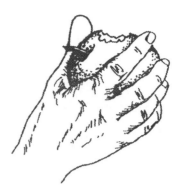

Every successful massage therapist I have spoken to has had to deal with some kind of physical or psychological problem that resulted from doing the work.

The most common physical problems are wrist injuries, back strain, neck and shoulder pain, and nodules (ganglia) in the fingers. In addition, some therapists suffer depression, some take on pain in places where their clients have it, and some "burn out" from the stresses involved in a massage practice.

There are practical ways you can avoid these problems. Successful therapists offered these tips from their experience:

Body Mechanics

Watch your body mechanics. Don't bend over when you work. Keep your spine straight and bend your knees. Let your force come from your hara, your abdominal center. Use the minimum number of muscles necessary for any particular motion. Make your body mechanics your first priority, even above the quality of work you do on your clients.

Exercise

Do yoga, tai chi, aikido, stretching, jogging, swimming, aerobics or some other exercise to improve your own bodily well-being. This helps not only to keep your body in good condition, but also to reduce the effects of stress.

Introspection

Involve yourself in psychotherapy, or meditation, and have a support group you can turn to in times of need. This will help you release your emotions, help you stay healthy, and promote your own growth.

Diet

Eat a balanced diet and drink plenty of water. You depend on your body as you would on a professional tool. You put good gasoline in your car, and keep the oil changed. Treat your body at least as well.

Attitude

Learn to let go. Life in the business world will bring you ups and downs, rewards and frustrations. Learn how to let go of the painful aspects. Letting go is not the same as denial or repressing your feelings. Accept people and situations as they are, let your emotions flow, and move on.

Receive Massage

Get massage on a regular basis. Three reasons: It promotes your overall health and well-being; you will learn techniques and awarenesses from receiving massage that will make you a better massage therapist; your credibility with your clients will be better if you "practice what you preach."

Specifics of Body Maintenance

Keep your wrists straight as much as possible while you work. Stretch your wrists before and after working. Use open fist, elbows or a T-bar to do deep work instead of fingers or thumbs.

If a nodule appears in a finger, try not to use that finger in your work for a week or two; apply pressure with the other fingers of that hand, but raise the finger with the nodule slightly so it is not used. If the nodule persists, work it with transverse friction to break it up. Consult a physician if the nodule will not recede.

Use a paraffin bath for sore hands, ice forearms or use liniment if inflamed.

Vacations and Days Off

Take days off. Success, when it finally comes, can be a shock to your system. If you find yourself very busy, make time to take care of yourself physically and emotionally.

Sometimes it is difficult to switch from the "I need all the clients I can get" consciousness to that of "I need to take time for myself." In the beginning, you do not have enough clients, and you are doing everything you can think of to get more. The time will arrive, however, when the clients will be coming. Allow yourself at that point to step back from your practice and make sure you are not wearing yourself out trying to achieve more "success" than you can stand.

14 Laundry and Linens

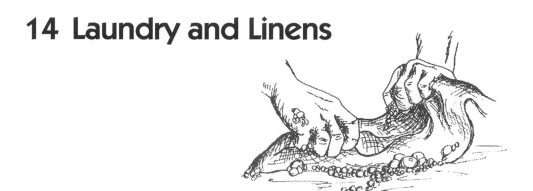

If you do Swedish massage, the issue of laundry is one you will face throughout your career. Unless you work in a setting where your employer takes care of laundry, you will have to make certain decisions about how to supply yourself with fresh linens to practice your trade.

Hire a Laundry Service vs. Do It Yourself

Depending on the laundry service you choose and what type of draping you use, having your laundry done for you can cost between $1 and $2.50 per client. Doing it yourself will bring the cost down dramatically, to between 10 cents and 50 cents per client.

If you hire a service, you will have to choose between furnishing your own linens and using theirs. If you use theirs, the cost will be higher. If you furnish your own, you will need twice as many as if you did your own wash, because at any given time, half your sheets and towels will be at the laundry.

Hiring a service makes the most sense in these situations:

1. You do not have a washer and dryer in your home or office. Trips to the laundromat can be very wearing when you are taking several loads per week.

2. You have a busy massage practice. If you are seeing lots of clients, then you are making enough money to afford paying a service to launder for you. If you have a busy practice, you probably do not have the time or energy to be dealing with the large amount of laundry your practice generates.

Choosing a Laundry Service

If you decide to use a laundry service, shop around. The prices charged by different services will vary quite a bit, as will the quality of their service.

Things to consider in hiring a service:

1. They may require you to use their sheets and towels, or they may be willing to sell you sheets and towels at wholesale prices. If you purchase the sheets and towels, the laundry will charge less to launder them than they would if they supply them.

However, any damaged linens will be your responsibility.

2. Be sure that this company can supply sheets and towels that you will like. See and feel samples before making an agreement.

3. Some massage oils can be difficult to remove from linens unless the company has the proper chemicals. Be sure they have experience with massage therapists and understand how to get these linens clean.

4. If you use a service, and they deliver a load of sheets and towels which are unsuitable in some way, you will be stuck with them unless the company is willing to make a special trip to remedy the problem. Find out how willing the company is to make sure problems will be taken care of and your needs will be met.

Finding Suppliers of Sheets and Towels

Buying a few linens at a time

If your practice is a casual one, meaning that you work on just a few clients a week, you will need a relatively small amount of linens, and should therefore purchase sheets and towels in the same way you do for personal use.

One option to consider is buying twin sheet sets. These include one fitted sheet, one flat sheet and one pillowcase, and sometimes can be found on sale for not much more than the cost of a single sheet. The fitted sheet on the table covered by the matching flat sheet creates a pleasant appearance.

Some therapists are quite particular about the linens they use, and this can be a very sensible attitude. The sheets and towels come in contact with a client's body, and you may want to create a luxurious impression by using colorful linens with a lush texture.

Buying in quantity

If you are most interested in presenting a clean (white) image, and keeping your costs to a minimum, consider purchasing sheets and towels through business channels. This is a decision to make when you begin to establish yourself in the field. It is not unlike a carpenter buying a set of tools—think toward the future and invest in a supply of sheets and towels you will be able to use for years to come.

Most companies that sell sheets and towels commercially are in the habit of selling at least 50 dozen at a time. The difficulty lies in finding a vendor who supplies linens commercially and is also willing to sell by the dozen. These are rare, but they do exist.

You will get some help looking in the yellow pages under "laundries." If your community has a Business-to-Business yellow pages, check under "linens." Occasionally, a commercial or institutional laundry will sell you one or two dozen odd or surplus sheets. These companies have large clients, and need to buy sheets by the gross for their own purposes. If they are willing to deal with you, you may be able to get a couple of dozen sheets from them at a discount price.

If you cannot locate any such businesses in your area, consider contacting someone who may have the connections you do not have. Your local hospital may be a wholesale purchaser of sheets and towels, and if you get in touch with the purchasing agent, she or he may be willing to resell a few dozen to you.

Choosing Sheets and Towels

Sheets

Whether you do your own laundry or use a service, you will still need to decide what size and quality sheets and towels to use. The thicker and more luxurious the linens, the more they will cost to buy and the more they will cost to launder.

Composition of sheets. The quality and comfort of sheets is determined by the "thread count." This is the number of threads used in a square inch of the fabric the sheet is made of. A higher thread count means a softer sheet. A thread count of 180 or higher usually signifies a good quality sheet. A thread count of 250 or more signifies a very luxurious sheet.

Also consider the fabric composition. The higher the percentage of cotton, the softer the sheet; the higher the percentage of polyester, the coarser the sheet.

Size of sheets. Keeping the size small helps a great deal in keeping the cost down at laundry time. Sheets come in a great variety of sizes, and the actual size of the sheets you receive may be a few inches different than the stated measurements.

If your goal is to create a luxurious feeling about your therapy room, and you are not being cost-conscious, buy large, thick sheets that will convey a sense of comfort and style. However, if your goal is simply to have a clean and pleasant sheet for your clients to lie on and under, consider the actual measurements of the sheets you need.

The normal size of a massage table is between 72" x 26" and 72" X 30". Two standard sheet sizes to consider are 72" x 42" and 75" x 54".

The actual size of the sheets you buy will be slightly smaller than the size stated on the package. This is partly because the stated size is "before hemming," and partly because it is accepted practice in the industry to have minor variations in sheet sizes. Therefore, a sheet that is called 72" long will actually be a few inches shorter than that, and will not quite cover the length of a massage table.

A 72" x 42" sheet is ideal for a table that has a face hole; it will cover the rest of the table and overlap a bit on all sides. It is also a good size to drape over a client, as it will cover most people from the neck down. A 75" x 54" sheet will cover the entire massage table, and will drape a few inches farther over the sides.

For a better looking image, you can leave a larger sheet draped over the table, concealing the legs. For each client, change the 72" x 42" or 75" x 54" sheet.

These smaller sheets are convenient to handle in laundry, and will take up a minimum of space in your washing machine. In fact, well over a dozen 72" x 42" sheets will fit into a normal washing machine at a time.

As you shop for sheets, you may hear a confusing mix of terms used to describe sheets — terms like "draw sheet," "twin sheet," "standard," and other terms. These names have general meanings, but they do not convey accurate information about the size of the sheets you will actually be buying. Keep in mind actual measurements only. Decide what size will be best for your style of draping and the image you want to create, and then shop with these requirements in mind.

Towels

The same considerations apply to towels as apply to sheets. The larger and more luxurious a towel is, the costlier it will be to purchase and launder. Keeping the size down is a big help.

Many standard sizes are available to fit almost any need. The size I find most convenient is 20" x 40". This is the size of a small bath towel. I find it meets my needs for draping very well, while taking up a minimum of space in the cabinet and the washer.

The quality of towels is measured in "pounds per dozen." This means, simply, how much does a dozen of these towels weigh? For a given size towel, the "pounds per dozen" figure will give you an idea of how thick and fluffy the towel is.

For the size I use, 20" x 40", a normal weight might be 6 or 7 pounds per dozen. I use a towel that weighs 8.5 pounds per dozen, because I want a soft and hefty feel to my towels. Towels like these are available for around $2 each, plus shipping, when purchased wholesale. However, it may be difficult to get a wholesale price on orders of less than 16 dozen.

If you are doing comparison shopping, remember that increasing thickness increases "pounds per dozen," and increasing size also increases "pounds per dozen." It helps to decide on the size you want, and then compare the different towels of that size based on the "pounds per dozen" figure. So long as you are comparing towels of the same size, the "pounds per dozen" figure will give you a good clue as to the thickness of the towel.

Tips for Do-It-Yourself Launderers

Doing your own laundry has advantages. First, you are in control of how many clean sheets and towels you have, and you know you will not run out unexpectedly, or have to rely on someone else to get your needs met.

Second, it is much cheaper to do your own laundry. Even factoring in the cost of a washer and dryer, in the long run doing your own laundry will probably cost only 10% to 20% as much as hiring a service.

Have the machines at your place

The most important consideration, if you plan to do your own laundry, is to have your own washer and dryer, in your home or in your office — whichever will be most convenient to your practice.

When your washer and dryer are convenient to use, you can throw in a load and be busy working, reading or relaxing. Throwing in a load becomes a routine activity and not a tedious chore, as it is when you have to leave your home or office to go to a laundromat. In addition, if the washer and dryer are for the exclusive use of your business, their cost can be deducted for income tax purposes (see Chapter 18).

Water dispersible oils

Most oil manufacturers now sell water-dispersible oils that are said to put an end to oil buildup in sheets and towels. These oils are a considerable help, and the oil removal process is now needed much less frequently than it was a few years ago. However, you may still find that oil accumulates in your linens, so the information below may one day come in handy.

Beating oil residues

Until recent years, there was no product generally available to remove oil residues from massage linens. A few years ago, a couple of products came on the market for removing oils from massage linens, Fresh Again and Sunfresh Soap. (For ordering information, see page 165)

Hints for success with Fresh Again

Fresh Again is the oil removal product I tried first. I have been happy with it, so I have stayed with it. Through experience, I have learned the following:

You do not need to use Fresh Again each time you wash. Use it to treat your sheets and towels when you notice a buildup of oil. You will notice either a rough texture, or the odor of cooked oil when the linens get hot in the dryer.

Shake well before pouring to mix the detergent fully. Use the hottest water you can. Use a larger amount of detergent for heavy oil stains. For persistent stains, soak the linens in hot wash water overnight and complete the wash in the morning.

If you have stubborn oil stains, try leaving the linens in a strong concentration of Fresh Again for several days. Another option is to use extreme heat to take the oil out. If your linen will fit into a crock pot, try soaking it for an hour or so on "high" in a concentration of Fresh Again. Otherwise, use an old pan to boil the linen in a solution of Fresh Again on your stove.

Use about 1/3 cup Fresh Again to one or two gallons of water, and boil the linen in this mixture at a low boil for at least five minutes. You will be amazed how much oil comes out of a soiled linen, even if this linen has just been soaked overnight in hot wash water. Although extreme heat can accelerate the wearing out of the stitching and fabric, it can save discarding a sheet or towel that may have a lot of life left in it.

15 Professional Associations
Profiles

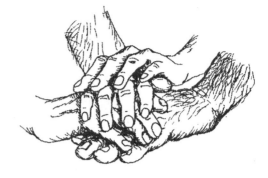

Associations of national interest are listed first. They are grouped into General Membership Organizations and Specialized Membership Organizations. At the end of this chapter, there is a listing of associations that are confined to one state or part of a state.

General Membership Organizations

American Massage Therapy Association (AMTA)

The AMTA is the oldest and largest national professional association for massage. It was founded in Chicago in 1943.

The AMTA has a program for curriculum approval/accreditation of massage schools. The requirement is a 500-hour program approved by the association, with a specified process of inspection and certification by AMTA.

Very active in the legislative arena, the AMTA lobbies for state and local laws. Some individuals within the AMTA work to have laws passed that require attendance at an AMTA-approved school, although this is not official AMTA policy.

Membership dues are $235 per year (some state chapters add a state fee), which includes professional and general liability insurance. Members receive a registry listing all members alphabetically and by state (published once a year), a quarterly magazine, and a newsletter. Each year the association sponsors one national conference and one national convention. State chapters sponsor state or regional conventions. Members have the opportunity to purchase group health, life and disability insurance, as well as AMTA pamphlets, books, media articles and products.

AMTA also maintains a referral service, supports the AMTA Foundation for research and community outreach, and sponsors a National Sports Massage Team.

Chapters exist in all 50 states, the District of Columbia, and the Virgin Islands, and some chapters have regional meetings. To join the organization, an applicant must 1) graduate from an approved school *or* 2) be licensed to practice in a state with standards acceptable to the AMTA *or* 3) pass the National Certification Exam.

For complete information, contact:

AMTA National Office
820 Davis St., suite 100
Evanston, IL 60201-4444
(708) 864-0123

Associated Bodywork And Massage Professionals (ABMP)

ABMP was founded in 1986. It is an international professional membership organization for massage, bodywork and somatic therapists, and is affiliated with 25 other professional associations.

Members include practitioners of Swedish massage, shiatsu, myomassology, Rolfing, Alexander, Feldenkrais, Hakomi, Trager, polarity, Rosen, on-site, Ortho-Bionomy, infant massage, reflexology, Hellerwork, and sports massage.

Members receive occurrence form professional liability insurance, premises liability insurance and independent contractor coverage. Members also receive a quarterly magazine, a newsletter for members, a Successful Business Handbook, a directory of schools and training programs, and a directory of suppliers that offer discounts to members. Members are also able to purchase discounted group health, life and disability insurance.

ABMP also maintains an 800-number for the public to call for therapist referrals, and works actively with legislative, municipal and regulatory committees to influence massage and bodywork regulations.

The ABMP has several levels of membership. Those who meet specified standards may join at the Professional Certified Level. This includes all benefits and costs $229 annually. Those with at least 100 hours training, including anatomy and physiology, are eligible for Practitioner Level membership, and those with at least 500 hours training are eligible for Professional Level membership. Membership at either of these levels costs $199 per year, and includes all professional liability insurance. Additional options include Certified (costing $99 for four years for U.S. residents), Associate and Student Level memberships.

The ABMP does not have state chapters, nor does it have association meetings. Members are encouraged to become involved in local organizations or specialty technique organizations.

In January, 1995, the ABMP announced the creation of a program to accredit schools that meet or exceed established standards of accreditation as developed by International Massage and Somatic Therapies Accreditation Council.

For complete information, contact the ABMP:

Associated Bodywork and Massage Professionals
28677 Buffalo Park Road
Evergreen, CO 80439-7347
(303) 674-8478

International Massage Association (IMA)

IMA was founded in 1994. Its growth in membership has been dramatic, and if current trends continue, IMA will become the nation's largest professional association for massage some time in 1997. The annual membership fee is $99.00, which includes professional liability and premises liability coverage, practice building materials, member discounts and low-cost Visa and MasterCard merchant accounts for its members. Associate membership costs $49 and includes all benefits except insurance.

The Association has an annual convention in Washington, DC.

A separate division of the IMA has been formed for movement teachers (such as yoga, Alexander, Feldenkrais, Trager, Pilates and the like). It is the International Movement Association. Its mailing address is the same as the one listed below but its phone number is different: (202) 332-0941.

For complete information about the IMA, contact:

International Massage Association, Inc.
3000 Connecticut Ave. NW, #102
Washington, DC 20008
(202) 387-6555

International Myomassethics Federation (IMF)

The IMF is an affiliate organization of the ABMP. The IMF seeks to promote all massage and bodywork disciplines, continuing education of practitioners, enhancement of public awareness of the benefits of natural health alternatives and adherence to a strict code of ethics.

Established in 1971 with 13 original members, the IMF now has approximately 1,000 members, with state affiliates, members at large and members in Canada and other countries. Members receive a quarterly newsletter, the option to purchase discounted liability insurance and other benefits.

For further information contact:

IMF Home Office
17172 Bolsa Chica, #23
Huntington Beach, CA 92649
(800) 433-4IMF or (714) 846-1849

Specialized Membership Organizations

American Oriental Bodywork Therapy Association (AOBTA)

The AOBTA is a membership organization for practitioners of oriental bodywork. It maintains a Council of Schools and Programs which approves curricula that meet AOBTA educational standards. Practitioners who have completed a prescribed 500-hour curriculum are eligible for Certified Practitioner Membership. The organization maintains a Code of Ethics and holds an annual convention.

Four levels of membership are Certified Instructor, Certified Practitioner, Associate Member and Student Member. Membership fees are $100 for Certified Instructor, $75 per year for Certified Practitioners, $50 per year for Associate Members and $30 per year for Student Members. In addition, the one-time application fee is $10 for students and $30 for all other applicants.

Members are eligible for professional liability and premises insurance through the Federation insurance program.

For full information, contact:

> AOBTA National Office
> Patricia Liantonio, Director of Administration
> 6801 Jericho Tpke
> Syosset, NY 11791
> (516) 364-5533

American Polarity Therapy Association (APTA)

Established in 1984, The American Polarity Therapy Association (APTA) is a non-profit organization that distributes educational material, registers practitioners, hosts educational conferences and publishes a regular newsletter. For further information about the association, polarity or trainings contact:

> American Polarity Therapy Association
> 2888 Bluff St., ste. 149
> Boulder, CO 80301
> (303) 545-2080

Association of Holistic Healing Centers (AHHC)

This is a non-profit membership organization created to support the evolution of health care centers that offer multi-disciplinary and multi-dimensional diagnosis and treatment, as well as wellness education programs.

AHHC offers networking to professionals interested in forming these centers, and provides a forum to share clinical outcomes and the practical aspects of center operation.

For further information, contact:

> Association of Holistic Healing Centers
> 109 Holly Crescent, ste. 201
> Virginia Beach, VA 23451
> (804) 422-9033 (Virginia)
> (602) 488-5502 (Arizona)

National Association of Nurse Massage Therapists (NANMT)

The NANMT was formed in 1987. In 1991 it had 87 members, and in 1994 had grown to over 500. The NANMT has recently been accepted into the National Federation for Specialty Nursing (a 350,000-member organization) and succeeded in having Massage Therapy named a nursing specialty. The organization is currently developing a certification model for Nurse Massage Therapists.

The NANMT is committed to bringing an increased awareness and acceptance of touch therapy to the mainstream medical and hospital community. It supports gaining insurance reimbursement for massage services, and also supports research into the health benefits of massage.

Members receive a quarterly newsletter, membership directory, and the chance to network with other Nurse Massage Therapists. Active membership requires an R.N. plus 500 hours of education in massage or bodywork. Active dues are $75 per year. Associate Supporting membership is $60 per year and student membership is $35 per year.

For further information, contact:

> Bobbi Harris, RN, LMT
> President NANMT
> P.O. Box 1268
> Osprey, FL 34229
> (813) 966-6288

The Guild of (financially) Accessible Practitioners

The Guild is a national forum offering information and support for making professional healing more financially accessible. The guild supports practitioners in clarifying their values. Members receive a quarterly newsletter. Membership is $35 per year, and membership on a sliding scale of $15 to $35 is also available if needed.

For further information, contact:

> The Guild of (financially) Accessible Practitioners
> Dan Menkin, Organizing Facilitator
> 3 Harvard Street
> Arlington, MA 02174-6017
> (617) 641-4469

Transformation Oriented Bodywork Network

Transformation Work involves acting as a facilitator for the client's healing process. Massage and bodywork practitioners who participate in the TOB-Network are dedicated to this type of work.

This is a member-driven network that will publicize trainings, provide a forum for therapists to communicate with each other, provide a membership directory and a newsletter. It is open to all graduates of a licensed massage school. Membership is $30 per year, and a packet of two sample newsletters plus information on the network costs $5.50.

For further information, contact:

Transformation Oriented Bodywork Network (TOB-NET)
Mickey McGinnis, Coordinator
P.O. Box 24967
San Jose, CA 95154-4967
(408) 371-6716

State and local organizations

State and local organizations tend to change addresses and phone numbers relatively quickly, so it is difficult to include current information about them in a publication of this nature.

Below is information about the organizations that responded to the author's request for information. Your local organization may not be listed here. As you network with other local practitioners or contact massage schools in your area, you may locate an organization in your home town — or you may start one.

Florida

Florida State Massage Therapy Association

FSMTA Central Office
1353 Palmetto Ave., #225
Winter Park, FL 32789=4949
(407) 628-2772

In existence since 1939, FSMTA has been active in the legislative arena, publishes its own magazine, and offers a host of member benefits.

Kansas

Kansas Association of Therapeutic Massage
An affiliate of International Myomassethics Federation
707 SE Quincy, suite A
Topeka, KS 66603
(913) 296-3232

Maine

Maine Massage Guild
Charlotte Davis, President
RR 1, Box 1875
Stonington, ME 04681
(207) 348-6684

Dues are $25 per year. The Guild promotes massage as a healing force, supports therapists and provides a network for body-oriented practitioners.

New York

New York State Society of Medical Massage Therapists
(NYSSMMT)
P.O. Box 1143
Port Washington, NY 11050
(212) NYS-SMMT

The oldest massage professional organization in the U.S., the NYSSMMT publishes a newsletter, holds meetings and workshops, promotes recognition of the field and protects the ethics of the profession.

Oklahoma

Body Work and Wellness Therapies Association
P.O. Box 60323
Oklahoma City, OK 73146-0323

An organization for those interested in massage, nutrition and other healing arts, BWWTA seeks to support the efficacy, legitimacy and professionalism of nontraditional as well as traditional health practitioners. Members receive a quarterly newsletter.

Pennsylvania

Pennsylvania Association of Massage/Bodywork Professionals
P.O. Box 317
Neffs, PA 18065

PAMBP is a grass-roots organization that wishes to help define educational standards in the state. Members are expected to serve on at least one committee. Membership fee is $25 per year.

Tennessee

Tennessee Massage Therapy Association
P.O. Box 52933
Knoxville, TN 37950-2933

TMTA has chapters in Memphis, Nashville, Chattanooga, Knoxville, Tri-Cities and Jackson. Contact the State office for membership information and local contact persons.

16 Insurance

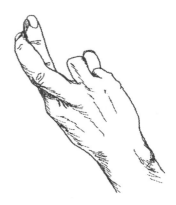

This chapter is about the types of insurance you can buy to protect yourself against certain risks. This chapter does not discuss having your work paid for by your clients' insurance, which is covered in Chapter 19.

Why Buy Insurance?

Insurance is risk protection. If you have no insurance, you bear all the financial risks of life alone.

The kinds of risks that insurance covers are illustrated by the following examples:

- If you are sued by a client and lose, you are responsible to pay the amount awarded to your client by the court.

- If a client slips and falls in your office, you might be required to pay for that injury.

- If you are sued by a client for any reason, you will have to pay your own legal fees for defending the suit.

- If your office burns down or is vandalized, you absorb the loss.

- If you are injured and cannot work for a period of time, you will have no assistance in meeting your financial obligations.

- If you fall ill and need medical attention, you will have to pay the full amount of the medical expenses.

Each of the examples above illustrates one type of risk for which the self-employed bodyworker can purchase insurance. Each kind of insurance is profiled in the next part of this chapter.

Kinds of Insurance Available to the Professional Bodyworker

Professional Liability Insurance

This insurance defends you against claims by clients that you harmed them in the course of performing your professional services.

In the medical and legal professions, this kind of insurance has become very expensive because of the large number of lawsuits alleging negligent injury.

In massage and bodywork, these suits are very rare, and the insurance is therefore relatively inexpensive.

Professional liability insurance is a benefit of membership in the AMTA, ABMP and IMA. The associations purchase group insurance policies, which allows them to pay very little for the insurance, compared to the amount they charge in dues. However, as an individual you probably could not buy the insurance on the open market any cheaper than the cost of membership in these associations. Discounted professional liability insurance is also available at an additional charge to members of the AOBTA, Rolf Institute, American Polarity Therapy Association, Trager Institute and Feldenkrais Guild.

Two general types of professional liability insurance are sold: "claims-made" insurance and "occurrence form" insurance.

A claims-made policy covers you for claims that are made while the policy is in force. "Claim" refers to the announcement by the client of their complaint against you.

An occurrence form policy covers you for incidents that occur while your policy is in force. "Occurrence" refers to the act you did that supposedly caused harm to the client.

The difference between these two types of policy comes up if you discontinue your insurance—for example, if you stop practicing massage. Say you retire from the practice of massage and discontinue coverage effective January 1, 2000. A client comes forth on February 1, 2001 and claims you injured her during a massage you gave her on June 30, 1999.

An occurrence form policy would cover you in this case, because the alleged injury *occurred* while the policy was in force. A claims-made policy would not cover you, because the *claim* was made after your insurance had lapsed.

If you plan to have a significant career in the massage or bodywork field, professional liability insurance is virtually a necessity. While you may think you do not need such insurance because you have no significant possessions to lose anyway, consider the broader question of how being uninsured might handcuff your future.

Spa owners, chiropractors and other massage employers will usually not hire an uninsured massage therapist. If the therapist is uninsured, then any client with a claim against the therapist would likely sue the employer, who does have insurance. An uninsured therapist is seen as an unnecessary risk. This is a career disadvantage you do not want to have.

Business Liability Insurance

Business Liability, or premises liability insurance, is "slip and fall" coverage. It protects you against suits that result from injuries people sustain on your business premises. The cause of these injuries might be icy steps, loose carpet, or any other cause of accidental injury.

Legally, you are liable for these injuries only if you do not keep your office in a reasonably safe condition for your clients. The legalities of how safe you need to keep it vary slightly from place to place. However, as a practical matter, any injury to a client is a potential problem, even if you are not ultimately legally responsible for it. If the client sues, you still will have to bear the expense of lawyer's fees to defend the action.

Business liability insurance covers both attorneys' fees to defend an action and any recovery that is ultimately awarded. It is included in the cost of membership in some professional associations, and can be purchased on the open market through insurance agents and insurance companies.

Fire, Theft, Vandalism, Earthquake Insurance

These types of insurance, also called "casualty" insurance, protect you against destruction of your business property by acts of nature or acts of human beings. Unless your office property is of high value, such insurance protection may be an expense you do not require.

Disability Insurance or Business Interruption Insurance

In the event you are unable to work due to accident or illness, disability insurance provides you with continued weekly income. You usually must be disabled for several weeks (or several months) before the policy will pay you a weekly income, and you can usually collect payments under the policy up to a maximum of one year.

Disability insurance is not cheap; a policy to provide you with $300 to $400 per week in the event of disability may cost around $1,000 per year to purchase. Base your decision whether or not to buy such insurance on how strong your need is to be sure of continued income.

Medical Insurance / Group Medical Insurance

Policies for medical insurance are available in many forms, from bare-bones to deluxe. The costs of such insurance range from high to exorbitant.

The least expensive coverage is referred to as "catastrophic illness insurance." This insurance will pay for most of the expense of a hospital stay, after a deductible of, for example, $2000. This is protection against being turned away from a hospital when you need care, and against being placed into bankruptcy by an illness. Such insurance may cost $500 to $2,000 per year, depending on your age and place of residence.

The most expensive coverage is major medical, which will cover a wide range of treatments, procedures and medications. The cost of this type of coverage seems to be going up weekly, and no one can tell where it will stop.

In-between are a wide range of compromise plans with varying price tags. AMTA and ABMP offer members opportunities to purchase discounted group health policies. Many other groups offer their members group health insurance of one sort or another. Some of these are bargains, and some are not. Speak to insurance agents and find out what type of coverage you realistically need before agreeing to any particular policy.

17 Laws You Should Know About and State Regulation of Massage

Many laws have some effect on bodyworkers. The first section of this chapter summarizes basic laws you should know about and legal principles you should understand.

The second section details state laws regulating massage, and also describes legislative activity in states that have not yet adopted laws regulating the practice of massage. A chart summarizing all state laws regulating massage appears on page 122.

Laws you should know about

Federal, State, County and Local governments. Most Americans live under the authority of four different governments. Each one has its own areas of major influence, in terms of what it offers you and what it requires of you.

The *Federal* government requires you to pay federal taxes on all the money you earn. The federal government also authorizes certain organizations to accredit massage schools, paving the way for the granting of financial aid for massage education. (Financial aid information is noted in schools' listing in the State-by-State Directory)

State governments sometimes enact laws regulating the practice of massage in the state. These laws are described in the second part of this chapter, and summarized on page 122. State governments sometimes require the payment of income taxes on the money you earn.

County governments occasionally pass laws concerning the practice of massage in the county. Such laws apply only in unincorporated areas of the county —that is, in areas which are not within the borders of a town or city that has a municipal government. The county government may also take over zoning and health requirements in unincorporated areas within the county, and has the power to levy some taxes.

County governments also keep track of business names ("assumed names" or "fictitious names") and issue certificates to businesses allowing them to use a business name.

City (or township or village) governments, also called *municipal* governments, regulate zoning, parking, health concerns, and the operation of businesses within the city limits. They have the power to decide what businesses can and cannot operate in the city, and what locations within the city are permissible locations for different types of businesses. Some cities have regulations for the practice of massage within the city limits. Some cities prohibit the practice of massage within city limits. Many cities have some form of municipal taxation.

If there is ever a conflict between the laws of different governments, the power structure works as follows: Federal law always has priority; state laws have priority over county and local laws; municipal laws control within the borders of the city, town or village; in unincorporated areas of the county, county law applies unless it is in conflict with state or Federal law.

County and Municipal Professional Licensing Laws. As mentioned above, laws specifically regulating the practice of massage can be enacted by state, county or local governments. In many areas, no regulatory law applies to the practice of massage, as neither the state, county nor city has enacted one.

Many local laws regulating the practice of massage require the applicant for a massage license to submit items like fingerprints, recent photo, recent employment history, references, and physician's certificate that he or she has no communicable disease. In addition, some have educational requirements.

Some representative municipal educational requirements are listed below:

Colorado Springs, CO 1000 hours; Des Moines, IA 1000 hours; Tucson, AZ 1000 hours (500 in-class hours); Ames, IA 750 hours at AMTA-approved school; Tempe, AZ 600 hours; Cedar Rapids, IA 500 hours; Davenport, IA 500 hours over a period of at least one year; Pueblo, CO 70 hours; St. Louis, MO 70 hours; St. Paul, MN, 40 hours.

As you can see, the range of 40 hours to 1000 hours is quite a broad one, and this reflects the situation within the nation as a whole concerning massage licensing.

Other Local Requirements. If your local government has a law regulating massage establishments, the law may have requirements for bathrooms, lighting, signs and other specifics concerning the office. If there is no such law, consider contacting the health department, fire department and the police department to see if there are any requirements you should know about before committing to a particular office space.

Business License. Business licenses are usually required by city governments. Occasionally a county requires a business license, and the state of Alaska requires such a license. It is used by the city government to keep track of who is performing what business activity, to generate money for the municipal treasury, and to make sure that zoning laws are being followed.

Zoning Laws. Most cities have a special map of the city that divides every location into one of several zones. (See Sample Zoning Map, page 56) A key explains the meaning of each zone. The zones create different kinds of neighborhoods — business areas, residential areas, industrial areas, and areas of mixed usage.

When you open a massage or bodywork practice, you will need to be sure you are locating your office in an area that is zoned for your type of business. You may find there is a dispute about the type of business you have — some zoning agencies classify massage as a profession, others consider it a health service, others call it a personal service, and others classify it as adult entertainment. The zoning board's classification decision can affect permissible locations for your office.

Local Taxes. Some local governments charge businesses a tax on business property. That means that they decide the value of the business property you own, and tax you a fixed percentage of that value each year. Some local governments also charge a sewer tax, which may be based on water usage or number of plumbing units.

Fictitious Name (or Assumed Name) Statement. If you use a made-up name for your business that does not include your own name, you should register that name with the county government. There is a fee, usually around $20, and you may be required to search through the county's record books to make sure that no one has already taken the name you are choosing. You may also be required to advertise the name in the legal classifieds of your local newspaper. Registering your fictitious name is a requirement for opening a checking account in the name of the business.

Taxpayer Identification Number. If you are a sole proprietor (see below) and do not have any employees, you can use your social security number on all tax documents. If you have employees, or if you incorporate or form a partnership, you will need to apply for a taxpayer identification number. Obtain form SS-4 from the Internal Revenue Service. For information on how to get the form, see the end of Chapter 18.

Business identity. In the eyes of the law, there are several possible "identities" for your business. The main ones are corporation, partnership and sole proprietor.

Corporations have a separate legal identity apart from the shareholders and employees. They can have tax advantages in some sophisticated situations, but if you are a self-employed bodyworker, it is not an advantage to incorporate.

Partnership is a special legal relationship in which the two or more partners can speak and act for each other. A promise by one binds the other, so if your partner makes a business deal and then fails to follow through, you can be held responsible for it. Partners usually share the partnership income, without regard to who actually did the work that generated the money.

Sole Proprietor means you, and you alone, run your business. In legal terms, there is no difference between you and your business. Your business income and personal income are simply added together to determine what your income is. Your business is treated legally just as it is in fact—as an extension of your life and a part of yourself.

Practically every bodyworker operates as a sole proprietor, and unless you have some good reason not to, you should too. Becoming a corporation or a partnership will not benefit you unless you are involved in some complicated or sophisticated business dealings. If you become involved in a group practice, the group may choose to incorporate. This is something the group will decide in consultation with a lawyer or accountant.

Contractual relationship. A contract can be oral or written. It is simply an exchange of promises in which each party agrees to do or give something of value to the other party. Once made, a contract is legally enforceable until it is ended by the parties who made it.

Written contracts are easier to enforce, because the exact terms of the agreement are on paper for all to see. Oral contracts can also be enforced, but the specifics must be proven by testimony about the agreement.

Simply opening a checking account involves making a contract. The bank agrees to hold your money and give it to you or the people you write checks to, according to certain rules the bank establishes. You agree to pay a set fee per check written, or keep a minimum monthly balance, and to pay prescribed penalties for writing checks that your account cannot cover.

As a massage therapist, contracts you are likely to enter into include agreements to work for others or to have others work for you, rental agreements for office space, contracts with the phone company for business phone service, and contracts for performance of services like printing, laundry and cleaning.

State Laws Regulating Massage

The following is an index to state regulation of massage as of January, 1995. In states that have governmental regulation of massage, this index lists their educational requirements, notes states that have adopted the National Certification Exam as their written exam, gives information about reciprocity, and gives the address and phone number for the licensing body. Additional requirements, such as health certificate, required fees, and continuing education requirements and not listed.

For states that do not regulate massage but have had legislative activity, a summary is given of the action that has taken place in the legislative arena.

Information of this nature necessarily goes out of date, since legislation regarding massage is changing rapidly. Fortunately, there are sources you can turn to that will provide periodic updates to this information.

For current information on massage laws that have been enacted, one resource is *Massage* Magazine, which prints a summary of current licensing laws toward the back of each issue. Another source of current licensing information is any of the massage schools located in a state. In addition, most professional associations keep abreast of licensing laws nationwide and can provide current information.

For up-to-the-minute developments about *attempts* to create new laws, see Touch Therapy Times. Jack Thomas, the editor of Touch Therapy Times, co-authored the part of this chapter on legislative developments in the various states. Touch Therapy Times reports monthly on legislative and legal issues relating to massage nationwide and is

the only source for accurate information on this subject. Subscriptions are $25 per year from Touch Therapy Times, 13407 Tower Road, Thurmont, MD 21788-1407 (301) 271-4812.

In states that regulate massage, information about reciprocity is noted in the listing. Reciprocity means that you may be able to become licensed in that state without a written exam if you are already licensed in another state. Generally, the state you are moving to will admit you to practice by reciprocity only if the state you are moving from requires equivalent educational training.

Sometimes a state will provide a list of other states it approves for purposes of reciprocity. More commonly, a state will consider requests for licensing by reciprocity on a case-by-case basis. This means the second state will take a look at all your documents and the information they receive from the state where you are already licensed. If your documents show your training matches their requirements, they will grant you a license.

In states that adopt the National Certification Exam as their written exam, passing the Exam in any location will satisfy the written test requirement. In effect, that amounts to automatic reciprocity as to the written exam. However, other licensing requirements must also be met to qualify for a license, such as specific educational requirements.

The current state licensing laws are summarized in a chart on page 122. The information in this section is meant to give fuller information about what is happening in individual states than can be contained in an explanatory chart.

Arkansas

State licensing, 500 hours required
Reciprocity is on a case-by-case basis

> Arkansas Massage Board
> P.O. Box 34163
> Little Rock, AR 72203
> (501) 682-9170

California

California does not have statewide massage regulation. The California Coalition for Somatic Practices has distributed 25,000 copies of a survey as a preliminary step toward creating a consensus concerning state regulation of massage and bodywork.

Licensing of massage practitioners in California is done only by city and county governments. A State of California law (Chapter 6, sections 51030 through 51034) gives authority to cities and counties to regulate massage. The law states what aspects of the practice may and may not be regulated. Section 51034 states that local laws may not restrict massage to same-sex massage only.

Some southern California jurisdictions exempt Holistic Health Practitioners from their massage laws. This is usually defined as someone with demonstrable training and experience in massage.

Massage schools in California are regulated by The Council for Private Postsecondary and Vocational Education, 1027 10th Street, fourth floor, Sacramento, CA 95814. All schools approved by the Council offer a minimum of 100 hours of instruction for their massage programs.

The following table of municipal and county licensing requirements was compiled in 1991. While most of this information is still accurate, it is the nature of such information that it slowly goes out of date. Nonetheless, this table provides a useful picture of the diverse state of massage licensing in California.

Aside from the educational requirements listed below, most cities have some practical requirements for a person who wants to practice massage. For example, some towns prohibit "outcall" massage, or house calls, and some regulate it separately and require a special outcall massage license.

The amount charged for business or professional licenses varies tremendously from place to place, from a few dollars to over two thousand dollars. Some towns require a business license but no professional credentials. Some regulate massage as "adult entertainment". Some prohibit the practice of massage altogether.

For updated information about local laws, inquire at the city hall or county government building in the county seat. If you cannot locate a city government, contact the League of California Cities, 1400 K Street, Sacramento, CA 95814.

1,000 hours (6): Orange, San Clemente, Santa Paula, Thousand Oaks, Tustin, Vista

600 hours (3): Fontana, Rialto, San Bernardino

500 hours (4): Brea, Cupertino, Palm Desert, Seal Beach

300 hours (1): Newport Beach

225 hours (1): Marina

200 hours (42): Alhambra, Auburn, Bakersfield, Big Bear Lake, Camarillo, Carlsbad, Carson, Chula Vista, Covina, Cudahy, Cypress, El Segundo, Fairfield, Glendale, Grover City, Hayward, Hercules, Highland, Imperial, Imperial Beach, Kern County, Laguna Beach, Loma Linda, Los Alamitos, Huntington Park, Marysville, Montebello, Ontario, Orange County, Placentia, Ridgecrest, San Bernardino County, San Buenaventura, Santa Barbara, Signal Hill, Solano Beach, Torrance, Twentynine Palms, Union City, Ventura County, West Sacramento, Yuba County.

180 hours (7): Atwater, Ceres, Dublin, Livingston, Merced, Modesto, Turlock

100 hours (20): Corona, Desert Hot Springs, Dublin, El Dorado County, Escondido, Fresno, Gardena, Hollister, La Mesa, Livermore, Merced County, Monterey, Monterey County, Novato, Palm Springs, Redlands, San Francisco, San Leandro, San Luis Obispo, Santa Monica.

70 hours (20): Alameda, Burlingame, Colma, Contra Costa County, Daly City, Half Moon Bay, Lakewood, Manteca, Milpitas, Pacifica, Palo Alto, Portola Valley, Richmond, San Mateo County, San Pablo, San Ramon, Santa Clara, Santa Clara County, Saratoga, Selma.

Any approved or recognized school (37): Adelanto, Arroyo Grande, Azuza, Beaumont, Belmont, Beverly Hills, Cloverdale, Encinitas, Eureka, Foster City, Fullerton, Glendora, Healdsburg, Imperial County, Lemon Grove, Millbrae, Napa, Oceanside, Oxnard, Pacific Grove, Pleasanton, Poway, Rancho Mirage, Sacramento County, San Bruno, San Diego County, San Marcos, San Mateo, Santa Rosa, Santee, Simi Valley, South Lake Tahoe, Stockton, West Covina, West Hollywood, Westmoreland, Whittier.

No educational requirement but other requirements (12): Anaheim, Bell Gardens, Burbank, Commerce, Culver City, Hemet, Long Beach, Los Angeles, Manhattan Beach, Riverside, Riverside County, Santa Fe Springs.

Colorado

In 1989, representatives of AMTA and ABMP, school owners, and several unaffiliated massage therapists came together to form a coalition to represent massage practitioners on licensing issues. These efforts resulted in a law defining "Massage Therapist" as a graduate of a state-approved school with at least 500 hours of education. One who meets this definition is exempted from the "massage parlor" law.

Massage regulation in Colorado is done by city and county governments, and approximately 15 county and municipal governments have laws regulating the practice of massage. At present, there is no plan to pursue state regulation of massage or bodywork.

Connecticut

State licensing, 500 hours at a school approved by comtaa *and* by an accrediting agency recognized by the U.S. Department of Education
National Certification Exam

Massage Therapy Licensure Program
Department of Public Health
150 Washington St.
Hartford, CT 06106
(203) 566-1284

Delaware

Voluntary certification, 500 hours or 300 hours plus two years practice after certification
Reciprocity is on a case-by-case basis
Certification exempts practitioners from the Delaware Adult Entertainment laws. Delaware's law is relatively new; regulations for certification were adopted in June, 1994 and the first practitioners were certified in December, 1994.

The state Department of Justice has sent letters to several uncertified practitioners instructing them to either apply for certification under the massage/bodywork law or apply for a license under the Adult Entertainment Law.

The state Joint Sunset Committee has scheduled review of the massage/bodywork program to determine whether it should be continued.

Delaware Committee of Massage Practice
Cannon Building, suite 203
P.O. Box 1401
Dover, DE 19903
(302) 739-4522, ext. 205

District of Columbia

A bill for licensure of massage therapists was approved by the D.C. Council in 1994 and will be sent to the U.S. House of Representatives for review in 1995. This legislation has a 500-hour educational requirement, which can be waived through a grandfathering provision to be in effect for two years. (Grandfathering means those already practicing can become licensed without meeting all the requirements of the new law)

Florida

State licensing, 500 hours required
National Certification Exam

Florida Department of Professional Regulation
Board of Massage
Northwood Centre
1940 N. Monroe St.
Tallahassee, FL 32399
(904) 488-6021

Georgia

Three massage regulation bills were introduced in 1992. These provided different options for massage regulation, from mandatory licensure to voluntary registration. The massage community had second thoughts about statewide regulation, the sponsor of one of the bills resigned under pressure, and none of the bills succeeded in the legislature.

Hawaii

State licensing, 570 hours required
Educational institution must be approved or licensed by a state department of education *or* approved by an accredited community college, college or university *or* approved by the AMTA *or* approved by the Rolf Institute.

The apprenticeship option in effect at time of publication allows 150 in-class hours and 420 apprenticeship; this alternative may be phased out in the near future.

Hawaii Department of Commerce and Consumer Affairs
Professional and Vocational Licensing Division
P.O. Box 3469
Honolulu, HI 96801
(808) 586-3000

Idaho

A legislative proposal for certification of massage therapists was introduced in 1994 but died in committee. Some interest exists in modifying the bill and resubmitting it in the 1995 session of the legislature.

Iowa

State licensing, 500 hours
No reciprocity

Iowa Massage Therapy Advisory Board
321 E. 12th St.
Lucas State Office Building
Des Moines, IA 50319
(515) 281-4422

Kansas

A coalition has been formed to consider development of laws regulating massage.

Louisiana

State licensing, 500 hours
National Certification Exam

Louisiana Board of Massage Therapy
11853 Bricksome Ave., suite A
Baton Rouge, LA 70816
(504) 295-8437

Maine

State registration as "Massage Practitioner" does not require specific educational standards or a written exam.

State certification as a "Massage Therapist" requires passing the National Certification Exam *or* graduation from a comtaa-approved school.

Bodyworkers are exempted so long as they do not use title "Massage Therapist"

Maine Department of Professional and Financial Regulation
Division of Licensing and Enforcement—Massage Therapists
State House Station #35
Augusta, ME 04333
(207) 582-8723

Maryland

The physical therapy profession in Maryland has tried to completely monopolize the practice of massage in that state. They have instituted legal proceedings against massage therapists, charging them with practicing physical therapy without a license. The AMTA has been a strong force in helping the massage community in Maryland fend off this challenge. Legal wrangling is somewhat complicated, including court challenges and legislative maneuverings. The outcome is still uncertain.

Eight times since 1987, bills have been introduced in the Maryland General Assembly to regulate the massage profession. Two of the proposals were approved by the House of Delegates, but at press time none had been passed by the entire legislature.

Scheduled for introduction in the 1995 session was a bill that would authorize the state Board of Nursing to regulate the massage profession through a Massage Therapy Advisory Council. This bill would also require that within five years, a certain number of credit hours in a higher education institution would be required of new applicants for licensure. If this educational requirement passes, is would be the first such law in the nation.

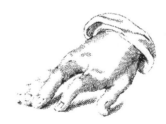

Massachusetts

In 1993, a task force with equal representation from the Massachusetts Health Officers Association and the Massachusetts Coalition of Professional Hands-On Practitioners completed two years of work by publishing a comprehensive manual on massage regulation for municipalities and counties.

In 1994 a massage licensure bill was introduced in the state legislature, was revamped because of opposition by some groups of bodyworkers, and eventually died in committee. The sponsor plans to file a new bill in 1995.

Michigan

A statewide massage licensure law was adopted in 1974 and modified in 1980, but it is legally defective and has never been implemented. Even though there is a licensing law "on the books," there is no license available in Michigan to those who practice massage or bodywork.

A coalition of bodyworkers was formed in 1992 to organize political activism in the state and lay the groundwork for future changes in the licensing law.

Those interested in massage licensing in Michigan may want to contact the Planning and Zoning Center, Inc., 302 S. Waverly Rd., Lansing, MI 48917 (517) 886-0555, and ask for *Planning and Zoning News* Volume 7, Number 9 (July 1989). This document outlines the history of massage legislation in Michigan and gives an organized presentation of ways municipal officials can recognize legitimate massage practitioners.

Minnesota

A coalition has been formed to consider development of laws regulating massage.

Mississippi

A bill to regulate massage was introduced in the House of Representatives in 1993 and died in committee. In 1994 a bill was introduced in the Senate. This measure also failed. Physical therapy interests have put the massage community on notice to expect opposition from the physical therapists "from now on."

Nebraska

State licensing, 1000 hours
National Certification Exam

> Nebraska Bureau of Examining Boards
> Department of Health
> 301 Centennial Mall South
> P.O. Box 95007
> Lincoln, NE 68509
> (402) 471-2115

Nevada

A massage licensing proposal died in the Senate Commerce and Labor Committee in 1991. A committee spokesperson said that mail and telephone contacts were "about 100 to 30 against the legislation."

New Hampshire

State licensing, 750 hours
Reciprocity on a case-by-case basis

> New Hampshire Department of Public Health
> Bureau of Health Facilities Administration
> 6 Hazen Drive
> Concord, NH 03301
> (603) 271-4592

New Jersey

In late 1993, New Jersey's massage therapists learned that an unnamed legislator was requesting information about massage and might be planning to introduce massage legislation. The identity of the legislator was never determined, and no legislation was introduced. However, the bodywork community formed a coalition to work toward the creation of a law regulating massage. At press time, preparations were under way to introduce legislation to regulate massage.

New Mexico

State licensing, 650 hours (may be 300 hours plus 350 hours Alternative Qualifying Experience)
National Certification Exam plus Jurisprudence Exam

> Reciprocity on a case-by-case basis (referred to as "by credentials")

> New Mexico Board of Massage Therapy
> P.O. Box 25101
> Santa Fe, NM 87504
> (505) 827-7013

New York

State licensing, 605 hours
Reciprocity is case-by-case and requires proof of practice for two years

> New York State Education Department
> Division of Professional Licensing Services
> Massage Unit, Room 3041
> Cultural Education Center
> Albany, NY 12230
> (518) 474-3817 (general info)
> (518) 474-3866 (practice issues)

North Carolina

A bill to regulate massage passed the House and was debated in a Senate committee in 1994. The measure failed. Physical therapy interests actively opposed the legislation.

North Dakota

State certificate of registration, 500 hours
Requires attendance at comtaa-approved school

North Dakota Massage Board
22 Fremont Dr.
Fargo, ND 58103
(701) 237-4036 (Albert Dahlgren)

Ohio

State licensing, 600 hours
Reciprocity is on a case-by-case basis, but an exam is still required.
In Ohio, a massage license is required for use of the title "licensed massage therapist" but is not required simply to practice massage. Practitioners who are not licensed probably cannot receive reimbursement from insurance companies.

Ohio State Medical Board
77 South High St., 17th floor
Columbus, OH 43266
(614) 466-3934

Oregon

State licensing, 330 hours
Reciprocity: Arkansas, Florida, Nebraska, New York, Utah, Washington (after 10/88)

Oregon Board of Massage Technicians
407-B State Office Building
800 NE Oregon St, #21
Portland, OR 97232
(503) 731-4064

Pennsylvania

A coalition has been working to develop legislation for statewide regulation of massage.

Rhode Island

State licensing, 500 hours at a comtaa-approved school or an equivalent academic and training program of 1000 hours
National Certification Exam

Rhode Island Department of Health
Room 104, Cannon Building
Three Capitol Hill
Providence, RI 02908
(401) 277-2827

South Carolina

A bill to regulate massage was introduced in the House in 1994. It did not pass, but was held over for possible consideration during the 1995 session.

Tennessee

Efforts are under way to introduce legislation regulating massage.

Texas

State registration (mandatory), 250 hours plus 50 hours internship

Texas Massage Therapy Registration
Texas Department of Health
1100 W. 49th St.
Austin, TX 78756
(512) 834-6616

Utah

State licensing, 600 hours at comtaa-approved school
Apprenticeship of 1000 hours is also available
Theory Exam and Laws & Rules Exam
Reciprocity is available to licensed out-of-state therapists whether or not their training was at comtaa-approved school. For purposes of reciprocity, National Certification Exam can substitute for Theory Exam.

Utah Department of Commerce
Division of Occupational and Professional Licensing
Herber M. Wells Building
160 East 300 South
P.O. Box 45805
Salt Lake City, UT 84145
(801) 530-6551

Washington

State licensing, 500 hours
National Certification Exam

Washington Department of Health
Professional Licensing Services
1300 SE Quince St.
P.O. Box 47869
Olympia, WA 98504
(206) 753-3199

Wisconsin

A coalition has been formed to consider development of laws regulating massage.

State Licensing Chart as of May 1, 1997

State	Type of Regulation	Education Required	NCE	Reciprocity
Alabama*	License	500/650/1000	**	
Arkansas	License	500 hours	no	case-by-case
Connecticut	License	500 hours/COMTAA	yes	
Delaware	Certification	500 hours or 300 hours plus 2 years of practice	no	case-by-case
Dist. of Columbia	License	500 hours	yes	
Florida	License	500 hours	yes	
Hawaii	License	570 hours or 150 hours plus 420-hour apprenticeship	no	none
Iowa	License	500 hours	yes	none
Louisiana	License	500 hours	yes	
Maine	Registration	COMTAA or NCE	yes	
Maryland*	Certification	500 hours	**	
Nebraska	License	1000 hours	yes	case-by-case
New Hampshire	License	750 hours	yes	case-by-case
New Mexico	License	650 hours or 300 plus experience	yes	case-by-case
New York	License	605	no	case-by-case
North Dakota	Registration	500 hours COMTAA	no	
Ohio	License	600 hours	no	case-by-case
Oregon	License	330	no	AK, FL, NE, NY, UT, WA
Rhode Island	License	500 hours COMTAA or 1000 hours	yes	
South Carolina	License	500 hours	**	
Tennessee	License	500 hours or NCE	yes	
Texas	Registration	300	no	
Utah	License	600 COMTAA or 1000-hour apprenticeship	yes	COMTAA not required for reciprocity
Virginia*	Certification	500 hours	yes	
Washington	License	500 hours	yes	

* Alabama's law provides that the educational requirement is 500 hours until 1/1/98, 650 hours until 1/1/02, and 1000 hours thereafter. Maryland's law requires 500 hours until 1/1/02, and 60 accredited college hours thereafter.

** The laws in Alabama, Maryland and South Carolina give the Board the power to adopt NCE or a different exam as the state's written exam. No decision as to the written test had been made as of press time.

18 Income Taxes

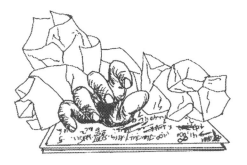

This chapter cannot give you all the information and advice you will need to prepare your income tax return. Instead, this chapter will:

1. Familiarize you with all of the key facts and ideas you need to understand about Federal income tax;

2. Explain what records you should keep for tax purposes, why you need them and how to keep them;

3. Guide you to all the resources you will need to do your own taxes, or to hire a professional to do your taxes for you.

The Big Picture

The following discussion gives you the basis of the federal tax laws that determine how much money you give the government at the end of the year.

This information is presented in condensed form, and on the first reading it may seem difficult to understand. This is only because the words are strange, not because the ideas are difficult.

Really try to "get" this big picture in your mind. Everything else in this chapter relates to this overall picture.

Some of the statements in this "big picture" would need additional explanation to be 100% accurate, so just use this information to understand the concepts at this point.

1. Employment income only

If you are an employee, and have no income from self-employment, your taxes will be very simple. You employer will give you a W-2 form showing income and withholding, and the forms the IRS sends you to fill out your taxes should be sufficient.

2. Self-employment income

Almost all massage therapists and bodyworkers, however, are completely or partially self-employed. When you are self-employed, your business profit and your other income are kept separate for some computations, and combined for others.

Business activity is reported on a separate IRS form, called Schedule C. In reporting your business activity on your Schedule C, you add all of the money you received during the year in your business, and you subtract your business deductions. (What you can subtract as business deductions will be discussed later).

If the money you *received* is a larger amount than your allowable *deductions*, you have a *profit*. We will call this your "business profit."

3. Self-employment tax

The business profit is subject to a self-employment tax. This is the self-employed person's equivalent of Social Security Tax. The amount of the self-employment tax for tax year 1994 was 15.3% on business profits up to $60,600, and 2.9% of amounts over $60,600.

4. Income tax

Income tax is completely separate from self-employment tax. To figure your income tax, begin by adding up your *personal* income for the year, such as interest and dividend income. Subtract from this your *personal* deductions. Your personal income minus personal deductions we will call your "personal gross income."

Add your *personal gross income* to your *business profit*, and you get the total amount subject to income tax, or your "taxable income." Income tax for tax year 1994, assuming you made under $70,000 was between 15% and 25% of your taxable income.

The following chart summarizes the above discussion:

Business earnings	Personal income
minus	*minus*
Business deductions	Personal deductions
equals	*plus*
Business profit	Business profit
	equals
Pay self-employment tax on business profit (15.3%)	Taxable income
	Pay income tax on taxable income (15% to 25%)

Notice that you pay both self-employment tax and income tax on your business profit. Personal (non-business) income is subject only to the income tax.

Deductions are beautiful

Once you grasp the overall picture of how taxes are figured, it becomes apparent that business deductions and personal deductions are money in your pocket. Since they reduce the total amount subject to taxes, they reduce the total taxes you have to pay.

Business deductions are especially helpful, since they reduce both the self-employment tax and the income tax. Personal deductions reduce only the income tax. Personal deductions include items such as charitable contributions, medical expenses, and the like.

Business deductions are discussed in some detail below. Become familiar with this information so that you have a clear understanding of what is deductible, and what records you need to keep to support your deductions.

Deductions are listed on "Schedule C" which is the form all self-employed persons file with their income tax returns. If your gross business receipts were under $25,000, you may be able to use Schedule C-EZ (see page 127). Otherwise, you must use the slightly more complicated Schedule C (see page 126).

What Can I Deduct?

In general, if it's a business expense, it's deductible. The expense must be for something "appropriate and helpful in developing and maintaining your trade or business" and the cost must be reasonable. That's it.

The following list demonstrates the most common deductible items. Other items not listed are deductible if they meet the "appropriate and helpful" test and are reasonable in amount:

- Business use of your automobile
- Office rental fees
- Painting or repair costs for office
- Your appointment book
- Business cards and any other business printing jobs
- Advertising
- Long-distance business phone calls (but not the base monthly service charge for the first residential line)
- Business travel expenses (cost of lodging plus 80% of cost of meals)
- Entertainment expenses
- Gifts to clients (up to $25 per client per year)
- Professional convention fees
- Continuing education expenses, including books
- Professional association dues
- Licensing fees
- Laundry expenses
- Costs of oil and other supplies
- Massage table and other equipment for treatment room (up to $10,000 in one year)
- Cassette player or disc player for treatment room
- Music for use in treatment room

Certain rules have been established for certain types of business deductions. Some of these rules that may affect your income taxes are the following:

SCHEDULE C
(Form 1040)

Department of the Treasury
Internal Revenue Service (99)

Profit or Loss From Business
(Sole Proprietorship)
► Partnerships, joint ventures, etc., must file Form 1065.
► Attach to Form 1040 or Form 1041.   ► See Instructions for Schedule C (Form 1040).

OMB No. 1545-0074

1994

Attachment
Sequence No. **09**

Name of proprietor

Social security number (SSN)

A Principal business or profession, including product or service (see page C-1)

B Enter principal business code
(see page C-6) ►

C Business name. If no separate business name, leave blank.

D Employer ID number (EIN), if any

E Business address (including suite or room no.) ►
City, town or post office, state, and ZIP code

F Accounting method: (1) ☐ Cash   (2) ☐ Accrual   (3) ☐ Other (specify) ►

G Method(s) used to value closing inventory: (1) ☐ Cost   (2) ☐ Lower of cost or market   (3) ☐ Other (attach explanation)   (4) ☐ Does not apply (if checked, skip line H)   Yes   No

H Was there any change in determining quantities, costs, or valuations between opening and closing inventory? If "Yes," attach explanation

I Did you "materially participate" in the operation of this business during 1994? If "No," see page C-2 for limit on losses.

J If you started or acquired this business during 1994, check here ► ☐

Part I   Income

1	Gross receipts or sales. **Caution:** If this income was reported to you on Form W-2 and the "Statutory employee" box on that form was checked, see page C-2 and check here ► ☐	1
2	Returns and allowances	2
3	Subtract line 2 from line 1	3
4	Cost of goods sold (from line 40 on page 2)	4
5	**Gross profit.** Subtract line 4 from line 3	5
6	Other income, including Federal and state gasoline or fuel tax credit or refund (see page C-2) ►	6
7	**Gross income.** Add lines 5 and 6 ►	7

Part II   Expenses. Enter expenses for business use of your home **only** on line 30.

8	Advertising	8	19	Pension and profit-sharing plans	19
9	Bad debts from sales or services (see page C-3)	9	20	Rent or lease (see page C-4):	
10	Car and truck expenses (see page C-3)	10	a	Vehicles, machinery, and equipment	20a
11	Commissions and fees	11	b	Other business property	20b
12	Depletion	12	21	Repairs and maintenance	21
13	Depreciation and section 179 expense deduction (not included in Part III) (see page C-3)	13	22	Supplies (not included in Part III)	22
			23	Taxes and licenses	23
14	Employee benefit programs (other than on line 19)	14	24	Travel, meals, and entertainment:	
15	Insurance (other than health)	15	a	Travel	24a
16	Interest:		b	Meals and entertainment	
a	Mortgage (paid to banks, etc.)	16a	c	Enter 50% of line 24b subject to limitations (see page C-4)	
b	Other	16b	d	Subtract line 24c from line 24b	24d
17	Legal and professional services	17	25	Utilities	25
18	Office expense	18	26	Wages (less employment credits)	26
			27	Other expenses (from line 46 on page 2)	27

28	**Total expenses** before expenses for business use of home. Ad	
29	Tentative profit (loss). Subtract line 28 from line 7	
30	Expenses for business use of your home. Attach **Form 8829**	
31	**Net profit or (loss).** Subtract line 30 from line 29.	
	• If a profit, enter on **Form 1040, line 12,** and ALSO on Sched see page C-5). Estates and trusts, enter on Form 1041, line 3.	
	• If a loss, you MUST go on to line 32.	
32	If you have a loss, check the box that describes your investme	
	• If you checked 32a, enter the loss on **Form 1040, line 12,** (statutory employees, see page C-5). Estates and trusts, enter	
	• If you checked 32b, you MUST attach **Form 6198.**	

For Paperwork Reduction Act Notice, see Form 1040 instructions

IRS form 1040
Schedule C,
page 1

Schedule C (Form 1040) 1994   Page **2**

Part III   Cost of Goods Sold (see page C-5)

33	Inventory at beginning of year. If different from last year's closing inventory, attach explanation	33
34	Purchases less cost of items withdrawn for personal use	34
35	Cost of labor. Do not include salary paid to yourself	35
36	Materials and supplies	36
37	Other costs	37
38	Add lines 33 through 37	38
39	Inventory at end of year	39
40	**Cost of goods sold.** Subtract line 39 from line 38. Enter the result here and on page 1, line 4	40

Part IV   Information on Your Vehicle. Complete this part **ONLY** if you are claiming car or truck expenses on line 10 and are not required to file Form 4562 for this business. See the instructions for line 13 on page C-3 to find out if you must file.

41 When did you place your vehicle in service for business purposes? (month, day, year) ► ...../...../.....

42 Of the total number of miles you drove your vehicle during 1994, enter the number of miles you used your vehicle for:

a Business ....   b Commuting ....   c Other ....

43 Do you (or your spouse) have another vehicle available for personal use? ☐ Yes ☐ No

44 Was your vehicle available for use during off-duty hours? ☐ Yes ☐ No

45a Do you have evidence to support your deduction? ☐ Yes ☐ No
b If "Yes," is the evidence written? ☐ Yes ☐ No

Part V   Other Expenses. List below business expenses not included on lines 8–26 or line 30.

46	**Total other expenses.** Enter here and on page 1, line 27	46

Ⓐ Printed on recycled paper

IRS form 1040
Schedule C,
page 2

SCHEDULE C-EZ
(Form 1040)

Department of the Treasury
Internal Revenue Service (99)

Net Profit From Business
(Sole Proprietorship)
▶ Partnerships, joint ventures, etc., must file Form 1065.
▶ Attach to Form 1040 or Form 1041. ▶ See instructions on back.

OMB No. 1545-0074

19**94**

Attachment
Sequence No. 09A

Name of proprietor | Social security number (SSN)

Part I General Information

**You May Use
This Schedule
Only If You:**
- Had gross receipts from your business of $25,000 or less.
- Had business expenses of $2,000 or less.
- Use the cash method of accounting.
- Did not have an inventory at any time during the year.
- Did not have a net loss from your business.
- Had only one business as a sole proprietor.

And You:
- Had no employees during the year.
- Are not required to file **Form 4562**, Depreciation and Amortization, for this business. See the instructions for Schedule C, line 13, on page C-3 to find out if you must file.
- Do not deduct expenses for business use of your home.
- Do not have prior year unallowed passive activity losses from this business.

A Principal business or profession, including product or service | B Enter principal business code (see page C-6) ▶

C Business name. If no separate business name, leave blank. | D Employer ID number (EIN), if any

E Business address (including suite or room no.). Address not required if same as on Form 1040, page 1.

City, town or post office, state, and ZIP code

Part II Figure Your Net Profit

1 **Gross receipts.** If more than $25,000, you **must** use Schedule C.
Caution: *If this income was reported to you on Form W-2 and the "Statutory employee" box on that form was checked, see **Statutory Employees** in the instructions for Schedule C, line 1, on page C-2 and check here* . . . . ▶ ☐ | 1

2 **Total expenses.** If more than $2,000, you **must** use Schedule C. See instructions . . . . . | 2

3 **Net profit.** Subtract line 2 from line 1. If less than zero, you **must** use Schedule C. Enter on **Form 1040, line 12**, and ALSO on **Schedule SE, line 2.** (Statutory employees **do not** report this amount on Schedule SE, line 2. Estates and trusts, enter on Form 1041, line 3.) . . . . . | 3

Part III Information on Your Vehicle. Complete this part **ONLY** if you are claiming car or truck expenses on line 2.

4 When did you place your vehicle in service for business purposes? (month, day, year) ▶ ..... / ..... / ....

5 Of the total number of miles you drove your vehicle during 1994, enter the number of miles you used your vehicle for:

a Business .... b Commuting .... c Other ....

6 Do you (or your spouse) have another vehicle available for personal use? . . . . ☐ Yes ☐ No

7 Was your vehicle available for use during off-duty hours? . . . . ☐ Yes ☐ No

8a Do you have evidence to support your deduction? . . . . ☐ Yes ☐ No

b If "Yes," is the evidence written? . . . . ☐ Yes ☐ No

For Paperwork Reduction Act Notice, see Form 1040 instructions. Cat. No. 14374D Schedule C-EZ (Form 1040) 1994

IRS form 1040 Schedule C–EZ

Education

You can deduct the cost of education, plus travel and meals expenses, if the education maintains or improves your professional skills, or is required by law for keeping your professional status.

Educational expenses are *not* deductible for training in a new field, or to meet minimum professional requirements.

In other words, once you are a practicing massage therapist, the expenses of continuing education are deductible, but the costs involved in becoming a massage therapist are not deductible.

Since expenses are deductible even if they are for education that "improves" your professional skills, you may be able to deduct a major educational expense, as long as you are already a practicing massage therapist. This is one advantage of taking a modest amount of training and practicing massage on the side before making a commitment to a more serious educational program.

Gifts

You can deduct the cost of gifts you give as part of doing business, up to a maximum of $25 worth of gifts to any one individual in one year. If there is a question whether something is a gift or entertainment (like football tickets) it will be considered entertainment.

Meal and Entertainment Expense

If you purchase meals or entertainment as a means of conducting business, you can deduct 80% of the cost of the meals and entertainment, including 80% of tips (as long as the costs are reasonable). You can also deduct 100% of your automobile costs for driving to the meal or entertainment. An example of meal and entertainment expense would be taking a chiropractor to lunch to discuss the possibility of cross-referrals.

Rent and other office expenses

Rental payments for your business office are fully deductible, as are other costs such as heat, electricity, insurance and the like.

Home office expenses

Rent and other costs for an office in your home are deductible if:

1. You use a part of your home exclusively for your business

2. You regularly see clients there as part of your business, and

3. Your home office is your principal place of business.

If your office is in a separate building on the property, such as a garage or coach house, you can take the home office deduction even if you do not regularly see clients there or it is not your principal place of business.

The rules for deducting the expenses of a home office have gotten tougher recently. In past years, the home office did not need to be your principal place of business in order to qualify. Under current (tax year 1994) rules, however, you are allowed this deduction only if your home office is the most important location for your business, or your spend more time seeing clients in your home office than you do in any other office.

If you qualify for a home office deduction, you can deduct a proportionate share of all household expenses from your taxable income. Such expenses include real estate taxes, mortgage interest, rent, utility bills, insurance, repairs, security systems and depreciation.

To determine the percentage of your home expenses that is deductible as a business expense, calculate the total square footage of your home, and the square footage of your home office. Divide the square footage of the office by the total square footage of the home, and you will get a decimal, for example .23. You then multiply your rent payments by .23 (or whatever number applies) to find the amount of your deduction for your home office rental.

If the rooms in your home are roughly the same size, and you use one room as an office, you can use a fraction instead of doing the square-foot computation. For example, if you have six equal-sized rooms and use one as an office, deduct one sixth of your combined rent, heat and electricity expenses as your home office expense.

The home office deduction cannot be larger than the amount of business income generated in the home office. In other words, the deduction cannot be used to create a business loss, only to offset income that you actually earned using that office.

Self-employment tax

You can deduct one-half of your self-employment tax from your gross income when you figure your income tax.

Start-up costs

If you are a practicing massage therapist, and you expand your business, or open a new office, the costs involved in doing so are ordinary and necessary business expenses, and are fully deductible.

However, if you decide to open a massage office *before* you earn any income as a massage practitioner, the costs involved in starting your business are "start-up costs" and these are *not* deductible.

This issue generally will not arise for a massage therapist or bodyworker, since opening an office without prior professional experience is not usually a realistic approach.

Travel

When you travel away from home for business, most of your expenses are deductible. Travel away from home means going for more than just a day's work, and must include going away long enough to need sleep or rest before coming home.

Deductible items

When traveling away from home on business, your deductible expenses include airplane, rail or bus tickets, automobile expenses, taxi fares, baggage costs, meals, lodging costs, cleaning and laundry expenses, telephone, telegraph, fax, tips, and other similar expenses related to travel.

Travel receipts

Keep receipts during your trip. If you travel by car, keep an envelope in the glove compartment, and put all receipts in the envelope. When you get home, staple them together and put them in the place where you collect all business receipts. At the end of the year, they will be together and easy to handle when you are totalling your deductions.

Optional methods for deducting meal costs when traveling

Meals can be deducted two ways — you may either deduct 80% of the amount you actually spend (so long as the amount is not lavish), or you may deduct the "standard meal allowance" which varies between $30 and $38 per day, depending on location (tax year 1994). For detailed information on the standard meal allowance, request Publication 463 free from the IRS. (see end of chapter)

When using the standard meal allowance, you do not need to produce receipts for your meals. For all other expenses, however, you need to have receipts to document your travel expenditures.

Mixed business and personal travel

If a trip is mainly business but partly personal, you can deduct the round trip travel expenses to get to your business destination, and the meals, lodging and incidental expenses that relate to the business portion of your trip. Any personal side trips, or expenses on days that were vacation days, are not tax-deductible.

If your trip was primarily for vacation and partly for business, no part of the expense is tax-deductible.

Business use vs. Personal use

If a particular expense has aspects of business and personal activity mixed together, remember that the test is whether it is "appropriate and helpful in promoting your business." If it meets this test, the fact that it also helps you personally is irrelevant; it is still deductible.

Some activities are personal and not business-related. For example, if you go to a bar on Saturday night hoping to meet someone who will become a bodywork client, you will not convince the IRS that your expenses are business-related.

However, if you go to the hardware store to get a wing nut to repair your massage table, that is a business trip, and it remains a business trip even if you also pick up a surge protector for your VCR while you are there.

If you pay attention to all the things you do for your business, you will see that much of your lifestyle actually is deductible. The cost of professional books, phone calls, entertainment, uniforms, and business laundry are all deductible expenses. You can also deduct the cost of traveling to shop for items for the business and to do errands for the business. You are entitled to proper business deductions, so plan for them, document them and take them.

Documenting deductions

The key to documenting deductions is keeping receipts, canceled checks, and in the case of automobile mileage, a log of business miles driven in your car.

What is documentation?

The IRS needs a paper record of any transaction you are claiming as a deduction. If you pay a bill for a business expense, keep the bill. When you get your canceled checks from your bank, save the ones that relate to business expenses.

Where to keep your documents

Create a space, in your office or your home, where you regularly keep a whole year's bills, receipts and canceled checks. It can be a drawer, a filing cabinet, a sturdy box, or any space that you can regularly keep these records. At the end of the year, you will take them out and organize them so they can be totaled and included in your tax return.

What to document

Keep all records of money spent on goods or services that relate to your business. These are items listed above under the heading "What Can I Deduct?", and any other items which are related to the operation of your business.

At the end of the year

When you go through your year's receipts and canceled checks, gather them into categories of deductions. This will make it easier for you or your accountant to make a final presentation of your business activity on your schedule C.

Schedule C contains a partial list of business deductions. These include: advertising, bad debts, car and truck expenses, depreciation, insurance, legal and professional services, office expenses, supplies, travel, meals, and entertainment. In addition, the form provides space for other expenses than the ones listed.

Use this list as a basis for organizing your receipts. Other categories you might use for organization purposes are printing and photocopying, telephone expense and gifts to clients. Receipts which do not fit into any other category can be labelled "miscellaneous."

Business use of your car

Are you a commuter?

Business use of your car is deductible, with one important exception: Commuting expense is not deductible. For tax purposes, commuting means traveling between your home and your main or regular place of work. The trip to your work and the trip home again are both considered non-deductible commuting. The IRS enforces this prohibition against deducting commuting expenses strongly and completely.

Perhaps you have no regular place of work; you may do house calls, or you may work in several different locations doing massage. In such a case, you are not a commuter. However, if you work principally in one office, that is your main or regular place of work, and the miles you drive to and from that place are not deductible... unless you have a valid home office.

If you have a home office, then travel between your home office and your workplace is not commuting, but business travel. The idea is that going from office to office is business travel, but going from home to office is commuting. With a home office, you get to decide whether it is your home or your office you are leaving from.

To qualify as a home office, your space in your home must be used exclusively for business and must be your principal place of business. However, you can work at other locations and still have your home office qualify so long as you see most of your clients at home. If you use a garage or out-building, the rules are more lax.

If you have a home office, step into your home office just before you leave on any other business trip. Then you are going from one place of business to another. When you return, step into your home office before doing anything else. Thus your return trip is from one office to another. In this way, none of your business driving is considered commuting. While this may sound a little shady, it is apparently entirely within the law, at least at the present moment.

It is possible the IRS would question this deduction if you were audited. If you wish to be more conservative, then deduct mileage expenses only on days when you see clients in your home office. If you are actually working in your home office on a particular day, there can be no legitimate question that travel from that office to some other business destination is business travel.

Two methods of computing automobile deduction

You may choose either of two methods to compute your deduction for business use of your car.

The methods are to use the standard deduction (29 cents in tax year 1994) for each mile driven for business, or to calculate actual expenses of operating your car for the year and to figure mathematically the amount of your deduction.

If you have a car that is not very expensive and costs little to operate, such as a Toyota tercel, you will come out ahead using the 29 cents per mile computation. If you have an expensive new car or one that required lots of expensive repairs this year, you may come out ahead using the actual computation method.

The standard per mile method is quite simple to use, and the actual cost method can become quite involved. I use the per mile rate on my tax return, because I don't enjoy keeping all the records necessary to use the actual cost method. Even if I am paying a little extra in taxes, for me it is worth it to simplify my record-keeping.

A brief explanation of both methods follows.

Standard deduction method—29 cents per mile (tax year 1994)

Keep a daily log of the use of your car. You should record business and personal use.

The best kind of record to keep lists the starting and ending odometer mileage for each business trip. This type of record shows each business trip individually, and also shows how many miles were personal use. It is also acceptable to list only the destination and the miles driven for each trip.

At the end of the year, total all the business miles and multiply the total by .29 to get the deduction for business use of your car.

Example: Your total business miles turn out to be 3,000.

$$
\begin{array}{r}
3000 \\
\times\ .29 \\
\hline
27000 \\
\underline{60000} \\
\$870.00
\end{array}
$$

Your deduction for business use of your car is $870. This figure is included on your Schedule C as your mileage deduction.

Actual cost method

Keep itemized records of all expenses related to operating your car. These include gasoline, oil, tires, lubrication, repairs and maintenance, insurance, license and registration fees and automobile club membership dues.

These actual costs will be added up at the end of the year. Another actual cost that can be included is the depreciation in value of your car during the year. The IRS has guidelines for computing depreciation.

Keep a log of business and personal miles, since you will need to figure the percentage of business use. At the end of the year, divide the year's total business miles by the year's total miles to arrive at the percentage of business use. Multiply the total of actual expenses by percentage of business use to determine your deduction.

For example, your total costs of operating your car for the year were $1758. In addition, your depreciation allowance was $2500. The total of these figures is $4258.

If your business use of the car was 20% of the year's total use, your calculation would be:

$$
\begin{array}{r}
4258 \\
\times\ .20 \\
\hline
\$851.60
\end{array}
$$

Your deduction for business use of your car is $851.60. This figure is included on your Schedule C as your mileage deduction.

Depreciation

Depreciation is one of the most complex concepts facing someone trying to understand income taxes. Fortunately, you can get along just fine without ever conquering this particular challenge.

In a nutshell, depreciation refers to spreading out the cost of a large expense over a period of years, and deducting part of the expense each year. This usually applies to heavy equipment which costs a great deal and lasts for many years. During each tax year, the owner takes a portion of the total cost as a deduction. The idea is simple enough, but the rules for putting it into practice can get confusing.

The government has given small businesses the option of avoiding the whole problem, by enacting a rule that any business expense up to $10,000 per year may be taken as a *deduction* entirely during that year.

Therefore, even if you purchase ten massage tables this year, you can take the whole deduction as a business expense during the year in which you spend the money.

In some cases, there can be tax advantages to using depreciation instead of taking the whole deduction. For example, if you make a large expenditure this year, and earn very little, a expenditure would be "wasted" if you took the whole deduction this year, because you would pay no taxes whether or not you take the deduction. Next year, when you have more income, you would like to be able to use part of the deduction to reduce you income taxes.

If you think that using depreciation could help you, send for IRS publication 534, Depreciation, or buy *Small-Time Operator*. See the end of this chapter for information on obtaining these items.

Estimated tax payments

If your total tax for last year was $500 or more, you are required to pay estimated tax for this year. This is paid in four equal installments, due April 15, June 15, September 15 and January 15.

Estimated taxes are paid on IRS form #1040-ES.

Your total estimated tax payments must be at least 90% of the tax you wind up owing for the year, or 100% of the tax you owed for the previous year. Unless your payments meet one or the other of these conditions, you can be assessed a penalty for underpayment of estimated taxes.

You are entitled to base your estimated tax payments on last year's taxes, even if you are making more this year than you did last year. However, if you under-pay your estimated taxes, you will have a large sum to come up with April 15th of next year. Not only will you have to pay the balance of last year's taxes, but you will also have to pay the first estimated tax payment for next year on the same day.

Hiring an accountant

Accountants are not cheap, but often they can pay for themselves in tax savings they find that you might miss. If you are motivated to do your own taxes, there is no reason you cannot do so. The resources listed below will give you all the information you need. With some time and study, you can learn what you need to know.

However, it can get complex, and unless you enjoy this sort of thing, consider hiring professional help. The non-CPA tax preparers may know just as much as an accountant, and may charge a little less.

Ask other therapists for recommendations for an accountant. When they recommend someone, ask why they like him (or her), or why they think he is a good accountant. If the reasons they give refer to things that matter to you in an accountant, consider using him.

Consider finding an accountant who will trade accounting services for massage. Use the yellow pages, and call accountants. Explain that you are just getting established, have a simple return, and would like to find an accountant who appreciates massage. You may catch someone in the proper mood to make an arrangement to trade services.

Consider, also, hiring an accountant to get you started with bookkeeping and tax systems you can understand, so that you can do your own taxes in future years. An accountant may be able to explain everything you need to know, and set you up with forms you will be able to use in future years.

Even if you use an accountant or tax preparer, keep your records clear and organized. If possible, keep them in categories that will make it easy to sort out at tax time. This will make the accountant's job easier, and may encourage him to keep his fees reasonable.

Getting further information

If you want help doing your own taxes, there are several good resources you can turn to.

1. One is a book, written by an accountant, for the purpose of helping small business owners take care of bookkeeping and taxes. It is well-organized, well written and inexpensive. It goes into more detail about depreciation, and a few other minor subjects, than this chapter, and has practical advice about book-keeping. The book is called *Small-Time Operator* and is available from:

   Bell Springs Publishing
   Box 640 Bell Springs Road
   Laytonville, CA 95454
   (707) 984-6746

2. Another good book is *Guide to Income Tax Preparation* by Consumer Reports Books. The 1994 edition sold for $13.99. Although it is over 600 pages long, it is very well organized, written in a style that is easy to read, and has a comprehensive index. It covers in detail any subject you would need to know about in order to do your tax return. When April 15 rolls around and you are up against a deadline, this book can be a comforting resource to have with you.

3. The final source of information is the IRS, and its information is available at no charge. The IRS will send you booklets explaining various aspects of your taxes, and is also available to answer questions by phone.

   IRS publications can be ordered by calling

   1-800-829-3676 (1-800-TAX-FORM)

The first publication to order is Tax Guide for Small Businesses, Publication 334. This contains the basics of record-keeping and taxes for small businesses, including filled-in forms.

The second publication to order is "Guide to Free Tax Services." This lists all the other IRS publications. Once you have this booklet, you can leaf through it to see what else is available and what you need.

Some of the subjects covered in these IRS publications are listed below. The IRS publication number is listed after each name. These can be ordered from the toll-free number listed above.

> Travel, Entertainment and Gift Expense 463
> Tax Withholding and Estimated Tax 505
> Educational Expenses 508
> Moving Expenses 521
> Reporting Income from Tips 531
> Self-Employment Tax 533
> Depreciation 534
> Business Expense 535
> Retirement Plans for the Self-employed 560
> Taxpayers Starting a Business 583
> Business Use of Your Home 587
> Alternative Minimum Tax for Individuals 909
> Business Use of a Car 917

All of these publications provide good detail, and are written in clear and readable fashion. However, they are written by the IRS, and will not necessarily tip you off to the best ways of getting the most out of your deductions.

To reach an IRS representative by phone, check your local phone book blue pages under Federal Government, Internal Revenue Service. Major cities have local offices. In other locations, call the IRS toll-free at: 1-800-829-1040.

19 Reimbursement For Your Service by Insurance Companies

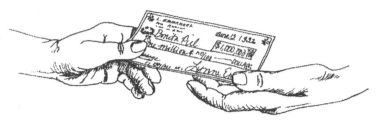

This chapter is written with the assistance of Christine Rosche, M.P.H., author of "The Insurance Reimbursement Manual" and publisher of "The Professional Bodyworker Newsletter." She also conducts seminars on insurance reimbursement for massage therapists, and consults on practice building and insurance. Information about reaching her and ordering her manual appears in the reference section on page 167.

The Current Status of Insurance Reimbursement for Massage

The issue of insurance reimbursement is a source of confusion for many in the massage industry.

In 1990, the AMTA surveyed its members about insurance reimbursement. Of those who answered the survey, 27% never participate in insurance billing. 9% have tried without success for insurance reimbursement. 34% report that they sometimes receive insurance reimbursement, and 20% receive reimbursement whenever they submit a claim.

Because of the lack of standardization in the massage industry, whether or not you are able to obtain insurance reimbursement for your services may depend on such factors as the legal status of massage in your state, the type of insurance company you are dealing with, and the kind of professional relationship you have with referring doctors.

In need of clarification

Most states do not license massage, and the ones that do have widely different laws (see page 122). Insurance plans differ greatly in whether and to what extent they cover massage therapy. Accordingly, there exist a variety of local answers to any questions about insurance reimbursement. In addition, in any one locality, the answers to questions about reimbursement are subject to change at any time.

This chapter will help clarify your status in the health care system, give you some information on the advantages and disadvantages of participating in insurance reimbursement, and some basic guidelines for obtaining insurance compensation for your services. Please be careful not to follow guidance from any non-experts in this area, as improper billing procedures can result in legal troubles for the therapist.

Advantages and disadvantages

Before we examine the specifics of the insurance compensation system, consider the effect on the massage profession of widespread dependence on insurance payments.

Insurance companies, especially in these days of managed care, have become aggressive in telling doctors, dentists, psychotherapists and chiropractors what treatments will be paid for under what conditions. Professionals who rely on insurance reimbursement are losing much of their freedom to practice as they see fit because they must conform to insurance company guidelines.

For the massage practitioner, working for insurance reimbursement means working by prescription of a doctor, usually a physician or a chiropractor. You work as an "adjunct therapist," carrying out the doctor's recommended treatment. In some types of practice, this can cast you in the role of a technician more than a therapist, as you may be told to work certain muscles only, or warm up an area for chiropractic adjustment. The type of client you work with can be determined by the kind of therapy you specialize in and your level of professional experience.

Another consideration is that you are likely to encounter at least some resistance by insurance companies to which you submit your claims for reimbursement. Insurance companies, like any other companies, make a profit by paying out less money than they take in. Most companies will pay legitimate claims, but they may require substantial paperwork to demonstrate that the claims are legitimate. Some companies resist even legitimate claims, requiring duplicative or excessive paperwork from the therapist.

The big advantages of working for insurance compensation are higher compensation and a stable client base. The average billable hourly rate for clinical massage is at least $60. The possibility of insurance compensation will also bring you clients who otherwise could not afford to use your services. These are very substantial advantages to an individual who is committed to the full-time practice of massage therapy.

It is up to you to decide whether the advantages to you outweigh the disadvantages, and you may not really know until you try it.

Your Role in the Health Care System

As a massage or bodywork practitioner working by doctor's prescription, your therapy is a part of the treatment plan of the referring doctor. He or she prescribes your services much the same as prescribing physical therapy or psychiatric care.

The doctor must provide a diagnosis in order to initiate the process. Diagnosis means identification of the patient's problem. So at the outset, it is apparent that this type of work is related to patients with problems, or symptoms, seeking relief. The problem can be a general one, indicating a need for relaxation massage, or a specific one, indicating a need for specific therapeutic techniques.

Relaxation Massage

Occasionally, a doctor will prescribe massage solely for its benefits in relaxing the client. Relaxation massage may or may not be reimbursable, depending on the patient's diagnosis and treatment plan.

Some chiropractors prescribe massage for patients who are too rigid to adjust, in hopes that the massage therapist will be able to help the patient release muscle tension, thus facilitating chiropractic care. A few medical doctors also prescribe massage for patients who are overly tense, as relaxation can help with a variety of medical problems that result from anxiety.

Medical Massage

Most prescriptions, however, are of a different sort, and involve what is commonly called "medical massage" or "clinical massage." This includes understanding of certain pathologies and knowledge of specific techniques that will be helpful in recovery from specific conditions and injuries. Certain schools specialize in medical massage, and other schools offer limited training in medical massage as part of their curriculum.

No *legal* requirement exists that you take a training in medical massage before working from a doctor's prescription. However, to attempt to do medical massage without proper training would be very ill-advised, and would lead to frustration for you and for the doctor.

Unless you have substantial training, you will not be able to understand the doctor's orders, and you will not know what to do to carry them out. Most doctors do not understand what massage therapists know and don't know, and therefore the responsibility to keep communication clear rests with you. Unless you are familiar with the terminology and procedures to be used in medical massage, problems will arise.

There is no industry standard for training in medical massage. Courses in pathology, medical terminology, neuromuscular therapy or trigger point therapy, and deep tissue massage are useful. Also consider programs that include rehabilitative exercises and treatments for specific injuries and conditions. The medical massage component of your education could easily take 500 classroom hours.

If massage therapists attempt to practice medical massage without proper training, doctors will view massage as an unprofessional modality, and will avoid creating a professional relationship with massage therapists.

Professional arrangements

A variety of professional arrangements are available to a massage therapist or bodyworker who wants to work with clients for insurance reimbursement.

1. Client pays therapist, and client then submits the therapist's bill to insurance company for reimbursement.

2. Therapist works by prescription of physician, and therapist deals directly with insurance company for reimbursement.

3. Therapist works closely with prescribing physician and physician's office handles insurance reimbursement. Physician may pay therapist by the hour or share insurance reimbursement proceeds, often 50-50. This arrangement is more common when massage therapists work in chiropractors' offices.

Number 3 is more common in states with no state-wide massage licensing law. Numbers 1 and 2 are more common in states that do license massage.

No matter which of these three arrangements you participate in, however, you should have a good understanding of insurance guidelines and the billing process. Even if the doctor's office does your billing, you should be able to supervise and assist the process, since the doctor's office person may not understand how to classify and bill for your services.

One procedure for billing services to insurance companies

1. Call the company for verification of coverage and limits

Call the client's insurance company before working with the client. Tell the company representative the client's policy number, and ask if that policy will cover payment for *soft tissue mobilization* or *neuromuscular re-education*. (If you use the term "massage," the insurance company will classify what you do as "relaxation massage" and will not cover it)

Ask the policy's limit of such payments, and write down the answer. Also write down the name of the person you spoke with and the date.

2. Billing the insurance company

When you submit your bill to the insurance company for payment, send it to the person you spoke to. Attach a copy of the prescription from the referring physician. In your bill, include the client's name, address, and policy number. Also include the date of the treatment, the length of time you spent, the type of work you did, and your fee. List your itemized fee for each procedure, and also your total fee.

Be sure to check if "procedure codes" are required for billing. Major Medical and Worker's Compensation carriers usually require that you show the code for the procedure you have performed. However, these codes are intended to be used *only* by licensed health care providers. Unlicensed providers may not use these codes when billing from their own office or when working unsupervised.

Bill amounts under $200 at a time. Larger amounts are scrutinized more carefully before being paid. If you do not receive payment within two to three weeks, call your contact person at the insurance company and politely ask if there has been a problem.

Keep a record of your treatments and amounts billed for each client. When you receive payment from the insurance company, note in your records which treatments have been reimbursed. Keeping accurate records will help you follow up on claims that are not promptly paid.

The Battle of the Forms

Some companies will require you to fill out detailed forms in order to obtain insurance compensation. If at all possible, negotiate with your referring doctor to have his or her insurance professional process these forms for you. It may well be worth paying a share of your professional fee to the doctor for the service of having the billing taken care of.

Even if the insurance person on the doctor's staff is too busy to take on your insurance work, consider using this person as a consultant or teacher, who can get you started by walking you through the forms and procedures, and explaining what you need to do and how things work.

Be aware that different companies operate differently. Some put up as many obstacles as they can to paying for your services, on the theory that any money they do not pay out is money in their pocket. It is worth it to them to pay their employee for putting up obstacles, if that results in paying out fewer claims dollars.

Other companies have no such strategy, and merely require accurate and orderly paperwork. With experience, you will get to know which is which. In time, you may even be able to be selective in working only for clients of insurance companies that pay for your services without undue paperwork requirements.

Record-keeping for insurance clients

If you are working on clients who are covered by insurance, you need to keep more complete records than you otherwise would for a massage practice. Your records should fit the model of charting patients in the medical health care system.

For each treatment, keep records of:

1. Length of treatment
2. Parts of body you treated
3. Type of treatment you used (i.e., deep friction, moist heat, trigger point therapy)
4. Changes you noted in client's condition
5. Goals for further sessions (if appropriate)
6. How this treatment fits into client's overall treatment plan

Record-keeping for insurance clients is also often called SOAP charting, which stands for Subjective, Objective, Assessment, Plan. These four elements should be in your client record for each session. Subjective refers to the physician's assessment and the client's statements about the condition. Objective refers to the specific muscles you work on and techniques you use. Assessment refers to your evaluation of the condition, and Plan refers to your opinion about what should happen next in this case.

If you decide you would like to make insurance billing a major part of your practice, consider studying it in depth in order to understand it more fully. Resources for further study and for assistance with record-keeping and billing can be found on page 167.

20 Keeping Client and Financial Records

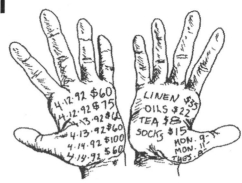

There are three basic kinds of records to keep, and they are all important.

Tax records

These are your records of all the money you earn and all the money you spend on deductible items. If you should be called on one day to demonstrate to the IRS the truth of all the entries in your tax return, you will need to produce accurate records of your income and deductions. These records should be kept at least three years after your return is filed, as your return can be audited up to three years after you file it.

Business records

These are the records you keep to give you a better understanding of your own practice. Different practices have different slow and busy times. Your practice may slow down for three weeks every August, which would make that a perfect time for your vacation in the Colorado Rockies. If you don't keep accurate records, you probably would never see that pattern, and might wind up staying in town during your slow season and leaving when clients will miss you more.

Client records

Client records allow you to better know and serve each client. Your records will let you know basic personal and medical information about each client, and will show you their history of receiving treatments from you. When appropriate, your records will give you an at-a-glance view of how your treatments affected specific problems or situations in your clients' lives.

This chapter discusses how to keep each of these three kinds of records, and suggests some ways to design your own record-keeping system that will make the whole process easier and more efficient. Sample forms appear at the end of the chapter. You may copy and use these forms, modify them to suit you, or create your own.

Record-keeping For Tax-Time

The records you need to keep are those proving your *income* and your *deductions*. Chapter Eighteen explains income and deductions.

The main things you should do to support proper tax record-keeping are 1) write down every payment you receive for your work in some type of ledger, 2) keep track of your automobile business mileage in a ledger, and 3) keep bills, receipts and canceled checks in one container until the end of the year, when you can sort them out and tally them up.

SHOE by Jeff MacNelly

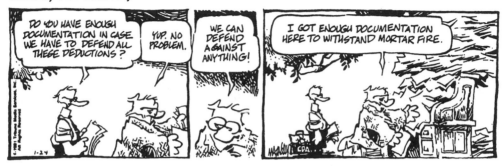

Recording income and business mileage

There is no required form for these records. The only requirement is that they be *accurate* and *complete*. If your car has a trip odometer, you can easily compute miles for each business trip by resetting the trip odometer to zero when you begin, and reading the trip odometer when you finish. Keep your log in the car, and record the mileage when you finish each business trip.

No matter what system you decide to use, take the time *each day* to record all of the day's business activity. Record the day's business mileage, and all income you receive each day. Get in the habit of recording each day's business activity before you go to sleep.

Records of Business Activity

Your records should show you your business activity for each day, each week, each month, and each year. It takes a minimum amount of effort to keep your records in good order, and the rewards can be substantial.

Charting your business activity not only gives you information about when you can expect seasonal ups and downs, but it also tells you whether your overall business activity is going up, going down, or staying about the same.

During some slow weeks, I could have become depressed or pessimistic about the progress of my practice. Instead, I glanced at my business activity chart, and I saw that last month I had a slow week and it was in-between two better weeks. Instead of thinking my practice was going sour, I realized I was experiencing a normal fluctuation and nothing was going wrong. That insight did a lot for my emotional health.

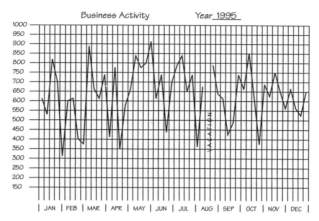

Business Activity   Year 1995

Charting your business activity can give you information about seasonal trends, usefulness of certain promotions, and short-term and long-term fluctuations in the volume of your practice. No other information costs so little in time or effort compared to the value it produces.

Keeping Client Records

If you or your clients are going to bill insurance companies for your services, you need to keep detailed records for each treatment you perform. See Chapter 19 dealing with billing insurance companies, and see page 167 for resources to help with record-keeping for insurance clients.

Even if you are not dealing with insurance billing, you should keep accurate records. For each client, you should have a completed intake form that includes the following basic information:

- Date of first treatment
- Client's name and address, with zip code
- Phone number
- Medical history (as much as you feel is necessary)
- Previous experience with massage or bodywork
- Current symptoms or problems
- Reason for seeking treatment

Date of first treatment will be useful to you later as you review your records on a particular client.

The address is necessary if you ever want to mail something to the client (such as a Christmas card, promotional flyer, or bill) or do a house call.

The phone number is necessary in the event of cancellation or change of plans on short notice.

Medical history gives you a better sense of how your treatment can fit into this person's whole picture, and can be useful in discovering contraindications for part or all of the treatment you will give.

Whether the person has previously had bodywork helps you to know how to approach this session.

Current symptoms or problems, and reason for seeking treatment give you information about what this client wants from you. Failure to get this information can result in doing a session that does not satisfy a client. They will not usually spontaneously tell you what they expect from your work.

If the client's care does not involve insurance billing, you may not need to keep further records for this client, except those necessary for business activity and tax purposes. If you do need to keep further records, you can use the back of the client's intake form, or create a separate file for records about continuing care clients.

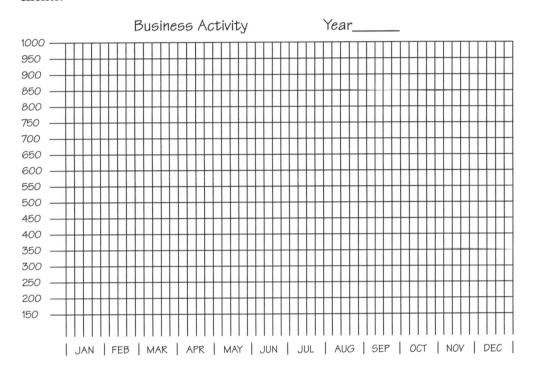

Client _____

Address _____

_____ Phone (_____) _____

Date of first treatment _____

Occupation _____

Medical History:
Previous major Illnesses:

Previous broken bones or other injuries:

Are you currently under a physician's care?

    Physician _____

    For what condition?_____

    Are you taking any medications? _____

Current Condition:
Areas of pain or discomfort:

Reasons for seeking massage:

Have you previously had massage or other bodywork? What type?

What do you do to manage your stress?

What is your routine of exercise?

Week of _____

Date	Client	fee	miles

21 Managing Your Money
Some Ideas On Financial Planning

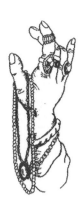

In the early years of your massage career, you will not have much money to manage. Spare dollars will go to necessities, and to improvements in your professional equipment.

In time, however, success will bring with it prosperity, and when it does, you will need to give at least a little thought to how to manage your money.

Savings

One of the hardest things for a self-employed person to do is to put money into a savings account. However, it is a very important habit to get into. Consider the following expenses you will have:

1. Quarterly estimated tax payments

2. Health insurance, auto insurance

3. Professional association dues

These expenses come quarterly, semi-annually, or annually. They can put a strain on your budget if you are living from month to month. Having a reserve in your savings (or checking) account makes life easier when these expenses come due.

Open a savings account at your bank. Start it with at least $100, and add whatever amounts you can. Avoid making withdrawals unless absolutely necessary. The fact that you have a few hundred dollars, or a couple of thousand dollars, can be very comforting when the mechanic tells you you need a transmission overhaul.

Beyond this issue of emergency reserves to meet unforseen expenses, you will also want to consider the larger financial reserves you will need to meet the major expenses you can expect sooner or later:

4. Buying a new car

5. Buying a home

6. Rearing children

7. Retirement

These are the expenses that require you to make, and save, substantial sums of money, and to manage that money in a way that gives you the most advantage out of it.

Long-range planning

As a rule of thumb, there are two critical points in the careers of many would-be massage therapists—two years into a career and five years into a career.

Many practitioners give up somewhere near the two-year mark. Either they failed to pursue any organized marketing approach, or they gave up before getting the benefit of the approach they were using.

Those who survive the two-year mark usually find some degree of success in the field. Another point often comes at the five-year mark, when the physical nature of the work may begin to take its toll, or the practitioner may decide to branch off into another kind of work.

Practitioners who stay with the work longer than five years can usually keep doing the work practically indefinitely. Some keep working into their seventies. If you are staying in the field longer than five years, you will do well to take up the study of estate planning and investment.

You can't live on Social Security

Consider what you will have to live on when you retire.

Social security may be enough to keep a roof over your head, and three very low-budget meals on the table, but it is not enough money to *live* on. Before you reach retirement age, you should have put aside enough to create your own retirement plan. The earlier you start, the easier it will be.

Kinds of Savings Plans

Savings plans can take many forms.

1. You can stockpile cash, but if you do so you earn no interest, and can lose everything in a theft or fire.

2. You can keep your money in a savings account, certificate of deposit, or money market account. These will earn interest, and your money will be basically safe.

3. You can choose a "tax shelter" keyed to retirement. While you must still pay self-employment tax on the money you put into your retirement plan, you do not pay federal income tax on this money. You pay income tax on the retirement money only when you receive it, at retirement. Tax breaks available to retired persons may help you pay lower taxes on your money at retirement time than you would now.

Tax Shelter Retirement Plans

In a nutshell, the great thing about tax shelter retirement plans is that they force you to keep your money invested until you retire. Because of high penalties for withdrawing money prior to age 59½, you are forced to keep your "nest egg" safe for your future.

This is both the advantage and the disadvantage of these plans—you lose the flexibility to deal with your money on a whim; you have fewer options now, but more security later.

The government makes this appealing by giving you a slightly better tax treatment if you put your money into a retirement plan. Consider the following example:

It is April 14th, and you are preparing your tax return for the previous year. You do all your computations, find out you owe $2,104 in income tax (we are ignoring social security tax in this example, because retirement plans do not change your social security tax).

If you use some money you have saved to make a contribution of $2,000 to a qualified retirement plan, your income tax bill will be reduced to $1,804. You therefore reduce your tax by $300 by placing $2,000 in a retirement plan. As long as you make this contribution by April 15, it counts as a deduction for the preceding year's taxes.

Save now, save later

To take the example a step further, consider the long-term effects of this decision. If you *do not* make the contribution to your retirement plan, you must spend $300 of the $2,000 on taxes. This leaves you with $1,700.

Assume that you keep this $1,700 invested at "average" interest rates for thirty years. Interest rates are always changing, but as a rule of thumb, you can figure that money will double itself every ten years. Therefore, in 30 years, an investment should grow to eight times the original amount. (After 10 years, the original investment will double; after 20 years it will double again, or be four times the original amount; after 30 years it will double a third time, and be eight times the original amount).

This rule of thumb tells us that $1,700 today will be $13,600 in 30 years.

Now consider the alternative where you put $2,000 in a retirement account. The same rule of thumb tells us that the $2,000 today will turn into $16,000 in 30 years. However, this $16,000 will be subject to income tax when you receive it at retirement. Current rates of income tax, 15%, would reduce that $16,000 to $13,600—exactly the same amount as if you had paid your $300 tax in the first place and left the $1,700 invested.

However, unless you are a person of incredible will power, you *will not* leave that $1,700 alone for 30 years to gain interest. What you will wind up with will be somewhat less than the $13,600 you know you can count on if you sock the money away in a retirement plan where you cannot reach it without substantial penalties.

In addition, tax breaks available to retired persons may make it possible for you to pay less than 15% tax on the money when you receive it at retirement. Any such breaks you get make it definitely advantageous to have your money in a retirement account.

Kinds of Retirement Plans

There are three kinds of retirement plans available to you as a self-employed person: The IRA (Individual Retirement Account), the SEP (Simplified Employee Pension Plan, a form of IRA); and the Keogh.

IRA

Easy to set up and widely available, an IRA allows you to shelter up to a maximum of $2,000 per year. IRA's are designed for people without large incomes, and if you are single and have an income over $25,000, or married and have a joint income over $40,000, you will lose the advantage of an IRA.

SEP

Also easy to set up and widely available, the SEP allows you to shelter up to 15% of your earnings (to a maximum contribution of $30,000 in any one year)

Keogh

Two types of plans exist, one which requires a set contribution each year, and one which does not. The maximum contributions are either 15% or 25% of income depending on the type of plan, up to a maximum of $30,000 per year. Keogh's are more complicated to set up, and can be more expensive to create and maintain than IRA's or SEP's.

IRA's and SEP's can be set up any time before April 15, and will still be valid for the previous year's taxes. Keogh's must be *set up* by December 31 in order to be valid for that tax year, although contributions can still be made until April 15 of the next year.

If you are interested in establishing one of these accounts, start with your local bank, savings and loan, or insurance advisor. Chances are, they can advise you and set up an account for you, often at no charge. Also check with your accountant or financial advisor. Once established, these accounts cannot be modified, so be very careful that you understand how your account will fit into your future plans.

V

Equipment
and Other
Professional
Resources

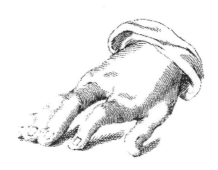

Networking, Marketing and Promotional Services

The Quiet Touch
1-800-946-2772
office address: 15294 S.W. 104 St., suite 1025, Miami, FL 33196

Accepts: Licensed Massage Therapists with current membership in AMTA, ABMP, IMA or you can get corporate discounts through The Quiet Touch from ABMP

Service Provided: The company makes agreements to provide massage services to clients in hotels, offices, health spas, the company's own massage offices and clients' homes. The company started in New York, spread quickly to New Jersey, Connecticut and Florida, and it expects to be in all 50 states soon.

Clients schedule appointments through the company office and participating massage therapists are told where and when to report to fill these appointments. The therapist receives 70% of the fee paid by the client. Therapists need not have their own office to participate. Therapists are charged an annual fee to participate.

ASSOCIATED MTs NEAR YOU^{SM}
From Quality of Work Life Services
1-800-747-0047
http://www.qwl.com/mts.html
E-Mail: mt@infohouse.com

Accepts: Present and Future Licensed Massage Therapists

Service Provided: This is a co-operative promotional, mentoring and advocacy network, created in NYC, 1992, to enhance the reputation, professional status and economic opportunities for licensed massage therapists. Currently in 13 states, the company maintains a website and places advertisements in national publications. Active members are included in print and online directories. They are entitled to a consultation with Bruria Ginton, LicMT, AMTA-RMT, Founding Director, can use the company logo and other promotional materials, and receive a quarterly newsletter.

In addition, members may also participate in co-operative promotions in which several massage therapists share the cost of a specific promotional effort. Active membership, open to qualified MTs, is $65.00 per year. Supportive membership, open to anyone, is $35.00 and Student membership is $25.00.

Massage Tables and Chairs

All of the following companies ship their products nationwide. They will all send you brochures or information packets about their massage tables and other products at your request.

Arnold Health Equipment Co.
4155 N. State Road 39
LaPorte, IN 46350
(219) 325-0582

Lightweight, portable, fixed height, inexpensive massage table

Astra Lite Tables
120 Manfree Rd.
Watsonville, CA 95076
1-800-368-5483
(408) 763-0397

Extremely lightweight, portable, fixed or adjustable height, inexpensive portable tables, bolsters, carrying cases

Blue Ridge Tables
Rt. 6 Box 490
South Industrial Park
Corinth, MS 38834
(601) 286-7007
1-800-447-2723

Lightweight, portable, adjustable height inexpensive table and accessories

Body Work Supply Company
3345 South 300 West, Unit B-3
Salt Lake City, UT 84115
(801) 467-9106

"Electric Lift" massage table with foot pedal for height adjustment during treatment, stationary and portable massage tables, bolsters, carrying cases

Colorado Healing Arts
P.O. Box 2247
Boulder, CO 80306
1-800-728-2426

Portable and non-portable tables, oils, sheets, bolsters and miscellaneous items

Creative Touch
1713 G Street #1
Sacramento, CA 95814
(916) 441-6759

Lightweight, adjustable height, oval massage tables

Custom Craftworks
P.O. Box 24621
Eugene, OR 97402
(503) 345-2712
1-800-627-2387

A selection of adjustable height portable tables; on-site chair reiki table, bolsters, carrying carrying cases, tableskate, wooden screens, cabinets and office accessories

G & A Manufacturers
1008 E. Fairview Bl.
Inglewood, CA 90302
(213) 412-0297 or 412-2467
1-800-822-5372

Stationary and portable tables, wooden or aluminum legs; very lightweight inexpensive portable, reiki/facial table, on-site chair, bolsters and carrying cases

Galaxy Enterprises, Inc.
5411 Sheila St.
Los Angeles, CA 90040
(213) 728-3980
1-800-876-4599

Lightweight, portable, adjustable height massage table

Golden Ratio Woodworks
P.O Box 440
Emigrant, MT 59027
1-800-796-0612

Full line of stationary and portable tables, spa tables, on-site chair, 14-pound on-site chair, covers, oils, bolsters, charts, books and other accessories. Top of the line table carries lifetime guarantee.

Greentree Massage Tables
7202 Treewater
Houston, TX 77072
(713) 530-1627

Portable, adjustable height lightweight, inexpensive table

Integrated Medical, Inc.
8100 Akron, ste. 320
Englewood, CO 80112
1-800-333-7617

Stationary massage table with electric motor for height adjustment during treatment

Living Earth Crafts
600 East Todd Road
Santa Rosa, CA 95407
In CA: 1-800-336-4114
Outside CA: 1-800-358-8292

Complete line of stationary and portable tables, including very inexpensive portable, on-site chair, desk-top face cradle, oils, linens, books, charts, music, videos, aromatherapy, pillows, body-cushion system, bolsters, carrying cases.

Matthew David Magnetic
Therapy and Massage Supplies
(Royal Pyramid International)
orders 1-800-325-7423
information (914) 769-4879

Massage treatment table with 48 1,000-gauss magnets built in

Mountain Laurel Massage Tables
RD1 Cone Hill Rd.
West Stockbridge, MA 01266
(413) 232-7937

Adjustable height portable tables, with optional built-in tilting face rest, carrying cases

New Generation Products
Montgomery Woods
6721 E. Akron St.
Mesa, AZ 85205
1-800-850-5552

Basic and deluxe lightweight adjustable height massage tables; carry case, fitted face cradle covers, oil pouch belt (lifetime guarantee except for vinyl)

Oakworks, Inc.
34 Main Street
P.O. Box 99
Glen Rock, PA 17327-0099
(717) 235-6807
1-800-558-8850

Complete line of stationary and portable tables, on-site chair, carrying cases, bolsters and sheets

Pisces Productions
50 Center Rd.
Petaluma, CA 94952
1-800-TABLE-33

Two models of portable, adjustable height tables, carrying cases, on-site chair

Prana Bodywork Tables
P.O. Box 228
Sharon, MA 02067
(617) 784-8535
1-800-458-1859

Adjustable height portable, futon massage table, carrying case, carrying strap, customization available

Robert Hunter Bodywork Tables
1104 NE 28th
Portland, OR 97232
(503) 249-0847
1-800-284-3988

Stationary and portable adjustable height tables, sheets, massage oil, carrying cases, customization available

SomaTech International
1730 Industrial Drive
Auburn, CA 95603
(916) 888-1518
1-800-655-4321

Full line of portable and stationary massage tables, ultra-light portable table, on-site chairs, hydraulically operated chairs, massage tools, body bridge, body support cushions, bolsters, full range of accessories

Somatron Corp.
3405 Ellenwood Lane
Tampa, FL 33618
(813) 960-2183
1-800-544-4294

Portable vibro-acoustic music body mats, stationary tables and recliners that direct music vibrations through the client's body during the massage

Stacy-Built Systems
P.O. Box 1032
Clinton, NC 28328
(919) 592-3237
1-800-356-8426

Stationary massage table with electronic lift for height adjustment during treatment; non-electronic stationary table; portable tables, carrying cases

Stronglite Massage Table Kits
255 Davidson St.
Cottage Grove, OR 97424
(503) 942-0130
1-800-BUY-KITS (289-5487)

Portable, lightweight adjustable height, inexpensive tables, on-site partially assembled tables and kits at substantially lower cost

Tatum's Custom Woodworks
Route 3, Box 114
Newberry, FL 32669
business: (904) 472-0020
residence: (904) 472-3847

Portable, adjustable height massage table, carrying case and bolsters.

Touch America
P.O. Box 1304
Hillsborough, NC 27278
(919) 732-6968
1-800-678-6824
FAX (919) 732-1173

Complete line of stationary and portable tables, spa products including a wet treatment table, acoustic music table, on-site chair, stool, sheets, workshop series on seated massage, sound and spa therapies, miscellaneous items

Ultra-Light Inc.
1745 Route 37 West
Toms River, NJ 08757
(908) 286-4322
1-800-999-1971

Extremely light portable table, adjustable legs available

Massage Oils

The following companies either manufacture or distribute massage oils. Most of these companies also sell other beauty, body-care, health-related or aromatherapy products. All companies listed below will send a catalogue on request.

The price listed next to the company name is the approximate price of a gallon of their least expensive massage oil including shipping charges (unless otherwise noted). Prices reflect a professional discount, if any applies. Some companies require a wholesale order, usually a four-gallon minimum.

Aroma de Terra
401 Euclid Ave., suite 155
Cleveland, OH 44114
(216) 566-8234

Botanical oils for use as massage or bath oils.
(16 ounce bottle $14.00 and up)

Barclay Labs ($25 plus S/H)
4780-A Caterpillar Rd.
Redding, CA 96003
(916) 244-4460

A light massage oil that will not go rancid, is stain resistant, coconut oil based, derived solely from plants; cruelty free, color and fragrance free.

Best of Nature ($30)
12 W. Front St.
Red Bank, NJ 07701
(908) 842-8987

A variety of scented and unscented oils, essential oils and aromatherapy blends, creams, lotions, liniments, books, bottles, pillows and massage tables

Biotone ($37)
4564 Alvarado Canyon Rd., #1
San Diego, CA 92120
1-800-445-6457
In CA: (619) 281-4228

Unscented, and scented massage oils, dual-purpose massage creme, deep tissue lotion, sports therapy creme and gel, pumps, Fresh Again detergent, essential oils, face cradle covers, cruelty-free

Charlie Sunshine's Secret Formula ($40 plus shipping)
88 Santa Marina
San Francisco, CA 94110
(415) 647-3973

Massage oil with a creamy texture like a lotion; 100% oil, will not disappear into the skin; recommended for deep tissue work.

The Crystal Rainbow Co. ($63.75)
P.O. Box 400
Milford, MI 48381
(313) 685-3628

Cold-processed sesame oil, unscented or blended with fragrances; aromatherapy supplies

Diamond Light Massage Products ($19)
14 Las Palomas
Orinda, CA 94563
(510) 253-0543

Sunfresh soap, valley of the sun natural massage oil
(10% discount on orders over $80)

Dr. Hauschka Products
59C North Street
Hatfield, MA 01038
1-800-247-9907

Dr. Hauschka line of specially prepared massage oils
(3.4 ounce bottle $11 to $14; minimum order $200)

Elements Plus
811 North Main, suite 201
Royal Oak, MI 48067
1-800-995-6404
(810) 544-6404

Activating massage oil, scented or unscented, replenishing massage lotion, restructuring creme, herbal formula

Everybody, Ltd. ($93.25)
1175 Walnut St.
Boulder, CO 80302
1-800-758-5675

Massage oils, lotions, essential perfume oils, skin trip, mother's special blend

Gaia Products ($45 plus shipping)
2452 East 24th St.
Brooklyn, NY 11235
(718) 389-8224

Unscented, scented, and custom blended massage oils, anatomy and physiology audio review tapes, essential oils.

The Heritage Store ($36)
P.O. Box 444-R
Virginia Beach, VA 23458-0444
1-800-726-2232
1-800-862-2923

Aura glow massage oil, from a formula prescribed by Edgar Cayce, consisting of peanut oil, olive oil, liquid lanolin, vitamin E and scent

Jacki's Magic Lotion ($46.60
258 "A" St., #7-A   plus shpg.)
Ashland, OR 97520
1-800-729-8428
1-503-488-1388

A 100% natural massage lotion and
moisturizer with a rich, smooth
texture, scented or unscented; free
samples available

Liberty Massage Products ($24)
8120 SE Stark St.
Portland, OR 97215
1-800-289-8427

Almond oil, variety of scented oils,
aromatherapy supplies

Myosoothe Products ($103.20)
124 East "F" St. #7
Ontario, CA 91764
1-800-841-0815

Pure base oils blended with selected
essential oils; blends for body massage,
muscle therapy, cellulite therapy

Pure Pro Massage Oils ($23.90)
955 Massachusetts Ave. #232
Cambridge, MA 02139
1-800-900-PURE (7873)

Four different base oils, sports blend,
apricot oil, gingered almond blend,
scented premium, citrus, peppermint,
white ginger

Rainbow Research Corp. ($42)
170 Wilbur Place
Bohemia, NY 11716
In NY: (516) 589-5563
Outside NY: 1-800-722-9595

Sports or moisturizing blend; contains
almond, olive and peanut oil, plus
Vitamin E, lanolin and paba

**Reign Dance Hawaiian
Massage Oils**
219 First Ave. south suite 405
Seattle, WA 98104
(206) 789-6429
1-800-221-1309

Hawaiian flower oils and combination
oils for all types of bodywork, deep
tissue work and healing work, plus
ceremonial oils
(9 ounce bottle $10.50 to $22.50)

**Third Millenium/Body
Care** ($30 plus s/h)
2195 Faraday Avenue, suite #F
Carlsbad, CA 92008
(619) 431-7181
1-800-776-6525

12 water washable formulations oils and
lotions, pain relieving massage lotions,
sterilizing cleanser, hand and body lotion (discounts for orders of 4 or more
gallons)

Total Sensations ($48 plus s/h)
Private Label Cosmetics
85D Mahan St.
West Babylon, NY 11704
1-800-446-4704
(516) 491-9010

Massage oil with gentle aromatic
fragrance

Uncommon Scents ($28)
380 W. First Ave.
Eugene, OR 97401
(503) 345-0952
1-800-426-4336

Massage oil blend, massage lotion, apricot oil, almond oil, coconut oil, cocoa butter, essential balm, tiger balm; customized scents available

Weleda, Inc. ($119)
P.O. Box 249
Congers, NY 10920
(914) 268-8572

Arnica massage oil, citrus massage oil, Calendula baby oil, essential oils

Massage Supply Stores and Catalogue Services

ASHA Book and Supply
1924 Cliff Valley Way, NE
Atlanta, GA 30329
1-800-726-0686
(404) 633-3100
Treatment tables, books, charts, linens, professional garments, hydrotherapy equipment, oils, lotions, office lighting, air control and water systems, electrotherapy instruments, magnetic healing supplies, aromatherapy and homeopathy supplies and business consultation services

Best of Nature
P.O. Box 3164
Long Branch, NJ 07740
1-800-228-6457
Massage tables, oils, lotions, liniments, essential oils, linens, self-massage tools, incense, books, bottles and pillows

Body Logic
5400 E. Mockingbird Ln. #210
Dallas, TX 75206
1-800-662-3306
(214) 826-BODY (2639) for information
Massage tables, oils, bolsters, aromatherapy supplies, paraffin bath, hot/cold therapy wraps, hand-held massagers, charts, books, video and audio tapes

The Body Shop
2051 Hilltop Dr., suite A-5
Redding, CA 96002
(916) 221-1031
1-800-736-6897
Massage Holster, jacknobber, aqua-relief pad, sunfresh soap

Body Therapy Assoc.
4442 Main St.
Philadelphia, PA 19127
1-800-677-9830
Massage tables and on-site chairs, futons, zafus, self-massage tools, bolsters, body support system, Solace natural hull pillows

Body Tools
15829 Haynes St.
Van Nuys, CA 91406
(818) 908-9155 or 1-800-845-6202
Self-massage tools, charts, skin brushes, cocoa butter, ayurvedic massage oils, incense, smudge sticks

Bodywork Emporium

338 North Highway 101	1451 Morena Blvd.	414 Broadway
Leucadia, CA 92024	San Diego, CA 92110	Santa Monica, CA 90401
(619) 942-9565	(619) 276-2608	(310) 394-4475

1804C Newport Blvd.	4529 Sepulveda Blvd.
Costa Mesa, CA 92627	Sherman Oaks, CA 91403
(714) 548-0220	(818) 990-6155

Large selection of massage tables and on-site chairs, massage oils and lotions, videos, books, charts, music and other supplies

Edcat Enterprises
P.O. Box 168
Daytona Beach, FL 32115
(904) 253-2385
1-800-274-3566
Large selection of anatomical and other charts, self-massage tools

Educating Hands School of Massage
Bookstore Catalogue
261 Southwest 8th Street
Miami, FL 33130
1-800-999-6991 (in Miami (305) 285-6991)
Extensive book selection, large selection of massage tables, large selection of massage oils and Chinese liniments, large selection of charts, audio cassettes, videos, hot and cold application equipment, self-massage tools, linen and hand cleaners, crystals, miscellaneous items

Hand Picked Products
75 Van Buren Street
San Francisco, CA 94131
(415) 333-7431
"Massage Heaven" T-shirts, note-cards, post-cards, holiday cards and tote bag, Charlie Sunshine's Secret Formula, analgesic balm, vitamins, posture pillows, bolsters, sunfresh soap, selected music tapes

Hands on Health Care Catalog
Acupressure Institute
1533 Shattuck Ave.
Berkeley, CA 94709
1-800-442-2232
(510) 845-1059
Books, reference charts, flash cards, videos, audio tapes, massage and self-massage tools, magnet devices, acupressure model, aromatherapy supplies, music, massage tables, on-site chair, on-site desktop support

Peacenergy
3420 Hidalgo, #314
Dallas, TX 75220
Books, book-keeping system, charts, aqua-cel packs, disposable face cradle covers, gift certificates, promotional items

Professional Development Catalogue
Sohnen-Moe Associates
3906 West Ina Road, suite 200-348
Tucson, AZ 75841
1-800-786-4774 or (602) 743-3936
Books and other material with an emphasis on practice building, practice management and self-care

Royal Pyramid International
414 Manhattan Ave.
Hawthorne, NY 10532
1-800-325-7423
Fax (914) 769-5043
Hydrocollators, paraffin bath, hot and cold applications packs, specialty treatment tables, Matthew David magnetic massage table and therapy items, electric massaging tools, lightweight and inexpensive portable massage table, extensive selection of charts and posters, homeopathic pharmaceuticals, large selection of anatomical teaching items

Zenith Supplies
Seattle, WA
(206) 525-7997
1-800-735-7217
Stationary massage table, selection of portable tables, on-site chair, curtain screen, step-stool, Hydrocollator, hot and cold packs, large selection of charts, pillows and back supports, massage oils and lotions, electric massaging tools, bolsters, Ma roller, paraffin bath, aromatherapy essential oils

Miscellaneous Massage Items

Table covers, sheets and related items:

Innerpeace
P.O. Box 648
Easthampton, MA 01027
1-800-949-7650
(100% cotton flannel sheets, face cradle covers, bolster slip covers and more)

Body Therapies
13423 Blanco Rd., suite #276
San Antonio, TX 78216
(512) 327-6632
(Cotton terrycloth and muslin massage table covers, towels, face cradle covers, bolsters and bolster covers)

Daffodil's Associates
12 Shelby Rd.
East Northport, L.I., NY 11731
1-800-368-3718
(Disposable 40" x 90" massage sheets)

Massage uniforms, aprons and half-aprons:

Utopia Uniforms
P.O. Box 170
Hollywood, FL 33022
1-800-741-7421

Printed items such as brochures about massage and gift certificates:

Caring Hands Patient Education
P.O. Box 373
Walnut Ridge, AR 72476
1-800-887-2420
(brochures, gift certificates, reminder cards, promotional items)

Hemingway Publications
P.O. Box 4575
Rockford, IL 61110
(815) 877-5590
(brochures, gift certificates)

Information for people
P.O. Box 1876
Olympia, WA 98507
1-800-754-9790
(brochures, compassionate touch book and video, gift certificates)

Touch of Heaven
P.O. Box 120561
Nashville, TN 37212
(615) 383-7077
(brochures, gift certificates, client intake forms, poster, music, thank-you notes, post cards)

Touch, Ink. MicroPublishing
225 Harrison
Oak Park, IL 60304
1-800-296-3968
(Touch, Ink. is a promotional newsletter aimed at massage clients. It is personalized with the name of the massage therapist on the front page, and contains informative articles about massage and related topics)

Products to remove oil from linens:

Fresh Again
  available from:

> **Biotone**
> 4564 Alvarado Canyon Rd., #1
> San Diego, CA 92120
> 1-800-445-6457
> (619) 281-4228

> **Golden Ratio Bodyworks**
> P.O. Box 440
> Emigrant, MT 59027
> 1-800-796-0612

Sunfresh Soap
  available from:

> **Diamond Light**
> Massage Products
> 14 Las Palomas
> Orinda, CA 94563
> (510) 253-0543

> **The Body Shop**
> 2051 Hilltop Drive #A5
> Redding, CA 96002
> (916) 221-1031

Assorted products and services:

Khepra Foot Balm — A preparation for use in massaging the feet, that creates a skin texture with a subtle resistance for better massage, eliminates foot odor, and conditions and refreshes the feet:

> **Khepra Skin Care, Inc.**
> 2525 IDS Center
> 80 South Eighth Street
> Minneapolis, MN 55402
> 1-800-367-9799

Myotherapi analgesic ointment—An ointment for temporary relief of minor aches and pains in muscles and joints, and for symptoms of sunburn, minor burns, insect stings and skin irritations:

> **Myo Laboratories, Inc.**
> Post Office Drawer 14174
> St. Petersburg, FL 33733
> 1-800-842-7374
> (813) 866-7455

"Thumper", a vertical percussion vibrator for use in massage:

> **Health Horizons Wellness Center**
> 4425 S. Harlem, suite 102
> Stickney, IL 60402
> (708) 795-0340

Body Support Systems—a contoured system of support that positions the body comfortably, prone, supine or laterally; useful for pregnancy, geriatric, disabled, on-site and seated massage:

> **Body Support Systems**
> P.O. Box 337
> Ashland, OR 97520
> 1-800-448-2400
> (503) 448-1172

Massage Table and on-site chair Selection Services (Service is free, and tables can be ordered at discount from retail):

> **Tablechoices** (All major brands)
> Mary Lou Clairmont
> (718) 339-9163

> **John Lentz** (Oakworks only)
> (413) 548-9763

Record-keeping and Insurance Billing Assistance

Insurance Billing Service
Guides and coordinates your process of billing massage services to insurance providers:

> **Parker Insurance Billing**
> 16172 Parkside Dr.
> Parker, CO 80134
> (303) 841-5520

Books for the clinical bodyworker:
The Insurance Reimbursement Manual by Christine Rosche, M.P.H.
This manual is several hundred pages long and sells for $62.95, postpaid, from Bodytherapy Business Institute, 10441 Pharlap Dr., Cupertino, CA 95014. The author is also available for telephone consultations. 1-800-888-1516

Hands Heal: Documentation for Massage Therapy: A Guide to SOAP Charting by Diana L. Thompson, LMP. $18.95 postpaid from Diana L. Thompson, Dealing Arts Studio, 916 N.E. 64th St., Seattle, WA 98115   (206) 527-9889 extension 7

Forms for Insurance Billing:

> **Carol Abernathy, LMT**
> 333 Jesse Jewell Pkwy, suite #5
> Gainesville, GA 30501
> (404) 503-9101

Computer programs that organize client and financial records and generate and track insurance billing:

> **Business Touch**
> 75-5778 Waiola Pl.
> Kailua-Kona, HI 96740
> 1-800-838-9690 or (808) 334-0873

> **The Therapist**
> L.G. Duffy Violante
> 297 Hull Ave.
> Clintondale, NY 12515
> (914) 883-7500 or 1-800-OB1-HELP

> **Tracking Plus**
> C & C Computer Support
> RR 3, Box 3700
> Factoryville, PA 18419
> 1-800-258-6382

Magazines, Journals, Newsletters and Books

Magazines

Massage Magazine covers a broad range of news and features of general interest to massage practitioners. Each issue also contains up-to-date nationwide licensing information. Published six times a year. Subscriptions 1-800-533-4263

Body Therapy provides articles of general interest to the massage community, and of special interest to those who practice both massage and aesthetics. Subscriptions (214) 526-0752

AMTA's *Massage Therapy Journal*, available by subscription to non-members, contains articles of interest to the general massage community, and items of special interest to AMTA members. Published four times a year. Subscriptions (708) 864-0123

ABMP's *Massage & Bodywork* Magazine, available by subscription to non-members, contains articles of interest to the general massage community, and items of special interest to ABMP members. Published four times a year. Subscriptions (303) 674-8478

In Business Calling itself "The magazine for environmental entrepreneuring," *In Business* presents information for the self-employed business owner from the "green" perspective. It contains some articles of interest to the self-employed bodyworker, such as tax updates, business planning advice, and the like. Subscriptions (JG Press) (215) 967-4135

Journals

The Journal of Soft Tissue Manipulation This is an international, multidisciplinary journal highlighting research, clinical change, aspects of the client/practitioner relationship, precautions and contraindications, and philosophical issues concerning massage and related disciplines. It is a publication of the Ontario (Canada) Massage Therapist Association. Subscriptions (416) 778-6682

Alternative Therapies in Health and Medicine This journal publishes research and clinical articles on the integration of alternative health care therapies with conventional Western medicine. Targeted toward physicians and primary care providers, it explores which alternative therapies can have the most validity in treating medical problems. Subscriptions (800)-M-LIEBERT

Newsletters

The Portable Practitioner The worldwide resource and networking guide for health and healing arts professionals, this is a quarterly newsletter that emphasizes travel, work and study overseas and in the US. Subscribers are able to place free classifieds and also have access to a job hotline. Subscriptions 1-800-968-2877 or (616) 347-8591

Touch Therapy Times Originally called Maryland Bodywork Reporter, this publication was started in response to the battle between physical therapists and the massage profession in Maryland. It originally reported on legal and political issues concerning the massage field in Maryland. Touch Therapy Times now covers legal, political and professional items of interest throughout the United States. Its coverage is reliably accurate and timely. Subscriptions (301) 271-4812

The Professional Bodyworker Newsletter is aimed at the clinical bodywork practitioner. It focuses on changes in state laws, insurance policies and practitioner interviews. Published twice a year. Subscriptions 1-800-888-1516

Books for Bodyworkers

The Ultimate Hand Book by Maja Evans, CMT, DH. This book focuses on self-care for the massage therapist or bodyworker, offering guidance on such subjects as physical, psychological and psychic self-care, burnout, abundance and success. Available from Laughing Duck Press (415) 221-5530

The Book by Cal Cooley, L.M.T. This book aims to coach you through passing the National Certification Exam or local certification tests. Most of the text covers anatomy. Also covered are improving your memory, massage styles and techniques, marketing and sample test questions. Spiral-bound, 150 pages plus appendix, also available in two-videotape format. Available from Southwest Myotherapies 1-800-263-9646

Textbooks

Many books are available describing different massage and bodywork techniques, but only two books have been listed here. These are comprehensive texts that describe not just one or more massage techniques, but seek to provide a professional level of education for the therapist.

Healing Massage Techniques by Frances M. Tappan, Appleton & Lange Publishers
Often used as a textbook by massage schools, this book covers purposes and history of massage, effects of massage, practice pointers, and descriptions of several systems of massage including Swedish, sports massage, infant massage, acupressure, jin shin do, shiatsu, polarity, bindegewebsmassage, reflexology, and others.

This book is often sold in massage school bookstores, or through mail order catalogues for massage professionals.

The Theory and Practice of Therapeutic Massage, Second Edition by Mark Beck, Milady Publishing Company.
This book covers the history of massage, basics of practice and ethics, anatomy and physiology, hygiene, massage techniques, hydrotherapy and heliotherapy, nutrition, exercise, and practice pointers. Available in hard cover only, for $31.95 plus tax, prepaid. It can be ordered from Milady Publishing, 1-800-836-5239.

Touch Research Abstracts

Touchpoints This is the quarterly publication of the Touch Research Institute, Tiffany M. Field, Ph.D., director. The publication reports on the work of the Touch Research Institute in scientifically documenting the health benefits of touch, and also provides information on programs sponsored by the Institute. Subscriptions are $10.00 per year. Touchpoints/Touch Research Institute, Department of Pediatrics (D820), University of Miami School of Medicine, P.O. Box 016820, Miami, FL 33101.

VI

Bodywork
Organizations
and
Trainings

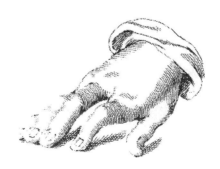

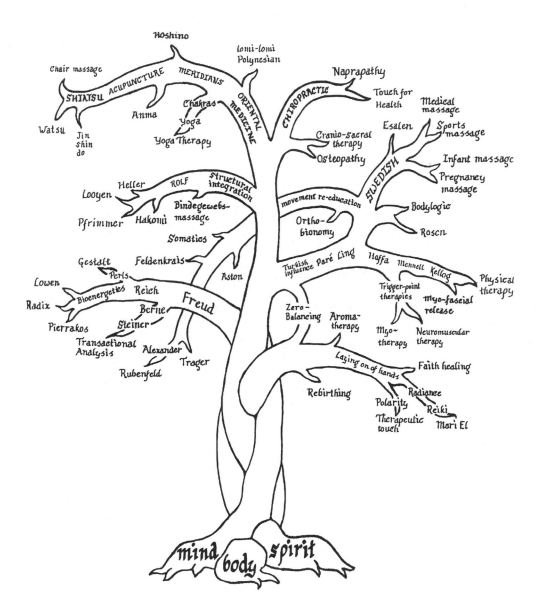

The Bodywork Tree ©1995

Based on a concept by David Linton

Bodywork Organizations and Trainings

For purposes of this Directory, "bodywork" refers to a body-centered therapy that is different from Swedish massage.

Some of the forms listed below are very similar to Swedish massage — for example, sports massage, Esalen, pregnancy massage. Some are entirely different from Swedish massage — for example, Alexander Technique, Reiki, Somatics Psychology.

For each form of bodywork, the listing includes a brief explanation of the nature of the work, the name and address of an official organization representing the form (if any) and a list of massage schools that include instruction in that form of bodywork. The schools may offer such instruction as part of their massage training program, or as continuing education, or as an advanced training. Refer to the school's listing in the State-by-State Directory for that information.

New forms of bodywork are continually created as imaginative and dedicated bodyworkers explore their own unique gifts and systematize their work. Some of the forms are thousands of years old (Shiatsu) and some are relatively new. All the forms listed below have been in existence since 1991 or before.

Acupressure

See Shiatsu, below

Alexander Technique

The Alexander technique is an educational method for improving coordination, and for developing awareness of unnecessary tensions in the body.

F. M. Alexander was an actor who had a problem with losing his voice. By studying his habitual movements in a mirror, he discovered ways he was using his body that created his vocal problem and was able to resolve the difficulty. He went on to create a system for enhancing balance, posture and the use of the body, which is called the Alexander Technique. Practitioners refer to themselves as teachers of the Alexander method and refer to sessions as lessons.

The following schools listed in the State-by-State directory offer some training in Alexander: 74, 78, 84, 94, 176, 205, 224, 240, 248.

AMMA® Therapy (or ANMA)

AMMA therapy is a method of restoring the flow of life energy in the body, and is used to treat a wide range of medical conditions. It combines Oriental medical principles with a Western approach to organ dysfunction. As taught by Tina Sohn at school #214, AMMA Therapy includes dietary plans, detoxification, herbs and vitamins, and therapeutic exercises.

Introductory and advanced trainings are offered at: School #214.

Introductory trainings are offered at: Schools #76 and #106.

Applied Kinesiology (see also Touch for Health)

Applied Kinesiology is a technique used mainly by chiropractors to gain diagnostic information through muscle testing and to strengthen muscles to aid in structural correction. Muscles are related to specific organs or systems through the acupuncture meridian network.

Training in this technique is offered at the following schools listed in the State-by-State directory: 25, 34, 88, 90, 99, 114, 136, 172, 188, 204, 205, 283, 290.

Aromatherapy

Aromatherapy involves working with aroma as a healing modality, usually in conjunction with massage, but not always.

For information about aromatherapy, conventions and evolving rules and standards, contact:

> American Aromatherapy Association
> P.O. Box 3679, South
> Pasadena, CA 91031
> (818) 457-1742

> International Society of Aromatherapy
> 728 Fentress Blvd.
> Daytona Beach, FL 32114
> (904) 274-5218

> The National Coalition of Certified Aromatherapist and Aromatologist
> Practitioners (NCCAAP)
> 7436 S.W. 117th Ave., suite 188
> Miami, FL 33183
> (305) 595-4776

The International Journal of Aromatherapy is published quarterly, covering issues and developments of interest to the practitioner. Subscriptions are $50 for four issues. Contact:

> International Journal of Aromatherapy
> 20780 Fortuna del Norte
> Escondido, CA 92025
> (619) 471-8765

The following schools listed in the State-by-State Directory offer training in aromatherapy as part of their curriculum: 2, 5, 12, 20, 21, 26, 36, 42, 51, 56, 64, 65, 70, 72, 73, 74, 77, 80, 97, 99, 101, 105, 109, 114, 122, 128, 135, 143, 146, 151, 173, 191, 194, 198, 202, 207, 209, 230, 234, 236, 240, 244, 245, 246, 252, 255, 271, 282, 283, 294, 298.

In addition, Aromatherapy trainings are offered at the following locations:

Aromatherapy trainings

> Aromatherapy Seminars
> 3379 S. Robertson Blvd.
> Los Angeles, CA 90034
> (213) 937-0600

> Body Naturals Center for
> Aromatherapy
> 333 New York Ave.
> Huntington, NY 11743
> (516) 351-6166

> Atlantic Institute of Aromatherapy
> 16018 Saddlestring Dr.
> Tampa, FL 33618
> (813) 265-2222

> Esthetec
> 580 Lancaster Ave.
> Bryn Mawr, PA 19010
> (215) 525-7516

Pacific Institute of Aromatherapy
P.O. Box 903
San Rafael, CA 94915
(415) 479-9121

Windrose Aromatics
12629 North Tatum Blvd., suite 611
Phoenix, AZ 85032
(602) 482-1814

The National Coalition of Certified Aromatherapist and Aromatologist
Practitioners (NCCAAP)
7436 S.W. 117th Ave., suite 188
Miami, FL 33183
(305) 595-4776

Aromatherapy Supplies

Aromatherapy supplies are available by mail from the following companies
(Some companies that supply massage oils also have aromatherapy supplies
—see the details of the listings under "Massage Oils", page 158):

Aroma de Terra
401 Euclid Ave., suite 155
Cleveland, OH 44114
(216) 566-8234

Aroma Land
Rt. 20, Box 29AL
Santa Fe, NM 87505
1-800-933-5267

Aromavera
3384 South Robertson Pl.
Los Angeles, CA 90034
213-280-0407

Aura Cacia, Inc.
P.O. Box 399
Weaverville, CA 96093
1-800-437-3301
(916) 623-3301

Best of Nature
12 W. Front St.
Red Bank, NJ 07701
(908) 842-8987

Body Logic
5400 E. Mockingbird Ln. #210
Dallas, TX 75206
1-800-662-3306
(214) 826-BODY (2639) for info.

Bodywise Spa Consultants
P.O. Box 64
Mill Valley, CA 94941
415-383-1050

The Essence
2041 Broadway
Boulder, CO 80302
1-800-621-4840

Essence Aromatherapy
211 Miller Ave.
Mill Valley, CA 94941
(415) 388-6970

Liberty Massage Products
P.O. Box 66068
Portland, OR 97266
1-800-289-8427

New Visions Center
P.O. Box 224
Allendale, NJ 07401
1-800-272-5683

Phytomed Inc./Original Swiss
Aromatics
P.O. Box 606
San Rafael, CA 94915
(415) 459-3998

Santa Fe Fragrance, Inc.
P.O. Box 282
Santa Fe, NM 87504
505-473-1717

Aston-Patterning®

Aston-Patterning aims to increase the body's grace, resiliency and ease of movement by releasing layers of tension throughout the body. It uses movement education, bodywork, environmental design and fitness training. For information about trainings and certification, contact:

>   Aston-Patterning
>   P.O. Box 3568
>   Incline Village, NV 89450
>   (702) 831-8228

Aston bodywork is also taught at School #33.

Bindegewebsmassage

Bindegewebsmassage is a type of connective tissue massage originated in Germany. It is an adjunctive therapy in the treatment of organic and musculo-skeletal disorders. The course is taught in a sequence of four 30-hour sections. For complete information, contact:

>   Patricia M. Donohue
>   Wholistic Pathways
>   152 N. Wellwood Ave., ste. 5
>   Lindenhurst, NY 11757
>   (516) 226-3898

Bindegewebsmassage is also taught at School #1.

Bioenergetics

Bioenergetics was created by Alexander Lowen, M.D., an outgrowth of his work with Wilhelm Reich, M.D. Bioenergetics is a way of understanding personality in terms of the body and its energetic processes. Bioenergetics therapy works with the mind and the body to release chronic stresses and chronic muscular tensions.

Dr. Lowen has written 14 books. An excellent introduction to bioenergetics is *Bioenergetics*, available at most bookstores and libraries.

For a brochure listing centers, workshops and books about bioenergetics, contact:

>   International Institute for Bioenergetic Analysis
>   144 E. 36th St.,
>   New York, NY 10016
>   (212) 532-7742

Bioenergetics is also taught at Schools #192 and #248.

Biokinetics/Hanna Somatics

Biokinetics uses a composite of techniques for rehabilitation through neuromuscular retraining. It is designed to release chronic muscular contraction and restore voluntary control of the muscular system. For complete information about Biokinetics and training, contact:

>   Biokinetics/Hanna Somatics
>   115 N. 5th St., suite 330
>   Grand Junction, CO 81501
>   (303) 245-4370

Body Logic^{SM}

Body Logic is a system of bodywork and body understanding developed by Yamuna Zake. It uses the principle of "space making" whereby space is created around joints and locked areas to allow the body to unfold and finds its own balance, enhancing freedom of movement, posture, strength and energy. For information on Body Logic, trainings and practitioners, contact:

> Body Logic
> 295 West 11th Street, apt. 1F
> New York, NY 10014
> (212) 633-2143

Body Logic is also taught at School #56.

Body-Mind (also see "Somatics")

"Body-mind" is a term used to acknowledge the intimate connection between the state of the mind and the state of the body. This is an awareness that is present in most forms of massage and bodywork, and many massage schools teach massage from a "body-mind" perspective. However, some forms make it the focus of the work. The programs listed below are designed as advanced programs for massage therapists, and focus on the body-mind connection.

> Bodymind Institute
> 11081 Missouri Ave.
> West Los Angeles, CA 90025
> (For information call Marv Treiger, PhD (213) 473-3855 or Jack Haer, PhD (213) 473-5737)

The course meets after working hours, 10 hours per week for five months. Curriculum includes connective tissue work, Reichian work, gestalt, movement re-education, and anatomy. Advanced trainings are also offered to those who complete the program.

> Body Synergy Institute, Inc.
> 305 Bangor Rd.
> Bala Cynwyd, PA 19004
> (215) 667-3070

Curriculum includes deep tissue bodywork, body reading, using a floor-length mirror as an educational tool, working with postural history and attitudes, and using your body with awareness and ease.

> School for Body-Mind Centering
> 189 Pond View Dr.
> Amherst, MA 01002
> (413) 256-8615

The school, founded by Bonnie Bainbridge Cohen, offers introductory and certification training programs in many locations. The course includes study of the body systems and how they support and initiate movement, as well as movement re-education to correct problems at their root level.

Somatic Therapy Institute
546 Harkle Road, suite B
Santa Fe, New Mexico 87501
(505) 983-9695

850-hour training and shorter intensives in body-mind integrative touch therapy.

Breema

Breema takes its name from the Kurdish mountain village of Breemava where it originated and was passed down from generation to generation. It is a comprehensive system of bodywork, done on the floor, with a variety of techniques ranging from simple
holding points on the body to techniques requiring flexibility and dexterity. This work
is taught at:

The Institute for Health Improvement
309 62nd Street
Oakland, CA, 94618
(415) 428-0937

Breema is also taught at School #36.

Chair Massage

See On-Site, below

Cranio-Sacral Therapy (also called cranial-sacral)

A technique for finding and correcting cerebral and spinal imbalances or blockages that
may cause sensory, motor or intellectual dysfunction.

Cranio-sacral techniques are taught at the following schools listed in the State-by-
State Directory: 5, 10, 12, 15, 25, 33, 36, 38, 42, 44, 51, 56, 72, 78, 82, 83, 85, 93, 96,
103, 105, 109, 122, 124, 135, 136, 145, 146, 157, 161, 163, 168, 170, 173, 174, 176,
177, 191, 198, 200, 203, 207, 209, 210, 222, 223, 224, 225, 227, 229, 243, 244, 248,
250, 252, 254, 268, 270, 290, 291, 295, 301, 311.

In addition, Cranio-sacral techniques are taught by the following institutions:

Colorado Cranial Institute
Peggy Daugherty-Davidson
1080 Hawthorne Ave.
Boulder, CO 80304
(303) 449-0322
Series of three-day trainings.

National Institute of Craniosacral Studies, Inc.
7827 N. Armenia Av.
Tampa, FL 33604-3806
(813) 933-6335

The Upledger Institute
11211 Prosperity Farms Road
Palm Beach Gardens, FL 33410
(407) 622-4334

Three- to five-day workshops in cranio-sacral therapy, somato-emotional release, visceral manipulation, muscle energy, fascial mobilization and principles of acupuncture.

Designer Massage™

A system of merging artistry and technique for a sensual therapeutic massage. After training in the Designer Massage method, students are offered a chance to purchase a complete marketing system.

Designer Massage
507 North Wilson Boulevard
Nashville, TN 37205
(615) 383-1952

Embodiment Training

This is not a training in a technique to use in your practice; it is for the personal growth of those who take the training.

Embodiment training is the work of Will and Lyn Johnson. Will is trained as a rolfer, and has created a work that adds a spiritual dimension to the work of rolfing. The goal of embodiment training is to relinquish the mind as means of identifying self, and to experience a purely energetic, sensory awareness of the body. Rolfing, movement, breath, diet, meditation and other practices are involved in the training.

The training is taken as sequences of three or seven-day intensives. For further information, contact:

The Institute for Embodiment Training
RR 2, Cobble Hill, B.C. V0R 1L0, Canada
(604) 335-0750

Equine Sports Massage

Massage or other bodywork can adapted to horses for the purpose of enhancing performance and preventing injuries. This field has recently been developed and shows signs of gaining rapidly in popularity, as breeders are interested in any techniques that can give them a competitive edge.

According to Jack Meagher, author of *Beating Muscle Injuries for Horses*, the practitioner applies techniques of human massage, especially sports massage, to horses. A pioneer in the fields of sports massage and equine sports massage, Jack Meagher turned to working with horses as a way of proving the value of sports massage techniques for athletes. By using the techniques on horses and achieving demonstrable results, he was able to rebut the contention that results with humans were due to psychological factors.

Beating Muscle Injuries for Horses, by Jack Meagher, helps to orient the practitioner to working on horses. It is available for $12.95 postpaid from Horse Muscle Injuries, 667 Weathersfield St., Rowley, MA 01969.

An instructional video about equissage™ is available for $49.95 postpaid from Equissage, P.O. Box 447, Round Hill, VA 22141, 1-800-843-0224. Equissage also offers week-long trainings in equine sports massage. For information about price and schedules, contact them at the above address or phone.

Week-long, one-day and two-day trainings are offered by Optissage, 7041 Zane Trail Road, Circleville, OH 43113, 1-800-251-0007.

Also offering training in Equine bodywork is Institute of Therapeutic Studies, 3401 W. Sunflower Ave., #125, Santa Ana, CA 92704, (714) 556-7730. Trainings from 100 hours to 1,000 hours are available.

In addition, the following schools listed in the State-by-State Directory offer training in equine massage: 73, 109, 125, 128, 172, 188, 191.

Esalen massage

Esalen is a variant of swedish massage pioneered at Esalen Institute in Big Sur, California. Esalen is the place where many therapies were tested or launched in recent decades, including gestalt therapy and rolfing. The unique brand of massage practiced there typically involves total nudity and long flowing stokes. Esalen is known for its original, honest, nurturing and probing atmosphere. Esalen massage tends to be nurturing, trance-like and meditative, allowing the greatest possible unfoldment to take place in the client. For information contact:

Esalen Institute
Big Sur, CA 93920
(408) 667-3000

Esalen massage is taught at the following schools listed in the State-by-State Directory: 12, 15, 16, 17, 27, 34, 36, 41, 42, 43, 44, 49, 51, 52, 54, 65, 72, 78, 81, 84, 112, 126, 133, 138, 146, 178, 182, 191, 203, 238, 252, 291.

Feldenkrais®

Moshe Feldendrais was an Israeli physicist who began developing this system in midlife. Feldenkrais work emphasizes having a coherent body image and thinking a movement through. The system is most effective for pain relief, and also promotes grace and ease of movement. For information about Feldenkrais work, teachers, and teacher trainings, contact:

Feldenkrais Guild
P.O. Box 13285
Overland Park, KS 66212-3285
(913) 492-1444

Some training in Feldenkrais is offered at the following schools listed in the State-by-State directory: 74, 78, 84, 87, 130, 146, 171, 173, 205, 224, 291.

Hakomi bodywork

Hakomi bodywork regards body, mind and spirit as one, and blends bodywork and psychotherapy into a simultaneous process. The work serves to lead a person to an awareness of limitations in his physical and psychological patterns, bringing the possibility of new openness and freedom.

The Hakomi Institute offers a 3½ day introductory workshop and a 1½ year training program.

Hakomi Integrative Somatics
P.O. Box 19438
Boulder, CO 80308
(303) 443-6209

Hakomi Integrative Somatics is also taught at School #237.

Hellerwork®

Hellerwork is an outgrowth of Rolfing (see below), created by Joseph Heller. It integrates movement and verbal communication with connective tissue work. Information about Hellerwork can be obtained from:

> Hellerwork, Inc.
> 406 Berry Street
> Mt. Shasta, CA 96067
> (916) 926-2500

The following schools offer partial or complete training in Hellerwork: #173, #301, #304.

Hoshino Therapy

A unique system of acupressure for the treatment of musculo-skeletal pain and sports injuries; physical fitness exercises are taught to complement the therapy. The training is offered in weekend workshops and intensives.

> Hoshino Therapy Clinic of Miami, Inc.
> 814 Ponce De Leon, suite 417
> Miami, FL 33134
> (305) 444-9984

Training in Hoshino Therapy is also offered at School #105.

Infant Massage

Infant massage instructors teach parents the art of infant massage. Trainings are offered to certify people as infant massage instructors. For information, contact:

> International Association of Infant Massage Instructors
> 2350 Bowen Rd.
> P.O. Box 438
> Elma, NY 14059
> 1-800-248-5432
> (415) 752-4920

> International Loving Touch Foundation, Inc.
> P.O. Box 16374
> Portland, OR 97216
> (503) 253-8482

Infant massage is taught at the following schools that are listed in the State-by-State Directory: 5, 23, 25, 87, 91, 93, 99, 101, 102, 105, 109, 110, 122, 124, 125, 130, 143, 146, 150, 152, 155, 156, 159, 160, 173, 176, 178, 200, 204, 207, 213, 228, 230, 234, 236, 250, 255, 256, 271, 274, 290, 291, 301, 303, 307, 309.

Jin shin do®

Jin shin do is a synthesis of acupressure theory, psychology and taoist philosophy, which helps release physical and emotional tensions. The Jin Shin Do Foundation publishes a directory of authorized teachers and registered acupressurists, and a newsletter. The foundation also has information about trainings, and a catalogue of charts, books, audio and video tapes.

Jin Shin Do Foundation for Bodymind Acupressure™
366 California Ave. #16
Palo Alto, CA 94306
(415) 328-1811

Jin Shin Do is taught at the following schools listed in the State-by-State Directory:
41, 76, 94, 125, 138, 146, 156, 231, 295.

LooyenWork™

Ted Looyen was a counselor who had a severe back problem that was helped by Rolfing.
He then set out to create a deep tissue therapy that was not painful, and he studied
several different systems. His synthesis is called LooyenWork, which uses connective
tissue techniques to release and separate adhesions in muscle fibers and fascial sheets.
The system also involves identifying the core issue of each individual and then using
deep pressure techniques to release accumulated holding patterns.

LooyenWork is taught through weekend intensives in various locations, and a 500-
hour certification program at the LooyenWork Institute. For more information about
the work or about trainings, contact:

The LooyenWork Institute
P.O. Box 1742
Sausalito, CA 94966
(415) 381-9025 or 1-800-332-3579

Lymphatic drainage (manual lymphatic drainage^SM or MLD®)

The lymphatic system is a vital part of the immune system in the body. Lymphatic
drainage massage assists the operation of the lymphatic system. The system was devised
in the 1930's by a Danish massage therapist, Dr. Emil Vodder, and is popular and well
established as a health modality in Germany and Austria. The organization certifying
practitioners and teachers is:

North American Vodder Association of Lymphatic Therapy™ (NAVALT®)
P.O. Box 861
Chesterfield, OH 44026
(216) 729-3258

The following individuals are certified by NAVALT to offer trainings in manual lymphatic drainage:

Howard Douglass
P.O. Box 861
Chesterland, OH 44026
(216) 729-3258

John F. Guarino
3313 Wyndham Cir. #4209
Alexandria, VA 22302
(703) 671-7790

Kathryn McKillip Thrift
11526 Coral Hills Dr.
Dallas, TX 75229
(214) 243-5959

Martha Zenger
5747 Birdwood Road
Houston, TX 77096
(713) 776-8533

The following school also offers a training in lymphatic drainage, though not a
Dr. Vodder training:

Dana Wyrick, BA, RMT, LMT
Wyrick Institute and Clinic
P.O. Box 99745
San Diego, CA 92109
(619) 273-9764

The following schools listed in the State-by-State Directory offer training in lymphatic
drainage massage: 2, 12, 14, 15, 17, 21, 23, 25, 28, 33, 34, 36, 38, 48, 50, 51, 56, 63,
64, 65, 66, 69, 72, 77, 80, 85, 87, 91, 97, 101, 102, 105, 106, 117, 122, 130, 135, 136,
138, 144, 146, 178, 189, 190, 192, 201, 208, 224, 229, 234, 236, 249, 252, 256, 283,
301, 302, 308, 312.

MariEL

MariEL is a way of working with energy, using the laying on of hands. It stimulates the
body to release repressed emotions, allowing personal transformation, which can result
in transforming emotional and physical diseases.

The originator and only teacher of MariEL is Ethel Lombardi. She gives trainings,
in which she attunes students to healing energy. For information about her trainings,
contact any of the following people, who sponsor trainings.

Diane Sherman
29 Linwood Circle
Princeton, NJ 08540
(609) 924-6328

Greta Rittenburg
3 Powder Horn Dr.
Acton, MA 01720

Medical Massage (clinical massage)

Working with injuries, pathologies and rehabilitation; working by physician's prescription. A program of instruction in medical massage is very desirable for a therapist interested in working in the health care system, and getting insurance reimbursement for
massage services. (See chapter 17)

The following schools, which are included in the State-by-State directory, offer instruction in medical massage or clinical massage: 11, 40, 42, 49, 56, 61, 70, 86, 89, 104,
121, 122, 124, 129, 130, 135, 137, 168, 172, 177, 179, 186, 189, 200, 216, 223, 226,
228, 229, 230, 237, 245, 256, 268, 283, 288, 298, 300, 301, 303, 305, 306, 307, 308,
309, 312.

Also offering certification in Medical Dysfunction is:

Kurashova Institute for Studies in Physical Medicine
P.O. Box 6246
Rock Island, IL 61201
(309) 786-4888

Myofascial Release

Myofascial release (MFR) is a technique for working with fascia as a means of achieving pain relief, restoring function and reducing stress. The system is taught in a series of seminars in various locations. It is designed to be used by massage therapists and physical therapists. For information about trainings contact:

> John F. Barnes' MFR Seminars
> Rts. 30 and 252
> Suite 1, 10 S. Leopard Rd.
> Paoli, PA 19301-1569
> 1-800-FASCIAL
> (610) 644-0136

The following schools offer training in myofascial techniques of one kind or another: 3, 14, 20, 42, 66, 78, 87, 93, 96, 112, 124, 126, 127, 128, 130, 143, 163, 174, 176, 188, 192, 200, 201, 210, 221, 224, 225, 227, 229, 232, 233, 234, 236, 245, 247, 257, 268, 272, 273, 294, 297, 300, 301, 316.

Myotherapy^{SM}

See Trigger Point Therapies, below

Neuromuscular Therapy

See Trigger Point Therapies, below

On-Site or Seated or Chair Massage

This refers to a 10 to 15 minute bodywork session, usually a shiatsu-based routine, done in a special chair in which the client sits facing toward the cushions, exposing the scalp, shoulders, neck, back and hips.

Originally pioneered as a modality for the workplace, it has expanded into many other environments, and is now becoming a fixed operation in storefronts, health food stores, airports and other locations, and may therefore need to be called "chair massage" or "seated massage" instead of "on-site."

Two companies conduct workshops on technique and marketing. These are:

> On-site Enterprises 1-800-999-5026
> Instructors certified and supervised by David Palmer
>
> Seated Massage Experience® 1-800-868-2448 / 1-800-TOUCH-4-U
> Workshops are taught by Raymond Blaylock

The following schools listed in the State-by-State Directory offer training in chair, seated or on-site massage: 3, 5, 15, 25, 29, 33, 36, 43, 44, 45, 48, 50, 56, 59, 66, 71, 77, 82, 83, 85, 101, 102, 104, 105, 106, 109, 114, 121, 128, 130, 143, 146, 151, 154, 159, 161, 164, 171, 172, 173, 176, 177, 178, 179, 180, 183, 191, 193, 194, 195, 197, 198, 200, 201, 202, 204, 205, 207, 212, 223, 225, 227, 228, 229, 230, 232, 234, 237, 246, 247, 248, 249, 251, 254, 255, 256, 257, 268, 283, 291, 294, 296, 298, 301, 303, 307, 308, 309, 312.

Oriental Modalities

The most commonly taught oriental modality is Shiatsu, which has its own listing in this directory, as do AMMA (ANMA) and Jin Shin Do. In order to supplement those listings, this section includes a general listing of schools that teach Oriental studies.

The following is a listing of schools that offer tui na, jin shin jyutsu, qi-gong, five element theory or Thai massage, or state that their curriculum includes Oriental or Eastern modalities:

5, 10, 15, 16, 25, 36, 39, 42, 53, 58, 67, 70, 72, 76, 77, 80, 81, 83, 84, 85, 86, 93, 94, 96, 104, 109, 110, 121, 124, 126, 134, 135, 138, 142, 143, 157, 164, 172, 173, 174, 177, 186, 188, 190, 205, 206, 207, 213, 214, 215, 228, 230, 244, 249, 254, 275, 286, 290, 291, 294, 302.

Ortho-Bionomy™

This system seeks to remind the body of its ability to find balance. The work involves positioning the client, working with points of tension in the body, and using movement. Results can include relieving pain, promoting emotional release, and improving structural alignment. For information, contact:

> Society of Ortho-Bionomy International
> P.O. Box 1974-70
> Berkeley, CA 94701
> 1-800-743-4890
>
> *or*
>
> Bay Area Ortho-Bionomy
> P.O. Box 7538
> Berkeley, CA 94707
> (510) 528-5657
>
> *or*
>
> Northwest Center for Ortho-Bionomy
> P.O. Box 70384
> Seattle, WA 98107
> (206) 783-5404

The following schools listed in the State-by-State Directory teach Ortho-Bionomy: 25, 64, 110, 146, 209, 231.

Pfrimmer Deep Muscle Therapy®

Pfrimmer Deep Muscle Therapy is a system of corrective treatment to aid in the restoration of damaged muscles and soft tissue. It is intended to be used as one aspect of treatment for a wide range of muscular and soft-tissue conditions. Information is available from the Therese C. Pfrimmer International Association of Deep Muscle Therapists at 1-800-484-7773, ext. 7368, or from either of the schools offering authorized Pfrimmer deep muscle therapy trainings: Schools #147 and #247.

Polarity

Developed by Dr. Randolph Stone, polarity focuses on the energy currents that exist in all life. The polarity therapist uses her hands as conductors of energy. The intention is to balance the electromagnetic energy in the body, toward the ultimate goal of uniting the body, emotions, mind and soul.

Polarity is commonly taught in massage schools, but programs also exist to teach polarity that have no connection to massage schools. Although many massage schools offer an introduction to polarity as part of their training, few offer a substantial amount of training.

The American Polarity Therapy Association (APTA) is a non-profit organization that distributes educational material, registers practitioners, hosts educational conferences and publishes a regular newsletter. For further information about polarity or about trainings contact:

American Polarity Therapy Association
2888 Bluff St., ste. 149
Boulder, CO 80301
(303) 545-2080

As of the publication deadline for this edition, the following schools offered trainings of 615 or more hours that are approved by the APTA as meeting their standards for becoming a registered polarity therapist:

Heartwood Institute
220 Harmony Lane
Garberville, CA 95542
(707) 923-5002

New Mexico Academy of Healing Arts
P.O. Box 932
Santa Fe, NM 87504
(505) 982-6271

Polarity Realization Institute
126 High Street
Ipswitch, MA 01938
1-800-497-2908

Polarity Wellness
10 Leonard St. #2-A
New York, NY 10013
(212) 334-8392

The following schools listed in the State-by-State Directory offer training in polarity: 5, 10, 15, 17, 20, 23, 25, 33, 42, 47, 51, 56, 58, 63, 65, 66, 73, 77, 80, 82, 87, 90, 93, 104, 105, 107, 110, 111, 112, 116, 117, 122, 125, 130, 134, 136, 138, 139, 144, 151, 154, 156, 158, 159, 160, 161, 170, 171, 172, 173, 174, 175, 176, 177, 183, 189, 190, 191, 192, 194, 203, 204, 207, 209, 210, 213, 215, 217, 218, 224, 229, 233, 234, 236, 237, 243, 244, 252, 254, 255, 256, 268, 282, 283, 290, 295, 301, 305, 308, 316.

Pregnancy Massage

Bodywork for the childbearing year; seminars for advanced certification conducted in various locations throughout the U.S. For complete information about courses, contact:

Somatic Learning Associates
8950 Villa La Jolla Dr., suite 2162
La Jolla, CA 92037
(619) 436-0418

An organization has been formed to certify pregnancy massage therapists, enhance the public image of pregnancy massage and provide a forum for continuing education, networking and referrals:

The National Association of Pregnancy Massage Therapy
P.O. Box 81453
Atlanta, GA 30136

Pregnancy massage, prenatal massage or massage for the childbearing year is taught at the following schools listed in the State-by-State directory: 1, 3, 21, 23, 26, 34, 36, 42, 45, 48, 56, 66, 72, 73, 77, 85, 88, 96, 99, 102, 110, 116, 122, 124, 130, 136, 139, 143, 146, 150, 155, 159, 160, 161, 172, 173, 176, 178, 184, 187, 193, 195, 201, 203, 207, 213, 228, 230, 234, 237, 248, 254, 256, 271, 274, 301, 302, 303, 308, 309.

Radiance Technique

The Radiance Technique Association was formerly The American-International Reiki Association, Inc. The Radiance Technique was formerly called The Official Reiki Program. For further information, contact:

Radiance Technique Association International, Inc
P.O. Box 40570
St. Petersburg Fl 33743-0570
(813) 347-3421

Radiance Technique is also taught at school #178.

Rebirthing

Rebirthing is a technique of conscious breathing that can help in releasing physical, emotional or mental blockages. It is best learned by participating as a client in rebirthing sessions with a certified rebirther. Several books are available that describe the process. The leading author on rebirthing is Sondra Ray.
Rebirthing is taught at schools #38 and #41.

Reflexology

Reflexology is a system of massaging the feet, or feet and hands, with the intention of affecting other parts of the body. The feet and hands are regarded much like maps of the body, with points on the feet and hands corresponding to organs and tissues in the body. It is thought that sensitivity or tenderness in the feet or hands indicates imbalances in the corresponding body part, and by working with the point on the foot or hand, beneficial results can be achieved in the corresponding body part.

It is more commonly practiced as a separate therapy in Europe, but there are a number of reflexologists in the U.S. and Canada as well who practice only reflexology and not massage. While many reflexologists spend an entire therapy session working only on the hands and feet (and sometimes ears), some spend approximately half of their time on the feet, and half on swedish massage.

Independent certification in reflexology is offered by:

American Reflexology Certification Board (ARCB)
P.O. Box 620607
Littleton, CO 80162
(303) 933-6921

The ARCB is a non-profit California corporation that certifies the competency of reflexology practitioners. It does not accredit schools or endorse curricula. To become ARCB certified, a reflexologist must be 18 years old or older, have a high school diploma or equivalent, live and practice in the United States, complete a "hands on" reflexology course beyond the introductory level, and pass the written, practical and documentation portions of the ARCB exam.

Reflexology training is usually a brief program. For information about trainings, contact:

Foot Massage Therapies Institute
P.O. Box 1254
Santa Rosa, CA 95402
(707) 544-8342

Laura Norman And Associates Reflexology Center
41 Park Ave.
New York, NY 10016
(212) 532-4404

International Academy for Reflexology Studies
P.O. Box 42798
Cincinatti, OH 45241-2432
(513) 489-9328
(600 hour training plus advanced programs)

International Institute of Reflexology
P.O. Box 12642
St. Petersburg, FL 33733-2642
(813) 343-4811

The following schools listed in the State-by-State Directory include reflexology in their massage curriculum: 1, 2, 6, 7, 8, 11, 12, 14, 17, 18, 20, 21, 22, 23, 25, 26, 28, 29, 33, 34, 36, 38, 39, 43, 44, 45, 47, 50, 53, 55, 56, 59, 62, 63, 63, 65, 66, 69, 71, 77, 78, 79, 80, 82, 83, 87, 88, 89, 93, 97, 99, 101, 102, 103, 105, 106, 107, 109, 110, 111, 112, 114, 116, 119, 122, 125, 130, 134, 136, 138, 139, 143, 144, 145, 146, 150, 151, 152, 154, 155, 157, 158, 159, 160, 161, 164, 165, 170, 171, 173, 176, 177, 180, 183, 184, 188, 189, 190, 191, 193, 194, 195, 200, 201, 203, 204, 205, 207, 210, 212, 213, 229, 230, 237, 238, 240, 243, 248, 249, 251, 252, 253, 254, 255, 256, 271, 282, 283, 290, 291, 293, 294, 295, 301, 303, 307, 309, 312, 314.

The following schools offer continuing education in reflexology: 25, 40, 48, 51, 63, 65, 72, 74, 76, 77, 85, 97, 107, 110, 122, 130, 142, 172, 173, 178, 190, 197, 198, 200, 202, 228, 236, 237, 244, 245, 246, 247, 256, 257, 268, 271, 273, 274, 301.

The following schools offer advanced trainings in reflexology: 5, 18, 40, 70, 102, 145, 193, 213, 230, 255, 272.

Reiki

Reiki is an energy process for restoring and balancing life energy and promoting healing and personal transformation. The practice involves a systematic process of attuning to and transmitting reiki energy. Further information can be obtained from:

Reiki Alliance
P.O. Box 41
Cataldo, ID 83810-1041
(208) 682-3535

Reiki is taught at the following schools listed in the State-by-State Directory: 2, 5, 14, 25, 42, 50, 64, 85, 88, 92, 93, 97, 116, 135, 158, 188, 207, 237, 244, 246, 249, 282, 301, 312, 316.

Rolfing®

Ida Rolf was the first to create, practice and teach a system of bodywork aimed toward working with the connective tissue of the body to achieve structural changes in the client. Her system, Rolfing, is taught by:

The Rolf Institute
205 Canyon Blvd.
Boulder, CO 80302

Some exposure to Rolfing is offered at the following schools listed in the State-by-State Directory: 11, 88, 101, 103, 109, 112, 125, 223, 295.

Rosen Method Bodywork®

Developed by Marion Rosen, this work emphasizes simplicity. The practitioner contacts contracted muscles and matches the muscle tension. The practitioner follows changes in the client's breathing as a means of guiding the client's inner process. The work can bring up buried feelings and memories, and can be a tool for pain relief and personal growth.

For further information about Rosen Method bodywork, trainings and practitioners, contact:

Rosen Method Professional Association
2550 Shattuck Ave., Box 49
Berkeley, CA 94704
(510) 644-4166

Some training in Rosen Method Bodywork is offered at schools #43 and #46.

Rubenfeld Synergy™

This method integrates elements of Alexander, Feldenkrais, gestalt and hypnotherapy into a body/mind therapy that helps clients contact and release energy blocks, tensions and imbalances. Rather than treating illnesses, the practitioner treats the psychophysical problems people carry with them. By dealing with the emotional body, the practitioner can often abate physical symptoms. For information, contact:

The Rubenfeld Center
115 Waverly Place
New York, N.Y. 10011
(212) 254-5100 (1:00 to 6:00 weekdays)

Seated Massage

See On-Site, above

Shiatsu or acupressure (see also Oriental Modalities)

Shiatsu is a Japanese bodywork which uses pressure to points on acupuncture meridians. Practice of shiatsu is usually accompanied by study of Chinese five-element theory and meridians, and it involves a way of looking at the body that is completely different from the "muscles, bones and blood" view of Western science, focusing instead on energetic awareness.

The following is a list of massage schools that offer instruction in shiatsu. They are listed in the order in which they appear in the State-by-State directory, and names have been abbreviated to save space. Some of these schools also teach acupressure, a related subject.

Massage schools offering shiatsu instruction: 1, 2, 3, 5, 7, 12, 15, 18, 20, 23, 25, 26, 30, 36, 39, 42, 44, 45, 49, 50, 53, 55, 56, 58, 60, 63, 64, 65, 67, 69, 71, 73, 76, 80, 81, 83, 86, 87, 88, 93, 94, 97, 102, 104, 105, 106, 107, 109, 110, 112, 116, 119, 121, 122, 125, 130, 131, 133, 134, 135, 136, 137, 138, 142, 143, 146, 150, 154, 157, 158, 160, 161, 171, 172, 173, 176, 178, 190, 191, 192, 193, 194, 195, 197, 198, 199, 200, 204, 205, 206, 207, 209, 210, 212, 214, 216, 217, 224, 228, 231, 233, 236, 237, 240, 244, 247, 248, 268, 270, 282, 290, 291, 296, 298, 300, 301, 302, 311, 312, 314.

Massage schools offering acupressure instruction (sometimes used as a synonym for shiatsu): 5, 7, 11, 15, 20, 21, 22, 23, 25, 29, 30, 39, 40, 41, 42, 43, 44, 45, 47, 53, 55, 58, 63, 65, 66, 67, 69, 70, 71, 72, 73, 74, 76, 77, 79, 80, 82, 85, 88, 93, 94, 97, 99, 105, 109, 114, 117, 138, 142, 143, 145, 146, 150, 155, 156, 163, 174, 177, 180, 188, 190, 191, 205, 227, 228, 229, 232, 238, 240, 250, 251, 291, 294, 303, 309.

Schools offering independent shiatsu training

Acupressure Institute
1533 Shattuck Avenue
Berkeley, CA 94709
(510) 845-1059
1-800-442-2232

Associates for Creative Wellness
Executive Mews, suite N-72
1930 E. Marlton Pike
Cherry Hill, NJ 08003
(609) 424-7501

Jin Shin Do Foundation for
Bodymind Acupressure
P.O. Box 1097
Felton, CA 95018
       or
366 California Ave. #16
Palo Alto, CA 94306
(415) 328-1811

Morris Institute of
Natural Therapeutics
3108 Rt. 10 West
Denville, NJ 07834
1-800-360-MINT

Meridian Shiatsu Institute
1 West Golf Club Lane
Paoli, PA 19301
(215) 647-5686

Aisen Shiatsu School
1314 South King Street, suite 601
Honolulu, HI 96814
(808) 596-7354

Centre de shiatsu Yuki Rioux inc.
8590 Sherbrooke est
Montreal, Quebec H1L 1B7
(514) 524-7818 or 354-2010

California Medical School of Shiatsu
1510 Coffee road, ste. Q
Modesto, CA 95355
(209) 544-0960
       or
4635 North First, ste. 202
Fresno, CA 93726
(209) 244-4707

International School of Shiatsu
10 South Clinton St., suite 300
Doylestown, PA 18901
(215) 340-9918

New York School for Shiatsu
and Reflexology
149 E. 81st. Street
New York, NY 10028

Ohashi Institute
12 West 27th Street, 9th Fl.
New York, NY 10001
(212) 684-4190
1-800-810-4190

The Shi'atsu Institute and
Therapy Center
347 Dolores St., suite #118
San Francisco, CA 241-9740
(415) 241-9740

Tsuko Therapy School
239 Seal Beach Blvd., Unit C
Seal Beach, CA 90740
(310) 493-0890

Santa Barbara College of
Oriental Medicine
1919 State Street, suite 204
Santa Barbara, CA 93101
(805) 682-9594

Shiatsu School of Canada, Inc.
547 College Street
Toronto, Ontario, Canada
M6G 1A9
(416) 323-1818

Somatics (also called Somatics Psychology or Somatic Therapy)

"Somatic" literally means "of or pertaining to the body." In the context of Somatics Psychology, it refers to the mind-body connection and make use of techniques to bring awareness of each to the other. It is therefore related to the form "Body-Mind" which is described above.

California Institute of Integral Studies offers an accredited masters in Body-Oriented Psychotherapy and Education. Within this degree program, specializations are available in Somatic Education and Somatic Psychotherapy. The curriculum is based on an examination of the body, in its psychological, social and political contexts. For information contact:

California Institute of Integral Studies
765 Ashbury St.
San Francisco, CA 94110
(415) 753-6100

The Lomi School offers a 10-day intensive professional training that includes psychotherapeutic techniques and meditative practices. Breath, movement, sound, touch, sitting meditation, Gestalt, Reichian and developmental theories are all presented. For complete information, contact:

Lomi Foundation
343 College Ave.
Santa Rosa, CA 95401
(707) 579-0465

The Neuromuscular Center offers a somatic movement therapy program training health and fitness professionals to understand functional anatomy in their own bodies. The work is based on Body-Mind Centering (See "Body-Mind" section, above). For complete information, contact:

The Neuromuscular Center
142 W. 23rd Street #1H
New York, NY 10011
(212) 242-1129

The following schools listed in the State-by-State directory offer training in Somatics or a similar approach: 103, 211, 217, 218, 283, 304, 312.

Sports Massage

Sports massage is an adaptation of Swedish massage. Its purpose is to prepare athletes for sporting activity and help them recover from the exertion of that activity.

Sports massage trainings vary in length dramatically, and there is no standard training length, although the American Massage Therapy Association and the United States Sports Massage Federation both have standards for approving trainings.

The following massage schools listed in the State-by-State Directory offer sports massage training as part of their massage school curriculum: 1, 3, 4, 8, 12, 20, 22, 23, 26, 28, 30, 33, 44, 45, 47, 53, 55, 56, 58, 61, 62, 63, 65, 66, 67, 69, 71, 73, 77, 78, 79, 80, 82, 84, 85, 87, 88, 89, 91, 93, 97, 99, 101, 102, 103, 104, 105, 106, 107, 109, 110, 111, 114, 119, 122, 124, 125, 126, 127, 128, 129, 130, 133, 134, 135, 136, 137, 139, 143, 144, 145, 146, 150, 151, 154, 157, 158, 159, 160, 161, 164, 168, 169, 170, 172, 173, 176, 177, 178, 179, 180, 182, 184, 187, 188, 189, 190, 191, 193, 195, 200, 201, 203, 207, 210, 212, 213, 218, 227, 229, 230, 233, 234, 237, 240, 241, 243, 247, 248, 249, 250, 251, 254, 255, 257, 270, 283, 290, 291, 294, 295, 296, 298, 300, 301, 302, 303, 305, 307, 308, 310, 312, 314, 316.

The following schools offer continuing education courses in sports massage: 15, 21, 25, 33, 37, 44, 48, 50, 59, 65, 72, 74, 76, 77, 81, 96, 105, 110, 111, 112, 135, 136, 142, 163, 168, 172, 173, 175, 176, 178, 183, 186, 189, 193, 198, 200, 201, 202, 209, 210, 229, 232, 234, 236, 237, 245, 247, 248, 256, 258, 268, 271, 273, 294, 312.

The following schools offer advanced trainings in sports massage: 5, 39, 40, 42, 56, 65, 70, 73, 84, 90, 102, 104, 109, 110, 130, 134, 143, 145, 188, 209, 213, 214, 244, 256, 272, 279, 294, 301.

Training in Russian Clinical Sports Massage is offered at Kurashova Institute, P.O. Box 6246, Rock Island, IL 61201 (309) 786-4888

Structural Integration (or Postural Integration)

This is a generic term for therapies that are related to Rolfing, in that they aim to improve the structure or posture of the client. See also Hellerwork and LooyenWork.

The following schools listed in the State-by-State Directory offer introductory or advanced structural or postural integration trainings: 1, 15, 29, 63, 70, 77, 79, 84, 93, 99, 101, 102, 104, 110, 114, 124, 139, 146, 168, 173, 213, 219, 270, 304, 305, 306.

The schools listed below offer independent structural integration or postural integration training.

Body Synergy Institute
305 Bangor Rd.
Bala Cynwyd, PA 19004
(215) 667-3070

The Boulder Center for Postural Integration
258 Brook Rd.
Boulder, CO 80302
(303) 443-1952

Florida Institute of Psychophysical Integration
5837 Mariner Drive
Tampa, FL 33609
(813) 286-2273
(Intensive residential program includes about 150 hours over a three-week period)

International Center for Release & Integration
450 Hillside Avenue
Mill Valley, CA 94941
(415) 383-4017
(Program takes about two years to complete)

Olson's Health Service
P.O. Box 170
Watford City, ND 58854
(701) 842-3296
(Two-day seminars held at various locations)

Soma Neuro-Muscular Integration
730 Klink St.
Buckley, WA 98321
(206) 829-1025
(300 hours of training over a 12-week period)

Therapeutic Touch (TT)

TT is a means of attuning to and directing the universal life energy. The goal is to release congestion and balance areas where the flow of life energy has become disordered. Removal of these blockages facilitates the person's intrinsic healing powers.

TT is most commonly taught to, and used by nurses. However, some massage therapists study TT and incorporate it into their work.

Several books are available on TT, including *Therapeutic Touch: A Practical Guide* by J. Macrae, Knopf, 1988; *The Therapeutic Touch* by D. Krieger, Prentice-Hall 1979; *Therapeutic Touch* by Borelli and Heidt, Springer Co., 1981.

Further information about TT can be obtained from:

Center for Continuing Education in Nursing
New York University, 429 Shimkin Hall
50 W. 4th St.
New York, NY 10012
(212) 988-5345

The following schools listed in the State-by-State Directory offer instruction in Therapeutic Touch: 1, 20, 92, 93, 104, 116, 122, 130, 173, 176, 177, 201, 207, 224, 246, 283, 295, 301, 303, 311.

Touch For Health (see also Applied Kinesiology)

This is a system for using applied kinesiology to aid the bodyworker. Applied kinesiology makes use of the fact that certain conditions result in weakening of specific muscles. Through muscle testing, the bodyworker gains information about the specifics of the client's condition. Further information is available from the Touch for Health Association:

Touch for Health Association
6955 Fernhill Dr.
Malibu, CA 90265
1-800-466-8342

The following schools listed in the State-by-State Directory offer training in Touch for Health: 2, 34, 38, 39, 54, 66, 73, 76, 83, 88, 96, 97, 105, 111, 135, 142, 146, 155, 173, 175, 176, 183, 197, 198, 200, 204, 224, 225, 236, 240, 244, 246, 252, 273, 290, 291, 307.

Trager®

Dr. Milton Trager, M.D., had a gift for bodywork from a young age, and developed his own system of bodywork which emphasizes gentle rocking of the client, and rolling body parts to encourage release and loosening and softening.

Some massage schools offer brief introductory trainings in Trager bodywork, giving the massage therapist a glimpse into the system. Such therapists often integrate a bit of the Trager awareness into their massage work. However, Trager practitioners practice only Trager, at least during a Trager session. Information about training as a Trager practitioner can be obtained from:

> The Trager Institute
> 10 Old Mill Street
> Mill Valley, CA 94941-1891
> (415) 388-2688

The following schools listed in the State-by-State Directory offer an introduction to Trager bodywork: 25, 46, 85, 88, 101, 104, 105, 106, 109, 111, 192, 194, 244.

Trigger Point Therapies (myotherapy^SM or neuromuscular therapy)

This refers to any or several systems of working with trigger points. Trigger points are tender congested spots in muscle tissue, which may radiate pain to other areas. Significant relief results when the trigger point is treated.

The techniques used in trigger point therapies are similar to those used in Shiatsu or acupressure, but trigger point therapies are based on western anatomy and physiology. Several institutions have refined the art of trigger point therapy into a self-contained modality, and teach their therapy in a non-massage context. These schools are:

> Bonnie Prudden™ School of Physical Fitness and Myotherapy
> 7800 E. Speedway
> Tucson, AZ 85710
> (602) 529-3979
> Nine-month, 1,300-hour program

> Institute of Myopathy
> 685 Placerville Dr.
> Placerville, CA 95667
> (916) 621-1775
> Three weekend trainings — basic, intermediate and advanced — offered at various locations in California.

> International Academy of NeuroMuscular Therapies
> C/O NMT Center
> 900 14th Ave N.
> St. Petersburg, FL 33705
> (813) 821-7167
> Four-weekend series for NMT certification, given at various locations (massage diploma or other professional training required before admission).

> Shaw Myotherapy Institute
> 6417 Loisdale Road, suite 309
> Springfield, VA 22150

St. John Neuromuscular Therapy Seminars
11211 Prosperity Farms Road
Palm Beach Gardens, FL 33410
1-800-232-4668
Seminars in various locations; home-study videos also available.

Many schools listed in the State-by-State directory offer training in trigger-point therapy. The lists that follow divide the schools into those that teach "trigger point," and those that teach "neuromuscular" technique or NMT.

Trigger point: 3, 4, 5, 10, 11, 20, 21. 26, 44, 63, 70, 72, 74, 78, 85, 91, 97, 104, 106, 107, 112, 130, 138, 143, 144, 146, 156, 168, 171, 173, 177, 179, 183, 188, 191, 204, 209, 214, 232, 233, 234, 244, 248, 255, 256, 257, 272, 288, 290, 291, 296, 300, 301, 305, 308, 314.

Neuromuscular or NMT: 1, 10, 15, 83, 84, 87, 89, 90, 91, 92, 93, 96, 99, 101, 102, 103, 104, 105, 106, 107, 109, 110, 111, 112, 114, 116, 121, 122, 124, 125, 127, 128, 129, 135, 139, 143, 157, 159, 160, 161, 172, 188, 190, 191, 194, 198, 201, 203, 207, 213, 215, 219, 223, 225, 227, 241, 243, 252, 254, 257, 273, 294, 300, 302.

Watsu™ (aquatic shiatsu)

Watsu (from "water" and "shiatsu") began when Harold Dull started floating people, applying the moves and stretches of the zen shiatsu he had studied in Japan. Physical and emotional blocks are removed by the work, which can be done even by small individuals since the client's body in water is buoyant. It is done in chest-high, 94-degree water.

Certification can be obtained by taking two week-long workshops (Watsu I and II) at:

School of Shiatsu and Massage (#30)
P.O. Box 570
Middletown, CA 95461
(707) 987-3801

Watsu is also taught at schools #5 and #25.

Zero-Balancing

Developed by Fritz Smith, MD, osteopath, Rolfer and acupuncturist, zero balancing works with the relationship between a person's physical structure and their energy. The practitioner works with fulcrums, points where structure and energy can be accessed together, to bring about change.

For fuller information about zero-balancing, trainings or practitioners, contact:

The Zero Balancing Association
P.O. Box 1727
Capitola, CA 95010
(408) 476-0665

Introductory training in Zero Balancing is also offered at the following schools listed in the State-by-State Directory: 15, 135, 163, 168, 198, 270.

Advanced Trainings

The following massage schools offer advanced trainings that may be taken independently of their massage training program. To qualify as an "advanced training," for inclusion in this list, a program must be longer than a weekend workshop. Weekend workshops are considered "continuing education."

Some of the advanced trainings listed below are brief, some are extensive. They range from a few days to 1000 hours. Some focus on one technique and others teach a combination of techniques.

The schools are listed by their sequential number in the State-by-State directory. Complete program information for these schools can be found in the State-by-State directory beginning on page 199. Contact the schools for complete and up-to-date information about their trainings.

2, 3, 5, 12, 14, 15, 17, 18, 19, 20, 21, 23, 25, 29, 30, 33, 34, 36, 37, 39, 40, 41, 42, 43, 44, 46, 48, 49, 51, 56, 58, 64, 65, 66, 70, 72, 73, 80, 81, 82, 84, 85, 86, 87, 90, 92, 93, 101, 102, 104, 109, 110, 112, 119, 123, 124, 126, 127, 128, 130, 133, 134, 135, 136, 139, 143, 145, 146, 156, 157, 163, 164, 167, 169, 170, 173, 177, 178, 184, 188, 190, 192, 193, 197, 198, 200, 204. 207, 209, 212, 213, 214, 215, 217, 219, 221, 224, 229, 230, 233, 234, 236, 237, 244, 247, 251, 253, 255, 256, 257, 258, 268, 270, 272, 273, 275, 276, 278, 279, 282, 283, 286, 287, 290, 294, 300, 301, 304, 316.

VII

State-by-State
Directory

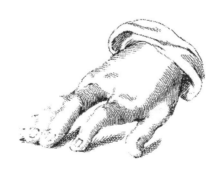

How to Use the State-by-State Directory

The following is true of listed schools, unless otherwise noted:

1. Schools' educational offering meet or exceed the requirements for licensing or other regulation *in the state in which they are located*. If a school prepares students for licensing in other states, that information is noted in the school's listing.

2. "Hours of training" means in-class hours unless otherwise noted. In-class time includes supervised practice time if a teacher is present during the practice session. An hour means at least 50 clock minutes.

3. "Cost" includes any *mandatory* fees collected by the school, such as registration fee and tuition. Also included is the cost of any books and supplies that students are required to purchase at the school. If books and supplies may be purchased outside the school, their cost is not included in the listing.

4. "Payment plan" when used in the financial aid category means the school allow students to pay tuition over time. In some cases, this is a no-interest or low-interest arrangement that can be a substantial benefit to the student. In other cases, the payment plan includes a high rate of interest or a hefty service charge, significantly increasing the cost of the program. No attempt has been made to distinguish between low and high-interest payment plans, so students are advised to consider the details of a school's payment plan.

5. "Accreditations/approvals" lists only those accreditations or approvals that are accepted by a governmental body, are pertinent to the school's approval for financial aid purposes, or have to do with college credit for course work. COMTAA refers to the AMTA's accrediting body. A few states require COMTAA approval in their licensing laws. ACCSCT (formerly NATTS) and ACCET refer to accrediting bodies that are approved by the U.S. Department of Education, and approval by one of these bodies triggers eligibility for federal financial aid.

6. Modalities and subjects taught includes subjects taught *in addition to* Swedish massage, Anatomy and Physiology. All schools listed teach those three subjects unless otherwise indicated.

7. Continuing Education and Advanced Trainings. These are sometimes difficult to distinguish from each other. For purposes of this guide, continuing education is a training of one or two weekends in length, or the equivalent. Advanced trainings are longer trainings designed to go into greater depth or teach a broader subject matter.

8. Accuracy of listed information. Every attempt has been made to assure that the information listed is accurate. When possible, information supplied was cross-checked in the school's catalogue. If no catalogue was supplied to the author, the notation "no catalogue" appears in the listing. Mistakes happen to even the most careful of us, so please forgive any inaccuracies in these listings. This information was current as of January 1, 1995. This kind of information changes, sometimes quickly, so please consult the individual schools to confirm or update any critical information.

Alphabetical List of Schools

The following list contains all 316 schools profiled in the State-by-State Directory. The Directory number of the school is at the left, and at the right is the number of *in-class* hours of instruction in the school's program.

Where there is no number listed for in-class hours, that school either did not furnish information for publication, or the number of in-class hours could not be discerned from the information furnished. This information was accurate as of January 1, 1995. Please contact schools for current program information.

97	Academy of Healing Arts	600
142	Academy of Massage Therapy	720 to 900
129	Academy of Somatic Healing Arts	660
98	Acupressure/Acupuncture Institute	—
39	Acupressure Institute of America	150
65	Advanced Training Massage Institute	100
32	Aesclepion Massage Institute, Inc.	48
310	Aesthetics University	—
131	Aisen Shiatsu School	—
1	Alabama School of Massage Therapy	620
298	Alexandar Sch. of Natural Therapeutics	600
147	Alexandria Sch. of Scientific Therapeutics	—
33	Alive & Well!	140 to 560
132	All Hawaiian School of Massage	—
133	Aloha Kauai Massage Workshop	370
99	Alpha School of Massage	500
100	America Duran Skin Care School	—
101	American Institute of Massage	600
40	American Institute of Massage Therapy	150
69	American Inst. of Massage Therapy, Inc.	609
140	American Inst. of Massage Therapy, Inc.	160
220	American Institute of Massotherapy, Inc.	—
231	Ashland Massage Institute	375
256	Asten Center of Natural Therapeutics	300 or 550
130	Atlanta School of Massage	620
102	Atlantic Academy	500
257	Austin School of Massage Therapy	300
311	Balanced Touch Institute of Massage	500
163	Baltimore School of Massage	500
164	Bancroft School of Massage Therapy	750
79	Banning Massage School	250
299	Bellevue Massage School	660
134	Big Island Academy of Massage	150 or 600
157	Blue Cliff Sch. of Therapeutic Massage	600
312	Blue Sky Educational Foundation	500
103	Boca Raton Institute	605
41	Body Electric School	100
81	Body Mind College	100 or 500
292	Body Music	296
49	Body Therapy Center	136 to 600
66	Body Therapy Institute	150 or 500
217	Body Therapy Institute	600
42	Body Tuneup National School	100 to 500
87	Boulder School of Massage Therapy	1,000
302	Brian Utting School of Massage	800
82	California College of Holistic Health	110 to 1,004

70	California College of Physical Arts	300 to 1,000
71	California Healing Arts College	150 or 566
26	California Institute of Massage	120 to 500
60	California Medical School of Shiatsu	—
27	Calistoga Massage Therapy School	100
313	Capri College	—
150	Capri College of Massage Therapy	510
43	Care Through Touch Institute	130
240	Career Training Academy	300 or 600
151	Carlson College of Massage Therapy	625
218	Carolina School of Massage Therapy	525
250	Carrie's Kadesh	900
232	Cascade Institute of Massage	565
63	Central California School	200 or 550
221	Central Ohio School of Massage	670
143	Chicago School of Massage Therapy	525
13	Chico Therapy and School of Massage	—
258	Christian Associates	300
88	Collinson School of Therapeutics	160
89	Colorado Institute of Massage Therapy	993
90	Colorado School of Healing Arts	546
91	Colorado Springs Academy	1,100
94	Connecticut Center for Massage	600 or 635
14	Conscious Choice School of Massage	100 or 150
104	Core Institute	500
92	Cottonwood School of Massage	500
203	Crystal Mountain Apprenticeship	675
252	Cumberland Institute	412 or 743
51	Cypress Health Institute	150
288	Dan Martin	300
3	Desert Institute of the Healing Arts	1,000
80	Desert Resorts School	100 to 720
34	Diamond Light	100
188	Dovestar Alchemian Institute	750
161	Downeast School of Massage	600 or 609
204	Dr. Jay Scherer's Academy	670
153	Dr. Welbe's College of Massage Therapy	—
185	Dr. Welbe's College of Massage Therapy	—
152	Dr. Welbes College of Massage Therapy	400
233	East-West College	405 to 1,064
105	Educating Hands School of Massage	624
289	Eleanor Scott, R.M.T.	300
52	Esalen Institute	—
106	Euro-Skill Therapeutic Training Center	600
259	European Health and Science Institute	—
260	European Institute	—

261	European Massage Therapy Institute	300	243	Lancaster School of Massage	500
107	Fabulous Fingers Academy	510	235	Lane Community College	—
213	Finger Lakes School of Massage	850	175	Lansing Community College	400
108	Florida Academy of Massage	—	244	Lehigh Valley Healing Arts Center	101
109	Florida Institute of Massage	624	149	Lewis Sch. & Clinic of Massage Therapy	—
110	Florida School of Massage	650	144	LifePath School of Massage Therapy	660
111	Florida's Therapeutic Massage School	500	29	Lifestream Massage School	128 or 400
294	Fuller School of Massage Therapy	200 to 500	115	Lindsey Hopkins Technical Ed. Center	720
2	GateKey Sch. of Mind-Body Integration	1,200	315	Lives Unlimited School of Healing Arts	—
262	Hands-On Therapy School of Massage	300 or 500	159	Louisiana Institute of Massage	300 to 500
263	Harmony Massage Institute	—	16	Loving Hands Inst. of Healing Arts	96 or 150
135	Hawaiian Islands School	160 to 1,000	54	Lupin Massage Institute	102
21	Healing Arts Institute	126	9	Lynne Darby	—
193	Healing Hands Institute for Massage	500	316	Madison School of Massage Therapy	582
83	Healing Hands School	100 to 1,000	116	Mandarin School of Chinese Medicine	530
166	Healing Touch Institute	160	6	Mary Beedle, R.N., B.S.	500
22	Health Awareness Academy	250	160	Massage Academy of the South	610
194	Health Choices Ctr. for the Healing Arts	475	245	Massage Arts and Sciences	120
172	Health Enrichment Center, Inc.	500	271	Massage Education Institute	300
148	Health Enrichment Ctr. Indiana Branch	—	168	Massage Institute of New England	728
264	Health Masters	—	272	Massage Resources, Inc.	300 to 550
241	Health Options Institute	200	74	Massage School of Santa Monica	150
265	HealthTouch	300	273	Massage Therapy Clinic & School	300
181	Heartland School of Massage	160	93	Massage Therapy Institute	594
15	Heartwood Institute	240 to 1,000	228	Massage Therapy Institute of Oklahoma	250 or 500
195	Helma Corp. Inst. of Massage Therapy	500	64	Massage Training Institute	200
205	Higher Knead	650	138	Maui Academy of the Healing Arts	450
222	Hocking College	approx. 600	44	McKinnon Institute	100 to 620
136	Honolulu School of Massage, Inc.	150 or 600	10	Medicine Mountain Massage	500
7	Hot Springs Sch. of Therapy Technology	500	17	Mendocino School of Holistic Massage	96 or 186
266	Houston Massage Ctr. Massage School	300	208	Mesilla Valley School of Therapeutic Arts	—
112	Humanities Center School of Massage	625	24	Messinger School of Massage	—
158	In-Touch Bodyworks	520	176	Michigan Institute of Myomassology	332
269	In-Touch School of Massage	—	223	Midwestern College of Massotherapy	600 or 630
196	Ingeborg Schlobohm	250	155	Millennium College of Massage	approx. 1,000
303	Inland Massage Institute	624	55	Milpitas Electrolysis College	100 to 600
206	Inochi Institute	660	178	Minneapolis School of Massage	136 to 440
137	Institute of Body Therapeutics	600	56	Monterey Institute of Touch	200 or 500
267	Institute of Cosmetic Arts	300	198	Morris Institute of Natural Therapeutics	520
72	Inst. of Psycho-Structural Balancing	120 or 500	274	MRC School of Massage	300
73	Institute of Therapeutic Studies	100 to 1,000	85	Mueller College of Holistic Studies	512
35	Integral Art of Massage Workshops	—	169	Muscular Therapy Institute	900
23	Integrative Therapy School	130 or 500	186	Myotherapy Institute	1,000–1,500
242	Intnl. Academy of Massage Sciences	128	290	Myotherapy Institute of Utah	600
84	International Professional School	120 to 1,000	236	National Health Care Institute	392
113	International Unisex Academy	—	45	National Holistic Institute	720
154	Iowa School of Natural Therapeutics	500	182	National Institute for Muscle Therapy	approx. 65
173	Irene's Myomassology Institute	382	224	National Institute of Massotherapy	600
114	Jacksonville School of Massage Therapy	510	275	Neuromuscular Concepts School	300
8	Jean's School of Therapy Technology	500	189	New England Acad. of Ther. Sciences	800
28	Jupiter Hollow School for Massage	100	190	New Hampshire Inst. for Ther. Arts	750
53	Just for Your Health	100 or 500	199	New Jersey School of Massage	—
174	Kalamazoo Center for the Healing Arts	120 or 520	18	New Life Institute of Massage Therapy	160
197	Kinley Institute for Massage	100	209	New Mexico Academy of Healing Arts	650
167	Kripalu Center	150	210	New Mexico Sch. of Natural Therapeutics	750
314	Lakeside School of Natural Therapeutics	500	304	New Perspectives Institute	1,250

215	New York Institute of Massage	675
191	North Eastern Inst. of Whole Health	750
276	North Texas School of Swedish Massage	300
179	Northern Lights Sch. of Massage Therapy	600
11	Northfield Clinic	500
75	Nova Institute	—
200	Ocean Massage Institute	520
225	Ohio College of Massotherapy, Inc.	552
226	Ohio College of Medical Arts	670
187	Omaha School of Massage Therapy	500
237	Oregon School of Massage	360 or 525
117	Orlando Institute School of Massage	500
95	Owens Institute of Massage	—
246	Owens Institute of Massage	100 to 500
184	Ozark Institute of Natural Therapies	600
19	Pacific Sch. of Massage & Healing Arts	110
286	Paul Frizzell	300
247	Pennsylvania School of Muscle Therapy	521
25	Phillips School of Massage	200
277	Phoenix School of Wholistic Health	—
4	Phoenix Therapeutic Massage College	645
248	Pittsburgh School of Massage Therapy	247
170	Polarity Realization Institute	180 or 600
162	Polarity Realization Institute	600
118	Port Charlotte School of Massage	—
96	Potomac Massage Training Institute	500
230	Praxis College	500 or 1,100
61	Quality College of Health Care Careers	150
5	RainStar School of Therapeutic Massage	100
46	re Source	—
145	Redfern Training Systems	150
119	Reese Institute, Inc.	600
296	Richmond Academy of Massage	208
120	Ridge Technical Center	518
238	Rogue Community College	46 credits
249	Rose Meta-Therapy	25 and up
307	S.W. Washington Massage Therapy Ctr.	550
36	San Francisco School of Massage	102 or 202
67	Santa Barbara Col. of Oriental Medicine	256
121	Sarasota School of Massage Therapy	540
122	Sarasota School of Natural Healing Arts	600
37	School for Self-Healing	160
86	School of Healing Arts	110 to 1,000
68	School of Intuitive Massage and Healing	—
278	School of Natural Therapy	300
30	School of Shiatsu and Massage	100 or 500
279	School of Therap. Advanced Relax (STAR)	300
305	Seattle Massage School	891
31	Sebastopol Massage Center	100
227	Self-Health School of Medical Massage	600
123	Seminar Network International, Inc.	600
76	Shiatsu Massage School of California	104 to 200
20	Sierra School of Health Sciences	110 or 500
57	Silicon Valley College	—
180	Sister Rosalind Gefre's School	550
306	Soma Inst. of Neuromuscular Integration	580
211	Somatic Therapy Institute	—
201	Somerset School of Massage Therapy	564
239	South Coast School of Healing Arts	330
251	South Dakota School of Massage Therapy	500
124	Southeastern School of Neuromuscular	500
77	Southern California School	100 to 1,150
125	Space Coast Massage Institute, Inc.	500
308	Spectrum Center School of Massage	534
171	Stillpoint Center	878
126	Suncoast School	500 or 600
216	Swedish Institute, Inc.	692
254	Tennessee Institute of Healing Arts	920
255	Tennessee School of Massage	500
280	Texas Massage Institute	—
281	Texas Massage Therapy Corp.	—
300	The Bodymind Academy	619
301	The Brenneke School of Massage	650
50	The Center for Body Harmonics	100
192	The Center for Transpersonal Body/Mind	175
165	The Central Mass. School of Massage	325
234	The Ewing Inst. of Therapeutic Massage	544
141	The Idaho School of Massage Therapy	—
268	The Institute of Natural Healing Sciences	300
270	The Lauterstein-Conway Massage School	300 to 800
156	The Louisville School of Massage	150 or 300
253	The Massage Institute of Memphis	500
207	The Medicine Wheel	650 to 1,000
214	The New Center For Wholistic Health	1,072
183	The Oasis School of Massage Therapy	100
229	The Oklahoma Sch. of Natural Healing	140 or 420
139	The Pacific Center	150 or 600
295	The Reilly School of Massotherapy	225 or 600
219	The Southeastern Sch. of Neuromuscular	500
78	The Touch Therapy Institute	150 to 1,000
285	The Winters School	300
38	The World School	123 to 600
62	Therapeutic Learning Center	200
282	Third Coast Center	300
202	Time-Out Professional Massage Sch.	100
47	Touching for Health Center	105 to 500
309	Tri-City School of Massage	576
58	Twin Lakes College	200 to 500
212	Universal Therapeutic Massage Inst.	520
291	Utah College of Massage Therapy	712
127	Venice School of Massage Therapy	500
293	Vermont Inst. of Massage Therapy	234
297	Virginia School of Massage	500
287	Wanda Yvonne Loggins	300
146	Wellness & Massage Training Inst.	700
283	Wellness Skills, Inc.	300 or 650
177	Wellspring Institute School	100 to 500
59	Western Col. of Therapeutic Massage	100
12	White River School of Massage	500
284	Williams Inst. School of Massage	300
48	Wind Walk Institute	100
43	Wood Hygienic Inst., Inc.	500

Alabama

No State licensing

School:

**#1 Alabama School of Massage Therapy
1776 Independence Court, suite 200
Birmingham, AL 35216
(205) 871-0441**

HOURS OF TRAINING: 740

IN-CLASS HOURS: 620

DURATION OF COURSE: six months days or nine months evenings

COST: $3,750

FINANCIAL AID: payment plan

MODALITIES AND SUBJECTS: deep tissue, sports massage, neuromuscular therapy, Zahourek system of kinesthetic anatomy, hydrotherapy, business skills, body-mind theory and applications, shiatsu, jin-shin-do, yoga, t'ai chi, bindegewebsmassage, TMJ dysfunction, structural integration, therapeutic touch, reflexology, cranial-structural integration, pregnancy and infancy massage, field trips

Alaska

No State Licensing

State Business License required, contact:

Department of Commerce and Economic Development
Business Licensing Section
P.O. Box D-LIC
Juneau, AK 99811-0800
(907) 465-2534

School:

**#2 GateKey School of Mind-Body
Integration Studies
4141 B Street, suite 302
Anchorage, AK 99503
(907) 561-7327**

HOURS OF TRAINING: up to 1,200

IN-CLASS HOURS: approximately one-third of total hours

DURATION OF COURSE: for 1,200 hours, approximately 15 months

DAY/EVENING/WEEKEND: program meets some days, some evenings, some weekends

COST: for 1,200 hours approximately $6,000.

YEAR FOUNDED: 1982

MODALITIES AND SUBJECTS: mind-body mapping, mind-body integration, Touch for Health, inner child intensive and retreat, t'ai chi, zen shiatsu, aromatherapy, lymphatic massage, yoga, Reiki, CPR, reflexology, kinesiology, office experience, business application, community presentations, community outreach

ADVANCED PROGRAMS: Individual advanced study programs can be designed.

Arizona

No State Licensing

Many cities regulate the practice of massage, and requirements for city licensing range from 100 to 1,000 hours.

For the city of Phoenix, contact:

Special Business Licenses
251 West Washington, 3rd floor
Phoenix, AZ 85003
(602) 262-6786

Schools:

**#3 Desert Institute of the Healing Arts
639 North Sixth Ave.
Tucson, AZ 85705
(602) 882-0899 or (800) 733-8098**

HOURS OF TRAINING: 1,000

DURATION OF COURSE: one year

COST: $7,647

FINANCIAL AID: payment plans, Pell grants, Stafford Loans, PLUS/SLS, approved for veterans' benefits

YEAR FOUNDED: 1982

ACCREDITATIONS/APPROVALS: COMTAA, ACCSCT

GRADUATES PER YEAR (APPROX.): 75 to 100

MODALITIES AND SUBJECTS: trigger point, rocking, shaking and rolling technique, myofascial strokes, treatments for specific conditions, hydrotherapy, body mechanics and self-care, clinic, plus electives.

Electives include addictions recovery, gerontology, massaging people with AIDS, massaging physically challenged clients, prenatal massage, sports massage, teaching aids, medical center externship, women in transition, experiential communications, journaling for ourselves, present your SELF, value oriented marketing, art of relaxation, movement integration, stretching and joint mobilization, t'ai chi, yoga, Anatomiken, corrective exercises, experiential anatomy, clinic, shiatsu, on-site, survey of healing modalities, communication skills, business and professionalism

ADVANCED PROGRAMS: 600-hour zen shiatsu program

#4 Phoenix Therapeutic Massage College
    2720 E. Thomas Road, suite C140
    Phoenix, AZ 85016
    (602) 955-2677

HOURS OF TRAINING: 735 (includes 90 hours supervised externship)

DURATION OF COURSE: day program 30 weeks, evening program 36 weeks

COST: $6,200 (includes massage table, books & supplies)

FINANCIAL AID: available for those who qualify

YEAR FOUNDED: 1981

ACCREDITATIONS/APPROVALS: COMTAA, ACCET, approved for veterans training

GRADUATES PER YEAR (APPROX.): 150

MODALITIES AND SUBJECTS: Maniken anatomy, vertebral anatomy, pathology, trigger point, cross-fiber friction, myo-fascial release, joint mobilization and stretches, sports massage, hydrotherapy, cryotherapy, client assessment, ethical/sexual issues, self-care, nutrition, AIDS awareness, CPR, career development, externship

UNIQUE ASPECTS OF SCHOOL OR CURRICULUM: community outreach program, including hospital and convalescent programs

CONTINUING EDUCATION: contact school

#5 RainStar School of Therapeutic Massage
    4130 N. Goldwater Blvd., suite 121
    Scottsdale, AZ 85251
    (602) 423-0375

HOURS OF TRAINING: Basic program 200

IN-CLASS HOURS: approx. 100

DURATION OF COURSE: 8 weeks day program or 16 weeks one evening per week plus four Saturdays

COST: $1,400

FINANCIAL AID: payment plans

MODALITIES AND SUBJECTS: health awareness, business, massage practicum

ADVANCED PROGRAMS: 300 and 500-hour advanced programs are offered. The total curriculum includes the following coursework: kinesiology, medical terminology, health/fitness/conditioning, lymphology, nutrition, watsu, pathology, sports massage, on-site, reflexology, trigger point, polarity, acupressure, shiatsu, infant massage, massage for dyslexia, hydrotherapy, light therapy, Eastern aromatherapy, deep tissue bodywork, Reiki, cranial-sacral therapy, Jin Shin Jyutsu, cryotherapy, ortho-dynamics, physical therapy, third party billing, ethics, stretching and facilitation, stress, first aid/CPR, marketing, bookkeeping, business success.

Arkansas

State Licensing: 500 hours

National Certification Exam not accepted

Schools:

#6 Mary Beedle, R.N., B.S.
    Massage Therapy Instructor
    815 E. Jackson
    Fayetteville, AR 72701
    (501) 443-0337

HOURS OF TRAINING: 500

DURATION OF COURSE: 8 months, weekends

COST: $2,700

YEAR FOUNDED: 1988

GRADUATES PER YEAR (APPROX.): 10 to 12

MODALITIES AND SUBJECTS: lomi lomi, deep tissue, treatment of pain, reflexology

CONTINUING EDUCATION: pain management, body posture for the massage therapist, exercises for the massage therapist

Note: Mary Beedle will be on break from teaching in 1995 and 1996 to be a family nurse practitioner. During that time the school will offer only continuing education/advanced workshops.

#7 Hot Springs School of Therapy Technology
    Body Wellness, Inc. Therapeutic Massage Clinic
    11323 Arcade Dr., suite D
    West Little Rock, AR
    (501) 221-2243 or (800) 844-0667

HOURS OF TRAINING: 500

DURATION OF COURSE: 4½ months, evenings and weekends

COST: $2,500

MODALITIES AND SUBJECTS: hydrotherapy, electrotherapy, heliotherapy, reflexology, acupressure, shiatsu, health service management skills, business practices, law, ethics

#8 Jean's School of Therapy Technology
    655 Park Ave.,
    Hot Springs, AR 71901
    (501) 623-9686

HOURS OF TRAINING: 500

DURATION OF COURSE: four to six months

COST: $2,400 (includes required books)

YEAR FOUNDED: 1985

ACCREDITATIONS/APPROVALS: veterans training program

PREPARATION FOR OUT-OF-STATE LICENSING EXAM: contact school

GRADUATES PER YEAR (APPROX.): 30

MODALITIES AND SUBJECTS: kinesiology, sports massage, deep tissue, hydrotherapy, heliotherapy, range of motion, reflexology, law, AIDS, business, pathology, electrotherapy

UNIQUE ASPECTS OF SCHOOL OR CURRICULUM: Students may enroll at any time, year round.

#9 Lynne Darby
Massage Instructor
Route 6, Box 737-C
Hot Springs National Park, AR 71901
(501) 262-3253

Contact instructor for program information

#10 Medicine Mountain Massage
4810 Central-Sunbay Resort
Hot Springs, AR 71913
(501) 623-3113 or (501) 525-8209

No Catalogue

HOURS OF TRAINING: 500

DURATION OF COURSE: 4 months to one year

DAY/EVENING/WEEKEND: evening and weekend programs available

COST: $2,700 (includes books)

FINANCIAL AID: vocational rehabilitation

YEAR FOUNDED: 1988

GRADUATES PER YEAR (APPROX.): 6

MODALITIES AND SUBJECTS: polarity, craniosacral, neuromuscular, Thai massage, trigger point, facials body masque, detox, environmental illness treatment, bach flowers, homeopathy

CONTINUING EDUCATION: contact school

#11 Northfield Clinic
Rt. 8 Box 1334
Texarkana, AR 75502
(501) 772-8622

No Catalogue

HOURS OF TRAINING: 500

DURATION OF COURSE: six months

DAY/EVENING/WEEKEND: evening and weekend programs available

COST: $3,000

FINANCIAL AID: contact school

YEAR FOUNDED: 1991

GRADUATES PER YEAR (APPROX.): 6

MODALITIES AND SUBJECTS: hydrotherapy, electrotherapy, exercise therapy, cryotherapy, trigger point, acupressure, reflexology, Rolfing, nutrition, ergonomics, health and hygiene, CPR, ethics, law, practice management

UNIQUE ASPECTS OF SCHOOL OR CURRICULUM: Class size is kept small and the school emphasizes clinical massage

CONTINUING EDUCATION: contact school

#12 White River School of Massage
48 Colt Square, suite B
Fayetteville, AR 72703
(501) 521-2550

HOURS OF TRAINING: 500

DURATION OF COURSE: days 6 months; summer intensive 4 months; weekends 10 months

COST: $3,425 (includes books) ($160 discount for tuition paid two weeks before classes start)

FINANCIAL AID: payment plans, approved for veterans training, some state assistance

YEAR FOUNDED: 1991

GRADUATES PER YEAR (APPROX.): 60

MODALITIES AND SUBJECTS: Esalen, sports massage, shiatsu, reflexology, integrative therapy, myo-fascial therapy, cranio-sacral therapy, hydrotherapy, spa treatments, hygiene, CPR, business and marketing skills

UNIQUE ASPECTS OF SCHOOL OR CURRICULUM: The course places equal emphasis on scientific techniques and intuitive process.

ADVANCED PROGRAMS: myo-fascial therapy, sports massage, shiatsu, manual lymphatic drainage

CONTINUING EDUCATION: aromatherapy, manual lymphatic drainage, yoga, herbology and others

California

No State licensing

Massage schools in California are regulated by:

The Council for Private Postsecondary and Vocational Education
1027 10th Street, fourth floor
Sacramento, CA 95814

All schools licensed by the Council offer a minimum of 100 hours of instruction for their massage programs.

Schools are listed by region (Far Northern, Sacramento Area, Napa and Sonoma Counties, Marin County, San Francisco, Berkeley & Oakland Area, San Jose & Santa Cruz Area, Fresno, San Luis Obispo Area, Bakersield, Santa Barbara, Los Angeles Area, Desert Hot Springs, San Diego Area).

Below, for easy reference, is a listing of all California schools in alphabetical order by school name. Some school names have been abbreviated to save space. Numbers identify the school's position in the full listing.

Acupressure Institute of America, Berkeley #39
Advanced Training Massage Institute, Santa Barbara #65
Aesclepion Massage Institute, Inc., San Rafael #32
Alive & Well! Institute, San Anselmo #33
American Institute of Massage Therapy, Inc., Costa Mesa #69
American Institute of Massage Therapy, Walnut Creek #40
Banning Massage School, Desert Hot Springs #79
Body Electric School, Oakland #41
Body Mind College, San Diego #81
Body Therapy Center, Palo Alto #49
Body Therapy Institute, Santa Barbara #66
Body Tuneup National School, Stockton #42
California College of Holistic Health, San Diego #82
California College of Physical Arts, Huntington Beach #70
California College of Physical Arts, San Juan Capistrano #70
California Healing Arts College, West Los Angeles #71
California Institute of Massage & Spa, Sonoma #26
California Medical School of Shiatsu, Fresno #60
Calistoga Massage Therapy School, Rohnert Park #27
Care Through Touch Institute, Berkeley #43
The Center for Body Harmonics, Santa Clara #50
Central California School, Los Osos #63
Chico Therapy and School, Chico #13
Conscious Choice School, Redding #14
Cypress Health Institute, Santa Cruz #51
Desert Resorts School, Desert Hot Springs #80
Diamond Light The Marin School, Mill Valley #34
Esalen Institute, Big Sur #52
Healing Arts Institute, Roseville #21
Healing Hands School, Valley Center #83
Health Awareness Academy, Citrus Heights #22
Heartwood Institute, Garberville #15
Institute of Psycho-Structural Balancing, Santa Monica #72
Institute of Therapeutic Studies, Santa Ana #73
Integral Art of Massage, San Francisco #35
Integrative Therapy School, Sacramento #23
International Professional School, San Diego #84
Jupiter Hollow School, Santa Rosa #28
Just for Your Health, San Jose #53
Lifestream Massage School, Napa #29
Loving Hands Institute, Fortuna #16
Lupin Massage Institute, Los Gatos #54
Massage School of Santa Monica, Santa Monica #74
Massage School of Santa Monica, North Hollywood #74
Massage Training Institute, Bakersfield #64
McKinnon Institute, Oakland #44
Mendocino School, Redwood Valley #17
Messinger School, Lockford #24

Milpitas Electrolysis College, Milpitas #55
Monterey Institute, Carmel #56
Mueller College, San Diego #85
National Holistic Institute, Emeryville #45
New Life Institute, Redding #18
Nova Institute, Los Angeles #75
Pacific School, Gualala #19
Phillips School, Nevada City #25
Quality College, Fresno #61
re Source, Berkeley #46
San Francisco School, San Francisco #36
Santa Barbara College, Santa Barbara #67
School for Self-Healing, San Francisco #37
School of Healing Arts, San Diego #86
School of Intuitive Massage, Santa Barbara #68
School of Shiatsu and Massage, Middletown #30
Sebastopol Massage Center, Sebastopol #31
Shiatsu Massage School, Santa Monica #76
Sierra School of Health Sciences, Chico #20
Silicon Valley College, Fremont #57
Southern California School, Riverside #77
Therapeutic Learning Center, Fresno #62
The Touch Therapy Institute, Sherman Oaks #78
Touching for Health Center School, Stockton #47
Twin Lakes College, Santa Cruz #58
Western College, Campbell #59
Wind Walk Institute, Berkeley #48
The World School, San Francisco #38

Schools:

California, Far Northern

#13 Chico Therapy and School of Massage
651 Manzanita Ct.
Chico, CA 95926
(916) 891-4301

Contact the school for program information.

#14 Conscious Choice School of Massage and
Integral Healing Arts
1648 Riverside Dr.,
Redding, CA 96001
(916) 241-4828

HOURS OF TRAINING: 110 (100 in-class); 165 (150 in-class)

DURATION OF COURSE: 110 hours fourteen-day intensive, two months evenings or two months weekends; 165 hours four week intensive, three months evenings or three months weekends.

COST: 110 hours $1,050; 165 hours $1,350

MODALITIES AND SUBJECTS: myofascial intervention, muscle testing, reflexology, lymphatic massage, mind/body/spirit relationships, Reiki, ethics, business practice

ADVANCED PROGRAMS: certified transformational hypnotherapist

#15 Heartwood Institute
220 Harmony Lane
Garberville, CA 95542
(707) 923-5002 admissions
(707) 923-5000 reception

HOURS OF TRAINING: massage practitioner 240; massage therapist 570; advanced massage therapist 750; holistic health practitioner 1,000

DURATION OF COURSE: 3 months, 6 months, 9 months, 12 months

COST: massage practitioner $2,043; massage therapist $4,493; advanced massage therapist $5,593; holistic health practitioner $7,093 plus room and board (costs listed include health fee, first aid/CPR instruction and manual, and student malpractice insurance)

FINANCIAL AID: payment plan

YEAR FOUNDED: 1978

ACCREDITATIONS/APPROVALS: COMTAA

PREPARATION FOR OUT-OF-STATE LICENSING EXAM: Oregon, Washington

GRADUATES PER YEAR (APPROX.): 30-40

MODALITIES AND SUBJECTS: Esalen, neo-Reichian, deep tissue, polarity, zen shiatsu acupressure and Oriental healing arts, kinesiology, pathology, successful business practices, ethics, therapeutic and professional skills, practicum, t'ai chi, yoga, exercise therapy, hydrotherapy, CPR, first aid, seated massage, bodymind integration, breath and transformation, Oriental traditions in nutrition, clinical pain relief, energy balancing, emotional release and process-oriented bodywork, breathwork, hypnotherapy, structural rebalancing

UNIQUE ASPECTS OF SCHOOL OR CURRICULUM: This is a residential school in a wilderness setting.

ADVANCED PROGRAMS: The school also offers a nine-month transformational therapist training and training as an addiction counselor, and allows self-directed learning called life exploration.

CONTINUING EDUCATION: NMT, sports massage, cranio-sacral therapy, lymphatic massage, TMJ dysfunction, counseling for bodyworkers, surviving sexual abuse, core zero balancing

#16 Loving Hands Institute of Healing Arts
639 11th St.
Fortuna, CA 95540
(707) 725-9627

HOURS OF TRAINING: holistic massage practitioner (HMP) 120; Seifukujitsu Japanese massage (SJM) 150

IN-CLASS HOURS: (HMP) 96, (SJM) 150

DURATION OF COURSE: 8 weeks each

DAY/EVENING/WEEKEND: day, evening and weekend programs available

COST: HMP $800 including books; SJM $850 including books

YEAR FOUNDED: 1989

ACCREDITATIONS/APPROVALS: approved for nursing CEU's

GRADUATES PER YEAR (APPROX.): 20 to 40

MODALITIES AND SUBJECTS: Esalen, reading and cleansing the energy field, massage theory and history, business, legal and ethical standards, massage practicum

UNIQUE ASPECTS OF SCHOOL OR CURRICULUM: Classes are kept small, and the training emphasizes ancient Oriental and Native American techniques and philosophies.

#17 Mendocino School of Holistic Massage and
Advanced Healing Arts
2680 Road B
Redwood Valley, CA 95470
(707) 485-8197

HOURS OF TRAINING: massage therapist (HMT) 120; advanced massage therapist (AHMT) 220

IN-CLASS HOURS: HMT 96; AHMT 186

DURATION OF COURSE: HMT — 3 weekends and three evenings over a three-month period; AHMT — 3 weekends over a three-month period

DAY/EVENING/WEEKEND: most classes meet from 1:00 p.m. Friday to 6:00 p.m. Sunday

COST: HMT $1,049; AHMT $995

YEAR FOUNDED: 1993

ACCREDITATIONS/APPROVALS: approved for nursing CEU's

GRADUATES PER YEAR (APPROX.): 50 to 60

MODALITIES AND SUBJECTS: HMT program includes integrative holistic massage, polarity, energy field anatomy and theory, relaxation and balancing techniques, organ revitalization, conscious breathwork, intuitive development, emotional point release, reflexology, counseling, mind-body principles, polarity yoga, self-care, body mapping, lymphatic drainage massage, Esalen, ethics, business

AHMT program includes MT program plus advanced coursework in polarity, relaxation techniques, reflexology, breathwork, core energy work, hypnosis for bodyworkers, counseling, lymphatic massage, and private instruction.

UNIQUE ASPECTS OF SCHOOL OR CURRICULUM: small classes, holistic orientation with emphasis on personal growth, rural setting, no charge for accommodations

ADVANCED PROGRAMS: rebirther training, holistic health practitioner

CONTINUING EDUCATION: contact school

#18 New Life Institute of Massage Therapy
1159 Hilltop Dr.
Redding, CA 96002
(916) 222-1467

HOURS OF TRAINING: 160

DURATION OF COURSE: approx. 12 weeks

DAY/EVENING/WEEKEND: day and evening programs available

COST: $1,350 ($1,100 without reflexology)

MODALITIES AND SUBJECTS: shiatsu, reflexology, hygiene, relaxing and stretching techniques, theory and history of massage, ethics and business practices

UNIQUE ASPECTS OF SCHOOL OR CURRICULUM: class size is limited to 10 students.

ADVANCED PROGRAMS: 130-hour reflexology training

#19 Pacific School of Massage & Healing Arts
44800 Fish Rock Road
Gualala, CA 95445
(707) 884-3138

HOURS OF TRAINING: 110

DURATION OF COURSE: two six-day sessions separated by one month of independent study and practice

COST: $1,500

FINANCIAL AID: payment plans

YEAR FOUNDED: 1978

ACCREDITATIONS/APPROVALS: approved for veterans' training, approved for nursing CEU's

GRADUATES PER YEAR (APPROX.): 36

UNIQUE ASPECTS OF SCHOOL OR CURRICULUM: Maximum class size of 12. Coursework is eligible for academic credit at Summit University of Louisiana.

CONTINUING EDUCATION: Transformational Bodywork Seminars

#20 Sierra School of Health Sciences
341 Broadway, suite 400-C
Chico, CA 95928
(916) 894-0118

HOURS OF TRAINING: 110, 500

DURATION OF COURSE: 110-hour course 3½ months evenings/weekends

COST: 110-hour course $900; 500 hours $3,835

YEAR FOUNDED: 1989

GRADUATES PER YEAR (APPROX.): 90

MODALITIES AND SUBJECTS: deep tissue therapy, polarity, sports massage, shiatsu, reflexology, aromatherapy, trigger point therapy, neuromuscular re-education, myofascial release, cross fiber techniques, health/hygiene/body psychology, Chinese medicine, therapeutic touch, energy generation, energy balancing, business ethics, massage law and history

UNIQUE ASPECTS OF SCHOOL OR CURRICULUM: Three different 110-hour trainings are offered — "sensitive Swedish massage" technician, Swedish massage/shiatsu/reflexology, and eclectic deep tissue massage. Two different 390-hour programs are also offered — acupressure therapy and eclectic deep tissue therapy. The list of modalities in the previous paragraph combines the offerings in all programs.

ADVANCED PROGRAMS: 350-hour teacher training

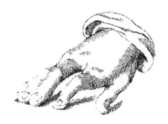

California, Sacramento Area

#21 Healing Arts Institute
112 Douglas Blvd.
Roseville, CA 95678
(916) 782-1275

HOURS OF TRAINING: 140; in-class hours: 126

DURATION OF COURSE: day class 3 weeks; morning or afternoon class 6 weeks; evening class 12 weeks

COST: $967.16 including books

YEAR FOUNDED: 1990

GRADUATES PER YEAR (APPROX.): 200

MODALITIES AND SUBJECTS: deep tissue, trigger point, reflexology, joint mobilization, stretches, lymphatic massage, massage for children, pregnant and elderly clients, business and ethics, stress management, deep relaxation techniques

ADVANCED PROGRAMS: acupressure certification training, hypnotherapy certification program

CONTINUING EDUCATION: deep tissue, sports massage, geriatric massage, manual lymphatic drainage, aromatherapy, marketing

#22 Health Awareness Academy
7525 Auburn Blvd., suite 3
Citrus Heights, CA 95610
(916) 969-4326

HOURS OF TRAINING: 275 (250 in-class)

DURATION OF COURSE: 4 to 6 months (students can go at their own pace)

DAY/EVENING/WEEKEND: day and evening programs available, plus weekend workshops

COST: $1,935 (includes books)

FINANCIAL AID: payment plan

YEAR FOUNDED: 1981

MODALITIES AND SUBJECTS: acupressure, reflexology, deep tissue, sports massage, business theory and creating a successful practice

UNIQUE ASPECTS OF SCHOOL OR CURRICULUM: emphasis on business skills, marketing, insurance billing and personal growth

#23 Integrative Therapy School
3000 T. St., suite 104
Sacramento, CA 95816
(916) 739-8848

HOURS OF TRAINING: 130 or 500

DURATION OF COURSE: 130-hour course 3 months, 500-hour course 9 months or 15 months

DAY/EVENING/WEEKEND: day and evening/weekend programs available

COST: 130 hours $1,183; 500 hours $4,435 (including supplies)

FINANCIAL AID: payment plan

YEAR FOUNDED: 1982

ACCREDITATIONS/APPROVALS: COMTAA, City and State Departments of Vocational Rehabilitation, approved for nursing CEU's

GRADUATES PER YEAR (APPROX.): 120

MODALITIES AND SUBJECTS: The 130-hour course includes reflexology, breath awareness, body mechanics, business practices. The 500-hour course adds acupressure, shiatsu, business and marketing, sports massage, nutrition, communication skills, polarity, muscle testing, medical considerations, student clinic

UNIQUE ASPECTS OF SCHOOL OR CURRICULUM: The curriculum emphasizes the physical, mental, emotional and spiritual aspects of bodywork.

ADVANCED PROGRAMS: advanced acupressure

CONTINUING EDUCATION: pregnancy massage, infant massage, lymphatic massage

#24 Messinger School of Massage
P.O. Box 1504
Lockford, CA 95237
(209) 727-0710

Contact the school for program information.

#25 Phillips School of Massage
P.O. Box 1999
Nevada City, CA 95959
(916) 265-4645

HOURS OF TRAINING: 200

DURATION OF COURSE: 6 weeks days; 8½ months evenings

COST: $1,200

FINANCIAL AID: payment plan

YEAR FOUNDED: 1983

ACCREDITATIONS/APPROVALS: approved for nursing CEU's

GRADUATES PER YEAR (APPROX.): 135

MODALITIES AND SUBJECTS: deep tissue, lymphatic massage, acupressure, shiatsu, reflexology, polarity, ortho-bionomy, aura, chakra and meridian balancing, body-mind awareness, vibrational healing, rocking, range of motion stretches, nutrition, applied kinesiology, self-health care, business practices

UNIQUE ASPECTS OF SCHOOL OR CURRICULUM: experiential learning through movement, meditation and guided visualization; community outreach program gives students and graduates volunteer service opportunity.

ADVANCED PROGRAMS: The school offers a student assistantship in which graduates assist students who are taking the program. The school also offers a 500-hour advanced certificate to students who take the 200-hour program, a 200-hour student assistant program, a 30-hour creative anatomy class, a one-week intensive on relaxing, and 80 hours of electives from the continuing education offerings.

CONTINUING EDUCATION: Programs include boundaries and relationships, chair shiatsu, couples massage, compassionate touch, drumming, expressive artistry in massage, Feng Shui, creative anatomy, exploration of movement, infant massage, ortho-bionomy, reflexology, table shiatsu, Thai massage, vibrational healing, watsu, craniosacral therapy, jin shin tao, Reiki, sports massage, introduction to Trager, and transformational breath.
Some continuing education programs are offered in exotic locations.

California, Napa and Sonoma Counties

#26 California Institute of Massage and & Spa Services
P.O. Box 673
Sonoma, CA 95476
(707) 939-8964

HOURS OF TRAINING:
Massage Technician (M/Tech): 150
Massage Therapist (M/Th): 500
Spa Services Certification (Spa): 100

IN-CLASS HOURS: M/Tech 120; M/Th 420; Spa 80

DURATION OF COURSE: M/Tech 14 weeks; M/Th one year; Spa 15 weeks

DAY/EVENING/WEEKEND: day or weekend programs available

COST: M/Tech $1,030; M/Th $3,985; Spa $895

YEAR FOUNDED: 1992

GRADUATES PER YEAR (APPROX.): 50

MODALITIES AND SUBJECTS: Massage programs: reflexology, body mechanics, yoga, conscious breathing, stretching, business practices, sports massage, trigger point therapy, shiatsu, pregnancy massage, ethics, kinesiology, pathology and medical terminology, massage without a table, communication skills. Spa program: aromatherapy, body scrubs, paraffin baths, seaweed and mud wraps, hydrotherapy, setting up a spa

UNIQUE ASPECTS OF SCHOOL OR CURRICULUM: The spa services course may be taken as part of the 500-hour certification.

CONTINUING EDUCATION: Some courses may be taken as continuing education by qualified practitioners.

#27 Calistoga Massage Therapy School
5959 Commerce Blvd., suite 13
Rohnert Park, CA 94928
(707) 586-1953

HOURS OF TRAINING: 100

DURATION OF COURSE: 7 weeks, evenings

COST: $750 (includes books)

YEAR FOUNDED: 1981

GRADUATES PER YEAR (APPROX.): 50

MODALITIES AND SUBJECTS: Esalen massage

UNIQUE ASPECTS OF SCHOOL OR CURRICULUM: Class size is kept to a maximum of 14 students, and the program emphasizes body sensitivity, intuitive awareness of client's energy blocks, and a spiritual awareness of the therapist's healing potential.

#28 Jupiter Hollow School for Massage
P.O. Box 8043
Santa Rosa, CA 95407
(707) 584-7903

HOURS OF TRAINING: 100

DURATION OF COURSE: alternate weekends for 12 weeks or 11-day intensive

COST: $1,000

YEAR FOUNDED: 1979

GRADUATES PER YEAR (APPROX.): 30-40

MODALITIES AND SUBJECTS: body mechanics, deep muscle work, foot reflexology, lymphatic-circulatory massage, terminology and treatment of sports-related injuries, business ethics and practices, marketing

#29 Lifestream Massage School
828 School St.
Napa, CA 94558
(707) 253-1359

No Catalogue

HOURS OF TRAINING: 170 or 500

IN-CLASS HOURS: 128 or 400

DURATION OF COURSE: 170 hours 4 months, 500 hours one year

DAY/EVENING/WEEKEND: day, evening and weekend programs available

COST: 170 hours $1,190

FINANCIAL AID: payment plans

YEAR FOUNDED: 1989

GRADUATES PER YEAR (APPROX.): 100

MODALITIES AND SUBJECTS: LifeStream massage, reflexology, seated massage, deep tissue bodywork, acupressure, spa treatments, structural transformation bodywork, joint mobilization

ADVANCED PROGRAMS: Advanced Certified Massage Technician, Structural Transformation Bodyworker

#30 School of Shiatsu and Massage at Harbin Hot Springs
P.O. Box 570
Middletown, CA 95461
(707) 987-3801

HOURS OF TRAINING: Training is offered in 50 and 100 hour segments. Certificates are given for 100-hour Practitioner Course and 500-hour Therapist Course.

DURATION OF COURSE: 50 hour segments 6 days; 100 hour segments 11 days

COST: Each 50-hour segment costs $600, inclusive of lodging and use of the facilities. There is a $50 reduction for registration 14 days in advance.

FINANCIAL AID: payment plan

YEAR FOUNDED: 1977

GRADUATES PER YEAR (APPROX.): 100 to 150

MODALITIES AND SUBJECTS: shiatsu, acupressure, watsu (aquatic shiatsu), rebalancing, deep tissue, sports massage, tantsu, NLP, healing intimate trauma, pain relief, wassertantzen

UNIQUE ASPECTS OF SCHOOL OR CURRICULUM: location at a hot springs retreat and resort, and availability of watsu (aquatic shiatsu)

ADVANCED PROGRAMS: The school offers a 100-hour instructor course and a 500-hour advanced body therapist course in addition to the 500-hour therapist training.

#31 Sebastopol Massage Center
     108 North Main St. #5
     Sebastopol, CA 95472
     (707) 823-3550

HOURS OF TRAINING: 150

IN-CLASS HOURS: 100

COST: $725

MODALITIES AND SUBJECTS: marketing, ethics, business practices, documented practice

UNIQUE ASPECTS OF SCHOOL OR CURRICULUM: Maximum of 12 students per class. Credit may be arranged for prior massage education.

California, Marin County

#32 Aesclepion Massage Institute, Inc.
     1314 Lincoln Ave., suite B
     San Rafael, CA 94901
     (415) 453-6196

HOURS OF TRAINING: 130

IN-CLASS HOURS: 48

DURATION OF COURSE: 3 months

COST: $1,250

FINANCIAL AID: (payment plans)

MODALITIES AND SUBJECTS: massage history, counseling skills

UNIQUE ASPECTS OF SCHOOL OR CURRICULUM: The course leads to certification as Massage Technician. However, many students pursue the program as a journey of self-discovery and growth, and regard the massage training as primarily recreational.

#33 Alive & Well!
     Institute of Conscious BodyWork
     100 Shaw Drive
     San Anselmo, CA 94960
     (415) 258-0402

HOURS OF TRAINING: 140 hours, 300 hours, 560 hours

DURATION OF COURSE: 140 hours 3-week intensive, 9 weeks or longer full-time; 560-hour program is at the student's pace.

DAY/EVENING/WEEKEND: Most classes meet evenings or weekends.

COST: 140 hours $1,145; 560 hours $4,536

FINANCIAL AID: payment plans, work-study

YEAR FOUNDED: 1986

GRADUATES PER YEAR (APPROX.): 50 to 75

MODALITIES AND SUBJECTS: Basic courses are kinesiology, Conscious BodyWork, conscious breathwork, counseling for bodyworkers, nutritional physiology, polarity, reflexology, establishing a business. Electives include Aston bodywork, on-site, massage ergonomics, bodywork for abuse survivors, brain function facilitation, carpal tunnel and wrist problems, cranial sacral therapy, deep tissue, energetic tune-ups, face and head massage, healing through sound, hip and pelvic mobilization, lymphatic and visceral massage, massage in hospital settings, neuro-muscular reprogramming, nutrition, chi kung, rocking and shaking, self-care, sports injury, Touch for Health/applied kinesiology

UNIQUE ASPECTS OF SCHOOL OR CURRICULUM: The focus is on the power of conscious attention as an agent of change within.

ADVANCED PROGRAMS: Aston massage certification course, integrative hypnotherapy certification course, advanced bodyworker (300 hours), conscious bodyworker (560 hours)

CONTINUING EDUCATION: All courses can be taken as individual electives.

#34 Diamond Light
     The Marin School of Massage
     P.O. Box 5443
     Mill Valley, CA 94942
     (415) 454-6651

HOURS OF TRAINING: 150

IN-CLASS HOURS: 100

DURATION OF COURSE: 6 weeks intensive or ten weeks (classes meet evenings and weekends)

Cost: $1,095 (up to $70 discount for early payment)

Year founded: 1987

Graduates per year (approx.): 40

Modalities and subjects: Esalen, lymphatic massage, prenatal massage, deep tissue, foot reflexology, laying on of hands, mediation, energy and chakra work, sound healing, transforming emotions, movement, working with the elements, hypnotherapy, hygiene and ethics, business practices

Unique aspects of school or curriculum: The focus includes emotional, spiritual and physical aspects of bodywork.

Advanced programs: deep bodywork specialization, spiritual healing certification, hypnotherapy certification

California, San Francisco

#35 Integral Art of Massage Workshops
2136 Sutter St.
San Francisco, CA 94115
(415) 267-7689

Contact the school for program information.

#36 San Francisco School of Massage
2209 Van Ness Avenue
San Francisco, CA 94109
(415) 474-4600

Hours of training: 102 Swedish massage; 100 advanced Swedish massage

Duration of course: 102 hours six weeks to 17 weeks; 100-hour advanced course 18 months

Day/evening/weekend: day and evening programs are available

Cost: 102-hour Swedish $875; 100-hour advanced Swedish $1,175

Year founded: 1969

Accreditations/approvals: approved for nursing CEU's

Graduates per year (approx.): 150

Modalities and subjects: Basic course includes Esalen, business, marketing, chair massage, breathwork, spa massage, energy work.
   Workshops are also offered, either as components of an advanced program or as continuing education. These include: aromatherapy, barefoot shiatsu, bodywork during pregnancy and after, breema, craniosacral massage, deep tissue massage, energy work, geriatric massage, light touch, lymphatic massage, massage for clients with physical limitations, nutrition, ki-gong, reflexology, shiatsu on a table, sports massage

Unique aspects of school or curriculum: The school offers 50 hours of continuing education free to those who take the basic course. The school puts emphasis on teachers with long experience in practice and teaching.

Advanced programs: 102-hour zen shiatsu course

#37 School for Self-Healing
1718 Taraval St.
San Francisco, CA 94116
(415) 665-9574

Hours of training: 160

Duration of course: two 8-day segments separated by approximately two months

Cost: $2,600 including books and materials

Financial aid: payment plans

Year founded: 1981

Modalities and subjects: development of kinesthetic awareness through movement, massage techniques for regeneration, joint mobility, digestion and the autonomic nervous system, breathing, the circulatory system and the heart, summary, discussion and homework, relationship between mind and body, muscles, integrating principles of kinesthetic awareness, introduction to tactile client assessment, forms of bodywork and vision improvement, introduction to visual evaluation of movement, evaluation and assessment, full activation of the nervous system, clients with neuromuscular ailments, vision, ethics and business development

Unique aspects of school or curriculum: The school is based on the method of Meir Schneider, Ph.D., who cured himself of congenital blindness. Classes are kept small to allow individual attention to each student

Advanced programs: Part II of the training includes practical work with clients. Also offered are apprenticeship and teacher training

#38 The World School of Massage and
Advanced Healing Arts
401-32nd Avenue
San Francisco, CA 94121
(415) 221-2533

Programs offered:
   Holistic Massage Therapist (HMT)
   Advanced Massage Therapist (AMT)
   Holistic Health Counselor (HHC)
   Master Bodyworker/Holistic Health Educator
      (MB/HHE)

Hours of training: HMT 123; AMT 123; HHC 256; MB/HHE 600

DURATION OF COURSE: HMT 3 months; AMT 5 months; HHC 6 months; MB/HHE 12 to 14 months

DAY/EVENING/WEEKEND: daytime and evening/weekend programs available

COST: HMT $1,007.69; AMT $1,200; HHC $3,050; MB/HHE $5,799.08 (prices include required books)

FINANCIAL AID: payment plans

YEAR FOUNDED: 1982

ACCREDITATIONS/APPROVALS: approved for nursing CEU's

GRADUATES PER YEAR (APPROX.): 200

MODALITIES AND SUBJECTS: Vibrational Healing Massage Therapy, philosophy, communication, business & ethics, individual coaching, cranial-sacral balancing, foot reflexology, Foot Bone Massage, lymphatic massage, educational kinesiology/Touch for Health, rebirthing, hypnosis, theory of healing, Holistic Fitness and Nutrition, death and dying, music and sound healing

UNIQUE ASPECTS OF SCHOOL OR CURRICULUM: The school offers Vibrational Healing Massage Therapy, developed by the school's founder, Patricia Cramer. The school's focus is on self-responsibility and communication, especially the internal communication with oneself and the belief that we create our bodies and our lives exactly as we want.

ADVANCED PROGRAMS: 600-hour Master Bodyworker/Holistic Health Educator program

California, Berkeley & Oakland Area

#39 Acupressure Institute of America
1533 Shattuck Ave.
Berkeley, CA 94709
(510) 845-1059 or (800) 442-2232

HOURS OF TRAINING: 150

DURATION OF COURSE: four weeks full-time, six months to one year part-time

COST: $975

FINANCIAL AID: payment plans, work trade

YEAR FOUNDED: 1976

ACCREDITATIONS/APPROVALS: approved for nursing CEU's

MODALITIES AND SUBJECTS: acupressure, reflexology, zen shiatsu, acu-yoga, Touch for Health, tui na, acupressure oil massage, barefoot shiatsu, the 12 organ meridians, five element theory, business practice and ethics, documented practice

UNIQUE ASPECTS OF SCHOOL OR CURRICULUM: Students can receive credit for some coursework done at other schools.

ADVANCED PROGRAMS: 200-hour specializations are offered in women's health, advanced shiatsu, sports acupressure, emotional balancing, arthritis and pain relief, traditional oriental therapy, and acupressure stress management. An 850-hour acupressure therapist program is also offered.

CONTINUING EDUCATION: contact school

#40 American Institute of Massage Therapy
1651 Tice Valley Blvd.
Walnut Creek, CA 94595
(510) 945-8976

HOURS OF TRAINING: 150

DURATION OF COURSE: days or evenings for 11 weeks or weekends for six months

COST: $1,007

FINANCIAL AID: payment plans

YEAR FOUNDED: 1979

ACCREDITATIONS/APPROVALS: approved for nursing CEU's, California State Department of Rehabilitation

GRADUATES PER YEAR (APPROX.): 80

MODALITIES AND SUBJECTS: ice and heat therapy, acupressure, Chinese and Japanese massage, communication skills, history, ethics, business practices, exercises, prana yama yoga, acupressure massage facelift

UNIQUE ASPECTS OF SCHOOL OR CURRICULUM: Class size is kept small and medical massage is emphasized.

ADVANCED PROGRAMS: advanced injury therapy (deep tissue, sports massage, reflexology)

CONTINUING EDUCATION: asian acupressure, reflexology, neuro-vascular acupressure, auditory neuro-muscular repatterning

#41 Body Electric School
6527A Telegraph Ave.
Oakland, CA 94609
(510) 653-1594

HOURS OF TRAINING: 100

DURATION OF COURSE: 16-day intensive

COST: $990

YEAR FOUNDED: 1984

GRADUATES PER YEAR (APPROX.): 50

MODALITIES AND SUBJECTS: Esalen, acupressure, bodywork for people with life-threatening illnesses, conscious breathing/rebirthing, successful business practices

UNIQUE ASPECTS OF SCHOOL OR CURRICULUM: The school is committed to exploring the healing potential of erotic energy. All sexual preferences are celebrated and all spiritual paths are honored.

ADVANCED PROGRAMS: deep tissue massage certification, Jin Shin Do

CONTINUING EDUCATION: healing the wounded healer

#42 Body Tuneup National School of Massage Therapy
1955 Lucile, Ste. D
Stockton, CA 95209
(209) 473-4993 or (800) 622-9766

HOURS OF TRAINING: Basic 100, advanced 100, additional programs to 500-hour total

DURATION OF COURSE: Basic course — 6 weekends or 10 weeks days or 14 weeks evenings; advanced course 6 weekends or 10 weeks days

COST: Basic 100-hour course $850 including workbooks; advanced 100-hour course $750

ACCREDITATIONS/APPROVALS: approved for nursing CEU's

MODALITIES AND SUBJECTS: Basic 100-hr course includes acupressure, aromatherapy, joint mobilization, shiatsu, Esalen, t'ai chi, body mechanics. Advanced 100-hr course adds myofascial work, business, deep tissue massage, joint mobilization and traction, prenatal and on-site massage.

ADVANCED PROGRAMS: advanced therapeutic massage (described above), sports massage (100 hours), paramedical massage (100 hours), massage in the chiropractic office, diagnosis in massage, aromatherapy, on-site, pre-natal massage, Thai massage

CONTINUING EDUCATION: polarity, lumbar sciatic pain relief, care giving massage for the elderly, wrist, forearm and shoulder massage, barefoot shiatsu, acuroma massage, Reiki, massage marketing, iridology, acupressure, insurance billing, caring touch massage, cranio therapy

---

#43 Care Through Touch Institute
2401 LeConte Ave.
Berkeley, CA 94709
(510) 548-0418

HOURS OF TRAINING: 180

IN-CLASS HOURS: 130

DURATION OF COURSE: 3-week intensive

COST: $1,200 (includes books)

FINANCIAL AID: payment plan

YEAR FOUNDED: 1990

ACCREDITATIONS/APPROVALS: Graduate Theological Union, Berkeley, CA, approved for nursing CEU's

GRADUATES PER YEAR (APPROX.): 36 to 40

MODALITIES AND SUBJECTS: Esalen, reflexology, acupressure, Rosen bodywork, business and ethics, special skills for working with children, the elderly, sick, disabled and abused, movement, breathing and introspection, theological reflection, pastoral ministry

UNIQUE ASPECTS OF SCHOOL OR CURRICULUM: The school teaches massage within the context of contemporary Christian spirituality. Students are prepared for work with the elderly, the poor, the dying, the physically disabled, AIDS patients and those recovering from addiction.
  A 25-hour weekend introduction "Massage: The Art of Anointing" is offered regularly.

ADVANCED PROGRAMS: supervised pastoral internship

#44 McKinnon Institute of Professional Massage and Bodywork
3798 Grand Ave.
Oakland, CA 94610-1594
(510) 465-3488

HOURS OF TRAINING: 100 to 620

IN-CLASS HOURS: 100 to 620

DURATION OF COURSE: 2 weeks to 3 months

DAY/EVENING/WEEKEND: days, evenings and weekend intensives available

COST: $9.00 per hour of class

YEAR FOUNDED: 1973

GRADUATES PER YEAR (APPROX.): 300 to 500 for all programs combined

MODALITIES AND SUBJECTS: Esalen massage, grounding the practitioner, body reading, subtle aspects of touch, sidelying and chair massage, cellular basis of health, medical terminology, business ethics, hygiene, meridian flow and release work, 5 element theory, movement and breath, shiatsu, acupressure, craniosacral therapy, sports massage, reflexology, deep tissue work, practice building

UNIQUE ASPECTS OF SCHOOL OR CURRICULUM: emphasis on the mind/body/spirit aspect of the work

ADVANCED PROGRAMS: advanced trigger point, techniques for specialized settings, deep tissue, unwinding

CONTINUING EDUCATION: shiatsu, acupressure, craniosacral therapy, subtle touch, sports massage, deep tissue, teacher training

#45 National Holistic Institute
5900 Hollis St. J
Emeryville, CA 94608
(510) 547-6442

HOURS OF TRAINING: 720

DURATION OF COURSE: day program 9 months, evening/weekend program approx. 12-15 months

DAY/EVENING/WEEKEND: day program and evening/weekend program available

COST: $6,859.95 (includes books, massage table and supplies)

FINANCIAL AID: federally guaranteed grants and loans available (contact admissions office)

YEAR FOUNDED: 1979

ACCREDITATIONS/APPROVALS: COMTAA, ACCET

GRADUATES PER YEAR (APPROX.): 500

MODALITIES AND SUBJECTS: acupressure/shiatsu, sports massage, massage for pregnant women, massage for people with injuries, seated massage, foot reflexology, deep tissue, energy massage, joint mobilization, rocking and shaking massage, body mechanics, customization of massage sessions, postural analysis, kinesiology, hydrotherapy, stress management, first aid, CPR, time management, communication skills, business skills, marketing, record-keeping, resume writing and interviewing

UNIQUE ASPECTS OF SCHOOL OR CURRICULUM: Students participate in a real-world clinic and receive extensive training in building a successful massage therapy practice. Students also work in a community non-profit agency assisting with case planning for people who could not afford massage therapy.

CONTINUING EDUCATION: free monthly programs for alumni

#46 re Source
Box 5398
Berkeley, CA 94705
(510) 841-4732

HOURS OF TRAINING: 200, 500 (approval pending), 1,000; program hours include home practice and student exchange

DURATION OF COURSE: Students proceed at their own pace

COST: 200 hours $850 plus cost of electives. Advanced trainings are comprised of individual courses.

YEAR FOUNDED: 1982

GRADUATES PER YEAR (APPROX.): 15

MODALITIES AND SUBJECTS: bodymind survey class, bodyreading, professional issues, professional practice workshop, anatomy games, experiments in massage

UNIQUE ASPECTS OF SCHOOL OR CURRICULUM: The school offers concurrent massage certification to students of Trager, Rosen method and ortho-bionomy. Coursework taken at other schools may apply toward 500 or 1000-hour certifications.

ADVANCED PROGRAMS: The healing relationship: obstacles to healing, ortho-bionomy, Trager beginning training

CONTINUING EDUCATION: All advanced coursework may be taken on a course-by-course basis as continuing education.

#47 Touching for Health Center
School of Professional Bodywork
628 Lincoln Center
Stockton, CA 95207
(209) 474-9559

HOURS OF TRAINING: 105, 200, 500

DURATION OF COURSE: 105 hours 3 months, 200 hours approx. 6 months, 500 hours up to 3 years

DAY/EVENING/WEEKEND: day and evening classes available

COST: 105 hours $856 including book, 200 hours $1,561 including book, 500 hours fee will vary but will not exceed $4,000.

FINANCIAL AID: payment plan

MODALITIES AND SUBJECTS: 105-hour course includes history and psychology of massage, massage theory and hygiene, business ethics and documentation. The 200-hour course adds anatomy and physiology, reflexology, advanced neck and shoulders, medical terminology, practicum. The 500-hour course adds advanced anatomy and physiology, clinical treatments, human behavior, indications/contraindications, massage theory practice, sports massage, introduction to other modalities, CPR, business practice, deep tissue, hydrotherapy, kinesiology, lymph drainage, polarity, reflexology, acupressure, assessment and treatment planning.

#48 Wind Walk Institute of Natural Healing
and Beauty
P.O. Box 2505
Berkeley, CA 94702
(510) 841-4569

HOURS OF TRAINING: 100

DURATION OF COURSE: two-week intensive or weekend classes

COST: $1,150 or $1,045 in advance

ACCREDITATIONS/APPROVALS: approved for nursing CEU's

MODALITIES AND SUBJECTS: passive joint work, pregnancy massage, chair massage, grounding for practitioner, subtle aspects of touch, body reading, business and marketing

UNIQUE ASPECTS OF SCHOOL OR CURRICULUM: Instruction is at wooded retreat center

ADVANCED PROGRAMS: 100-hour master's in massage therapy

CONTINUING EDUCATION: reflexology, herbal medicine, sports massage, lymphatic drainage, Native American sacred stone massage, sacred drum-making

California, San Jose & Santa Cruz Area

#49 Body Therapy Center
368 California Ave.
Palo Alto, CA 94306
(415) 328-9400

HOURS OF TRAINING: 136 to 600

DURATION OF COURSE: 136 hours 3 months, evenings/weekends

COST: 136 hours $1,125

MODALITIES AND SUBJECTS: 136-hour course includes client-therapist relationship, Esalen, introduction to other body therapies, general business practices.

ADVANCED PROGRAMS: 120-hour clinical deep tissue training, 175-hour advanced massage and bodywork training, 121-hour beginning shiatsu training, 121-hour intermediate shiatsu

#50 The Center for Body Harmonics
2340A Walsh Ave.
Santa Clara, CA 95051
(408) 727-1939 or (800) 700-1993

HOURS OF TRAINING: 100

DURATION OF COURSE: six weeks weekends or three weeks weekdays

MODALITIES AND SUBJECTS: deep tissue stretches, reflexology

CONTINUING EDUCATION: shiatsu, chair massage, sports massage, lymphatic drainage massage, Reiki

#51 Cypress Health Institute
P.O. Box 2941
Santa Cruz, CA 95063
(408) 476-2115

HOURS OF TRAINING: 150

DURATION OF COURSE: Wednesday evenings and Saturdays for 10 weeks

COST: $875

YEAR FOUNDED: 1982

ACCREDITATIONS/APPROVALS: approved for nursing CEU's

GRADUATES PER YEAR (APPROX.): 75

MODALITIES AND SUBJECTS: Esalen, polarity, counseling for bodyworkers, business practices

UNIQUE ASPECTS OF SCHOOL OR CURRICULUM: Emphasis is placed on proper body mechanics, and class size is limited to 14 students.

ADVANCED PROGRAMS: craniosacral therapy, intermediate and advanced polarity, lymphatic drainage massage

CONTINUING EDUCATION: deep tissue therapy, aromatherapy, reflexology

#52 Esalen Institute
Coast Rt. 1
Big Sur, CA 93920
(408) 667-3000

Contact the institute for program information.

#53 Just for Your Health College of Massage
2075 Lincoln Ave., suite E
San Jose, CA 95125
(408) 723-2570

HOURS OF TRAINING: 100 or 500

DURATION OF COURSE: 12 days to 5½ months

DAY/EVENING/WEEKEND: day and evening programs available

COST: 100 hours $850; 500 hours $4,300 (both include books and supplies)

FINANCIAL AID: payment plans and some assistance

MODALITIES AND SUBJECTS: deep tissue, reflexology, acupressure, nutrition, magnetic fields, focusing, sound and color therapy, professional ethics, business practices, Chinese medicine, shiatsu, acupressure, Tuina, t'ai chi, pediatric massage, sports massage, student apprenticeship

#54 Lupin Massage Institute
Lupin Naturist Club
20600 Aldercroft Hts. Rd.
Los Gatos, CA 95030
(408) 353-2250

HOURS OF TRAINING: 120

IN-CLASS HOURS: 102

DURATION OF COURSE: three weeks to three months

COST: $950 (couples $665 each)

FINANCIAL AID: payment plan

MODALITIES AND SUBJECTS: physics and metaphysics of the human body, Esalen, business practices and ethics, Touch for Health, Lomi Lomi

UNIQUE ASPECTS OF SCHOOL OR CURRICULUM: Located at Lupin Naturist Club

#55 Milpitas Electrolysis College
500 E. Calaveras Blvd. #202-204
Milpitas, CA 95035
(408) 946-9522

No Catalogue

HOURS OF TRAINING: 100 to 600

DURATION OF COURSE: 3 weeks to one year

DAY/EVENING/WEEKEND: day and evening programs available

COST: $750 to $3,550

FINANCIAL AID: available only for students taking electrology and massage courses

YEAR FOUNDED: 1982

GRADUATES PER YEAR (APPROX.): 53

MODALITIES AND SUBJECTS: shiatsu, reflexology, sports massage, acupressure

#56 Monterey Institute of Touch
27820 Dorris Dr.
Carmel, CA 93923
(408) 624-1006

HOURS OF TRAINING: massage practitioner 200; massage therapist 500

DURATION OF COURSE: 200-hour course varies from 5-week intensive to 18 weeks part-time; 500-hour course takes one to two years.

DAY/EVENING/WEEKEND: day and evening programs available

COST: 200-hour program $1,100 (includes books); 500-hour program contact school

YEAR FOUNDED: 1983

GRADUATES PER YEAR (APPROX.): 100

MODALITIES AND SUBJECTS: 200-hour program includes polarity, shiatsu, self-care and movement awareness, range of motion, reflexology, sports massage, intuitive massage, business practice and ethics, supervised internship. 500-hour program adds clinical massage, body handling, hand/wrist/forearm care, CPR/emergency medical practice, advanced massage,

advanced anatomy and physiology, plus electives from continuing education offerings.

UNIQUE ASPECTS OF SCHOOL OR CURRICULUM: The school stresses movement to help students do massage without creating stress in their own bodies.

ADVANCED PROGRAMS: Three different 100-hour programs are available to graduates of 200-hour course; intermediate massage, advanced massage, and specialized massage (specialized massage may be craniosacral therapy or sports massage). Taking all three advanced 100-hour programs qualifies student for 500-hour certificate.

Continuing education programs offered include: body logic, massage for couples, prenatal massage, intuitive massage, pathology, soft tissue release, chair massage, skilled touch for the seriously ill, movement awareness, advanced massage, lymphatic and visceral massage, Hawaiian massage, healing and meditation, massage in the chiropractic setting, cranial-sacral therapy, aromatherapy

#57 Silicon Valley College
41350 Christy St.
Fremont, CA 94538
(510) 623-9966

Contact the school for program information.

#58 Twin Lakes College of the Healing Arts
1210 Brommer St.
Santa Cruz, CA 95062
(408) 476-2152

HOURS OF TRAINING: 200, 300 or 500

DAY/EVENING/WEEKEND: day and evening programs available

COST: 200 hours $1,198 (can vary with electives chosen); advanced classes are priced individually

YEAR FOUNDED: 1982

GRADUATES PER YEAR (APPROX.): 100

MODALITIES AND SUBJECTS: The 200-hour course includes two elective massage classes (choices: integrative Swedish, polarity I and II, acupressure I and II, shiatsu I and II, subtle body energywork) counseling and communications skills, internship/practice, and a massage-a-thon event.
The 300-hour program adds advanced anatomy, advanced professional studies, CPR/first aid.
The 500-hour program adds a concentration of study in one of the following: integrative Swedish & sports massage, integrative Swedish & deep tissue, Oriental & ayurvedic massage, or Oriental & acupressure, shiatsu, or polarity.

UNIQUE ASPECTS OF SCHOOL OR CURRICULUM: Graduates of other state-licensed massage programs may be eligible for advanced standing in the 300 or 500-hour programs. The school also offers a certificate program for women only.

ADVANCED PROGRAMS: hypnotherapy

#59 Western College of Therapeutic Massage
2002 White Oaks Rd., #3
Campbell, CA 95008
(408) 244-8350 or (408) 371-8200

HOURS OF TRAINING: 100

DURATION OF COURSE: 10-day intensive or three evenings per week for three months

COST: $795

YEAR FOUNDED: 1983

GRADUATES PER YEAR (APPROX.): 90

MODALITIES AND SUBJECTS: reflexology, hot & cold packs, deep tissue massage, business aspects of massage, professionalism

UNIQUE ASPECTS OF SCHOOL OR CURRICULUM: Scheduling can be flexible to adapt to the needs of the individual student.

CONTINUING EDUCATION: deep tissue massage, sports massage, on-site

California, Fresno

#60 California Medical School of Shiatsu
4635 N. First St., suite 202
Fresno, CA 93726
(209) 544-0960

Contact the school for program information.

#61 Quality College of Health Care Careers
1570 N. Wishon Ave.
Fresno, CA 93728
(209) 266-7356 or (209) 497-5050

HOURS OF TRAINING: 150

DURATION OF COURSE: 18 weeks, two evenings per week

COST: $2,350

FINANCIAL AID: payment plan

YEAR FOUNDED: 1994

MODALITIES AND SUBJECTS: clinical therapeutic massage, deep friction, rocking, joint mobilization, sports massage

UNIQUE ASPECTS OF SCHOOL OR CURRICULUM: 75 of the 150 program hours are supervised practice on patients who are receiving chiropractic treatment.

CONTINUING EDUCATION: physical therapy aide, chiropractic assistant programs

#62 Therapeutic Learning Center
3636 N. First, suite 160
Fresno, CA 93726
(209) 225-7772

HOURS OF TRAINING: 200

DURATION OF COURSE: 14 weeks (2 evenings per week plus Saturday)

COST: $1,500 (includes required texts)

YEAR FOUNDED: 1986

GRADUATES PER YEAR (APPROX.): 48

MODALITIES AND SUBJECTS: shiatsu, reflexology, sports massage, overview of forms of bodywork, posture, body reading and palpation, range of motion and stretching, stress reduction, health, hygiene, draping, business administration, law, ethics

UNIQUE ASPECTS OF SCHOOL OR CURRICULUM: Maximum of 16 students at any one time. Emphasis is on holistic health.

CONTINUING EDUCATION: contact school

California, San Luis Obispo Area

#63 Central California School of Body Therapy
Administration: 448 Woodland Dr.
Classroom: 2030 10th Street
Los Osos, CA 93402
(805) 528-7519

HOURS OF TRAINING: 200 or 550

DURATION OF COURSE: 200 hours 3 months; 550 hours 10 months

COST: 200 hours $850; 550 hours $4,375

FINANCIAL AID: payment plans

YEAR FOUNDED: 1991

ACCREDITATIONS/APPROVALS: COMTAA

MODALITIES AND SUBJECTS: acupressure, reflexology, guided imagery, principles of nutrition, business ethics and record keeping, evaluation skills, communication dynamics, body mechanics/movement, lymphatic massage, deep tissue sculpting, introduction to structural integration, cross fiber friction, trigger point therapy, therapeutic stretching, mobilizations, naturopathic adjunct therapy, joint structure and function, polarity therapy, reflexology, sports massage, health in the 90's, business management

UNIQUE ASPECTS OF SCHOOL OR CURRICULUM: The school allows practitioners with 120 or more hours of massage education to apply for advanced placement in the 550-hour program

CONTINUING EDUCATION: reflexology, polarity therapy, naturopathic adjunct therapy, acupressure

California, Bakersfield

#64 Massage Training Institute
1527 19th St., suite 428
Bakersfield, CA 93301
(805) 632-2823 or 631-1966

HOURS OF TRAINING: 200

IN-CLASS HOURS: 100

DURATION OF COURSE: 10-day intensive or six weekends, evening program also available

COST: registration fee $100, tuition $850

YEAR FOUNDED: 1993

MODALITIES AND SUBJECTS: body psychology, movement awareness, counseling skills, nutrition, AIDS, avoiding sexual harassment, business practices, 100 intern/extern hours

UNIQUE ASPECTS OF SCHOOL OR CURRICULUM: The curriculum is holistically oriented and emphasizes both professionalism and personal growth.

ADVANCED PROGRAMS: shiatsu certification course, Swedish/shiatsu combination course

CONTINUING EDUCATION: aromatherapy, t'ai chi, lymphatic drainage, ortho-bionomy, Reiki, kinesiology

California, Santa Barbara

#65 Advanced Training Massage Institute
Business office: 330 Mohawk Road
Classroom location: 31 Parker Way
Santa Barbara, CA 93109
(805) 966-1414

HOURS OF TRAINING: 200 including 100 clinical hours

DAY/EVENING/WEEKEND: day, evening and weekend courses available

COST: $650

FINANCIAL AID: payment plans

MODALITIES AND SUBJECTS: Esalen, passive exercises, sports massage, deep-tissue therapy, postural balancing, stress management, nutrition, polarity therapy, reflexology, shiatsu, acupressure, medical terminology, communication, business skills

ADVANCED PROGRAMS: Neurosomatics, deep tissue therapy certification, sports massage certification, hypnosis trainings

CONTINUING EDUCATION: sports massage, deep tissue therapy I and II, neurosomatic bodywork I and II, advanced body reading, marketing and action plan, lymphatic massage, acupressure, reflexology, polarity therapy, aromatherapy

#66 Body Therapy Institute
835 N. Milpas St.
Santa Barbara, CA 93103
(805) 966-5802

HOURS OF TRAINING: 200 or 500

IN-CLASS HOURS: 150 or 500

DURATION OF COURSE: 200-hour program one month intensive or 14 weeks; 500-hour program approximately 18 months

DAY/EVENING/WEEKEND: day, evening and weekend programs available

COST: 200-hour program $1,000; 500-hour program $3,500

YEAR FOUNDED: 1985

GRADUATES PER YEAR (APPROX.): 100

MODALITIES AND SUBJECTS: The 200-hour course includes acupressure, polarity, joint articulations, rocking technique, abdominal organ massage, movement skills, centering, seated massage, interpersonal skills, pregnancy massage, nature retreat, nutrition, practicum, community outreach.
  The 500-hour program includes polarity therapy, deep tissue/sports, anatomy, lymphatic drainage, reflexology, Touch for Health, myofascial release and holodynamics.

ADVANCED PROGRAMS: 50 and 100-hour segments in the 500-hour program may be taken as individual advanced trainings or continuing education.

#67 Santa Barbara College of Oriental Medicine
1919 State St., suite 204
Santa Barbara, CA 93101
(805) 682-9594

HOURS OF TRAINING: 256

DURATION OF COURSE: 8 months, evenings

COST: $1,250

YEAR FOUNDED: 1987

GRADUATES PER YEAR (APPROX.): 10 to 12

MODALITIES AND SUBJECTS: shiatsu, acupressure, sports massage, point location

UNIQUE ASPECTS OF SCHOOL OR CURRICULUM: The shiatsu training is part of the school's 3-year Masters Program in acupuncture and Oriental medicine.

CONTINUING EDUCATION: Chinese diagnostic technique

#68 School of Intuitive Massage and Healing
     1911-D de la Vina
     Santa Barbara, CA 93101
     (805) 687-2917

Contact the school for program information.

California, Los Angeles Area

#69 American Institute of Massage Therapy, Inc.
     2156 Newport Ave.
     Costa Mesa, CA 92627
     (714) 642-0735

HOURS OF TRAINING: 1,009 (609 plus 400 hours clinical SportsMassage internship)

DAY/EVENING/WEEKEND: day and evening programs available

COST: $5,160

FINANCIAL AID: payment plans

YEAR FOUNDED: 1983

ACCREDITATIONS/APPROVALS: COMTAA, approved for nursing CEU's

PREPARATION FOR OUT-OF-STATE LICENSING EXAM: Washington

GRADUATES PER YEAR (APPROX.): 20 every nine months

MODALITIES AND SUBJECTS: sports kinesiology, functional muscle testing, conterstrain, PNF stretches, sports pathology and psychology, immediate injury care, pre-event massage, post-event massage, training and conditioning, restoration/rehabilitation, pathology, nutrition, psychology and philosophy, hydrotherapy, acupressure, shiatsu, reflexology, Chinese and Russian techniques, remedial exercises, lymphatic drainage, Thai stretches, hygiene, CPR/first aid, medical ethics, clinical practice, business practices and marketing

UNIQUE ASPECTS OF SCHOOL OR CURRICULUM: Graduates receive dual certificates as massage therapist and sports massage specialist.

#70 California College of Physical Arts
     18582 Beach Boulevard, suite 14
     Huntington Beach, CA 92648
     (714) 964-7744

     32332 Camino Capistrano, suite 206
     San Juan Capistrano, CA 92675
     (714) 240-7744

HOURS OF TRAINING: 300 to 1,000

DURATION OF COURSE: 3 months to 12 months

DAY/EVENING/WEEKEND: day, evening and weekend classes available

COST: registration fee $75, each 100-hour segment $775

FINANCIAL AID: Pell grants

YEAR FOUNDED: 1980

ACCREDITATIONS/APPROVALS: ACCET

GRADUATES PER YEAR (APPROX.): 100

MODALITIES AND SUBJECTS: The first 300 hours include history, theory and ethics of massage, hydrotherapy, nutrition, trigger points, professionalism, joint movement, injury care, introduction to holistic theory.

Advanced programs include sports massage, clinical massage, externship, oriental health systems, botanical modalities, acupressure, aromatherapy, choreography, color modalities, geriatric massage, massage for the physically challenged, music modality, postural re-education, practitioner's well-being, reflexology, symptomatic assessment, visualization modality

UNIQUE ASPECTS OF SCHOOL OR CURRICULUM: Placement department is actively involved with the medical community. Externships are available with athletic teams.

Programs offered: massage technician (100 hours), massage therapist (100 hours), advanced massage therapist (100 hours), sports massage therapist I (100 hours), sports massage therapist II (100 hours), clinical massage therapist I (100 hours), clinical massage therapist II (100 hours), massage practitioner (600 hours), myotherapist (700 hours), holistic health practitioner I (1,000 hours), holistic health practitioner II (1,200 hours), massage instructor (600 hours)

CONTINUING EDUCATION: contact school

#71 California Healing Arts College
     12217 Santa Monica Blvd., suite 206
     West Los Angeles, CA 90025
     (310) 826-7622

HOURS OF TRAINING: 150 (all class hours) or 650 (566 class hours, 84 internship)

DURATION OF COURSE: 150-hour course 8 weeks (day + Saturday or evening + Saturday classes available); 650-hour course adds 42 weeks, evenings

COST: 150-hours $1,525 including books; 650-hours $5,575 including books

YEAR FOUNDED: 1988

MODALITIES AND SUBJECTS: 150-hour course includes hygiene, on-site, foot reflexology, herbology, nutrition, oscillation, deep tissue therapy, sports massage, business ethics and practice, CPR/first aid. The 650-hour course adds pathology, kinesiology, acupressure, shiatsu, internship, and advanced courses in business, deep tissue, oscillation herbology, and anatomy and physiology.

#72 Institute of Psycho-Structural Balancing
1131 Olympic Boulevard
Santa Monica, CA 90404
(310) 450-8301

HOURS OF TRAINING: massage technician 120; massage therapist 500

DURATION OF COURSE: 120-hour course 3 to 10 weeks depending on format

DAY/EVENING/WEEKEND: day, evening and weekend programs available

COST: 120-hour course $1,035 including books and supplies

YEAR FOUNDED: 1980

PREPARATION FOR OUT-OF-STATE LICENSING EXAM: 500-hour program may prepare students for some state licenses — contact school for specifics.

GRADUATES PER YEAR (APPROX.): 330

MODALITIES AND SUBJECTS: 120-hour course includes t'ai qi chuan, Esalen massage, body psychology, self-massage, joint mobilization, energy balancing. 500-hour course adds acupressure, advanced circulatory massage, anatomy and physiology, business and professional ethics, CPR/first aid, deep tissue, emotional dynamics of the body, human energy systems, hydrotherapy, hygiene, pathology, electives (see continuing education).

UNIQUE ASPECTS OF SCHOOL OR CURRICULUM: Holistic approach to body/mind integration, use of T'ai Qi to enhance body mechanics of practitioner

ADVANCED PROGRAMS: 1,000-hour professional bodyworker program, polarity certification

CONTINUING EDUCATION: acupressure II, Chinese herbology, cranio-sacral therapy, lymphatic drainage massage, internal organ and post-surgical intervention massage, polarity, pregnancy massage, reflexology, sports massage, trigger point therapy, tui na, aromatherapy, deep tissue

#73 Institute of Therapeutic Studies
3401 W. Sunflower Ave. #125
Santa Ana, CA 92704
(714) 556-7730

HOURS OF TRAINING: 100, 200, 500, 1,000

DURATION OF COURSE: 100-hour class 9 weeks; 1,000-hour program 15 to 18 months

DAY/EVENING/WEEKEND: day, evening and weekend classes available

COST: 100 hours $885, additional 100-hour segments $860; 1,000-hour program $5,325

YEAR FOUNDED: 1989

ACCREDITATIONS/APPROVALS: approved for nursing CEU's, department of vocational rehabilitation

GRADUATES PER YEAR (APPROX.): 50

MODALITIES AND SUBJECTS: sports massage, stretching, Touch for Health, acupressure, t'ai chi, aromatherapy, shiatsu, Oriental herbology, Western herbology, iridology, geriatric massage, prenatal/postnatal massage, massage in chiropractic setting, massage in hospital setting, post-surgical massage, business/administration, advertising/marketing, supervised field work, clinical applications, CPR, cadaver tutorial

UNIQUE ASPECTS OF SCHOOL OR CURRICULUM: All programs are build on the core 100-hour training. Additional trainings are advanced massage technician 200 hours; massage therapist sports massage specialty 500 or 1,000 hours; massage therapist hospital/clinic 500 or 1,000 hours; massage therapist holistic practitioner 500 or 1,000 hours.

ADVANCED PROGRAMS: 100, 600 and 1,000-hour trainings in equine massage

CONTINUING EDUCATION: Many elective courses may be taken as continuing education

#74 Massage School of Santa Monica
1334 Third St., suite 303
Santa Monica, CA 90401
(310) 393-7461 or (310) 453-2386

MSSM Extension
6422½ Coldwater Canyon
North Hollywood, CA 91605
(818) 763-4912

HOURS OF TRAINING: Massage Therapist 150

DURATION OF COURSE: 12 weeks

DAY/EVENING/WEEKEND: day and evening programs available

COST: $1,082 (includes book)

FINANCIAL AID: payment plan

YEAR FOUNDED: 1979

GRADUATES PER YEAR (APPROX.): 240

MODALITIES AND SUBJECTS: ethical, legal and business aspects of massage practice, hygiene, nutrition, self-care

UNIQUE ASPECTS OF SCHOOL OR CURRICULUM: flexible schedule, classes start monthly

CONTINUING EDUCATION: functional anatomy, pathology, deep tissue work, sports massage, trigger points, advanced Swedish, acupressure, reflexology, Feldenkrais, Alexander, hydrotherapy, nutrition, aromatherapy, energy work, human relations, business for bodyworkers, massage movements, tests review

#75 Nova Institute
3000 South Robertson Blvd., 3rd floor
Los Angeles, CA 90034
(310) 840-5777

Contact the school for program information.

#76 Shiatsu Massage School of California
2309 Main St.
Santa Monica, CA 90405
(310) 396-4877

HOURS OF TRAINING: 104, 150, 200

DURATION OF COURSE: 3 to 7 months

DAY/EVENING/WEEKEND: day and evening programs available

COST: 104 hours $1,090; 150 hours $1,550; 200 hours $2,050

YEAR FOUNDED: 1983

ACCREDITATIONS/APPROVALS: approved for nursing CEU's

GRADUATES PER YEAR (APPROX.): 120

MODALITIES AND SUBJECTS: shiatsu, anma, traditional Chinese medicine theory, Do-in, CPR/first aid, ethics/legal/business issues, pain and orthopedic evaluation, clinical study

CONTINUING EDUCATION: Jin Shin Do acupressure, Sotai method for sports injuries, East meets West, Touch for Health, foot reflexology, Tuina Chinese massage, basics in nutritional metabolism, basic sports massage, Oriental philosophy, culture and history

#77 Southern California School of Massage
9980 Indiana Ave., suite 7-8
Riverside, CA 92503
(909) 353-8012

HOURS OF TRAINING: 100 (massage technician); 250 (massage specialist); 500 (massage therapist); 1,000 (holistic health practitioner); 1,150 (massage instructor)

DURATION OF COURSE: 100-hour course may be taken in 10-day intensive format or 5 weekends. Other programs are completed at the student's pace.

DAY/EVENING/WEEKEND: day, evening and weekend classes are available

COST: 100 hours $745; 250 hours $1,895; 500 hours $3,295; 1,000 hours $5,295

YEAR FOUNDED: 1984

ACCREDITATIONS/APPROVALS: approved for nursing CEU's

MODALITIES AND SUBJECTS: history, ethics, acupressure, acupressure facelift, body wraps, cellulite massage, integral body balancing, all about headaches, structural kinesiology, energy systems, mind/body dynamics, deep tissue, CPR, aromatherapy, tui-na, sports massage, Thai massage, pregnancy massage, hospital massage, color therapy, on-site, polarity, reflexology, powder massage, manual lymphatic drainage, face reading, healing with charcoal, ear acureflex, nutrition, social psychology, hydrotherapy, business and marketing, health, hygiene

CONTINUING EDUCATION: All courses may be taken on an individual basis as continuing education.

#78 The Touch Therapy Institute
5170 Sepulveda Blvd. #240
Sherman Oaks, CA 91403
(818) 788-0824

HOURS OF TRAINING: 150, 500, 1,000

DAY/EVENING/WEEKEND: day and evening programs available

YEAR FOUNDED: 1990

MODALITIES AND SUBJECTS: 150-hour course includes ethics, basic communication skills, history and business management, hygiene and nutrition, beginning movement, CPR, practice massage.
   500-hour course adds functional anatomy, kinesiology, Feldenkrais, fieldwork project, advanced communication skills, hydrotherapy, body reading, breath and toning, myofascial reorganization massage plus 102 hours of electives (acupressure, reflexology, connective tissue massage, Esalen, Alexander, sports massage trigger point, nutrition, herbology, chakra massage, pathology)
   1,000-hour training adds fascial anatomy, myofascial reorganization, reichian core contact and craniosacral work.

CONTINUING EDUCATION: contact school

California, Desert Hot Springs

#79 Banning Massage School
66-705 E. 6th Street
Desert Hot Springs, CA 92240
(619) 329-5066

HOURS OF TRAINING: massage specialist 250

DURATION OF COURSE: 10 weeks

COST: $1,770 (includes books)

YEAR FOUNDED: 1989

GRADUATES PER YEAR (APPROX.): 28

MODALITIES AND SUBJECTS: deep tissue massage, reflexology, lymph massage, hydrotherapy, sports massage, structural kinesiology, hygiene, ethics, massage theory, business

UNIQUE ASPECTS OF SCHOOL OR CURRICULUM: Banning is a Christian school and the curriculum includes medical missionary work. Banning is in a rural setting in the mountains

---

#80 Desert Resorts School
13090 Palm Drive
Desert Hot Springs, CA 92240
(619) 329-1175 or (800) 279-1175

HOURS OF TRAINING:
massage technician (M.tech) 100
massage therapist (M.Th) 250
acupressure therapist (AT) 120
holistic health practitioner (HHP) 250
M.Tech is a prerequisite for M.Th (total 350)
M.Tech, M.Th and AT are prerequisites for HHP (total 720)

DAY/EVENING/WEEKEND: day and weekend programs available

COST: M.Tech $750; M.Th $1,485; AT $1,040; HHP $1,490

YEAR FOUNDED: 1991

GRADUATES PER YEAR (APPROX.): 120

MODALITIES AND SUBJECTS: shiatsu, tui na, manual lymphatic drainage, aromatherapy, sports massage, deep tissue, polarity, reflexology, history and theory of massage, business and ethics, kinesiology, aromatherapy, communication skills, hydrotherapy, nutrition, holistic theory, advanced anatomy, massage clinic, sports events

UNIQUE ASPECTS OF SCHOOL OR CURRICULUM: Program is spa oriented and provides travel opportunities, including study in China and Ironman in Hawaii.

ADVANCED PROGRAMS: HHP program (see above)

CONTINUING EDUCATION: contact school

California, San Diego Area

#81 Body Mind College
4050 Sorrento Valley Blvd. #1
San Diego, CA 92121
(619) 453-3295 or (800) BDY-MIND

HOURS OF TRAINING: 100 or 500

DURATION OF COURSE: 100-hour course 3-week intensive or 6 weeks; 500-hour course requires approximately one year

DAY/EVENING/WEEKEND: day, evening and weekend programs available

COST: 100 hours $600; 500-hour program $4,000 (consists of five segments which can be taken individually)

YEAR FOUNDED: 1988

ACCREDITATIONS/APPROVALS: approved for nursing CEU's

GRADUATES PER YEAR (APPROX.): 40 to 50

MODALITIES AND SUBJECTS: 100-hour program includes Esalen, body mechanics, t'ai chi, energy work, body-mind theory, legalities, guidelines for setting up a successful practice

UNIQUE ASPECTS OF SCHOOL OR CURRICULUM: Class size limited to 12

ADVANCED PROGRAMS: The 500-hour and 1,000-hour advanced trainings are made up of modules which may be taken individually. These include advanced body therapy, personal body clearing, personal emotional clearing, personal mental/belief clearing, integration, business practicum, supervised practice, body-mind integration, psycho-spiritual aspects of healing, practitioner development tools, nutrients in food and supplements, counseling skills and practicum, research project

CONTINUING EDUCATION: shiatsu, physical activity & support work for beginners, herbology, healing touch, sports massage, hypnotherapy, Thai massage, releasing the past

---

#82 California College of Holistic Health
5005 Texas St. suite 205
San Diego, CA 92108
(619) 260-0363

HOURS OF TRAINING: 110 to 1,004

DURATION OF COURSE: 2 weeks to one year

DAY/EVENING/WEEKEND: evening classes only

COST: 110 hours $675, 1,000 hours $5,250

FINANCIAL AID: payment plans

YEAR FOUNDED: 1988

GRADUATES PER YEAR (APPROX.): 185

MODALITIES AND SUBJECTS: deep tissue, passive joint mobilization, structural release, sports massage, acupressure, advanced therapeutics, aesthetics, hypnosis, on-site, cranio-sacral, nutrition, polarity, reflexology, professional development, psychology, business management, CPR/first aid, pathology, personal fitness training program

ADVANCED PROGRAMS: The total curriculum is divided into five courses: massage technician (110 hours), massage science (250 hours), massage therapy

(250 hours), massage arts (250 hours) and personal fitness trainer (150 hours). Each course may be taken individually as advanced training.

#83 Healing Hands School of Holistic Health
11064 Pala Loma Drive
Valley Center, CA 92082
(619) 742-3449

HOURS OF TRAINING: 100, 500, 1,000

DURATION OF COURSE: 100 hours 3 to 13 weeks; other courses proportionally longer

DAY/EVENING/WEEKEND: day, evening and weekend courses available

COST: 100 hours $420 ($380 prepaid); additional courses individually priced

MODALITIES AND SUBJECTS: body mechanics, deep tissue manipulation, communication skills, Oriental healing techniques, shiatsu, tui na, hypnotherapy technician training, teacher training, drug and alcohol recovery practicum, structural organization, neuromuscular therapy, reflexology, subtle touch: transformational bodywork, herbal body wrap workshop, on-site, the compassionate communication—a bridge to empathy, geriatric massage, cranio-sacral therapy, Touch for Health, herbology, yoga

UNIQUE ASPECTS OF SCHOOL OR CURRICULUM: The 100-hour program includes basic Swedish massage, anatomy and physiology. All other courses are offered individually and counted toward advanced certifications

#84 International Professional School of Bodywork
1366 Hornblend St.
San Diego, CA 92109
(619) 272-4142 or (800) 748-6497

HOURS OF TRAINING: 120 (level I), 270 (level I + II), 600 (level I + II + III), 1,000 (level I + II + III + IV)

DURATION OF COURSE: 120 hours 3 weeks or 12 weeks; 1,000 hours 12 to 18 months

COST: application fee $100; 120 hours $835, 270 hours $1,880, 600 hours $4,170, 1,000 hours $6,950

YEAR FOUNDED: 1977

ACCREDITATIONS/APPROVALS: COMTAA, Department of Vocational Rehabilitation, approved for veterans' training, approved for nursing CEU's

GRADUATES PER YEAR (APPROX.): 200

MODALITIES AND SUBJECTS: Level I includes Esalen, deep tissue work, passive joint manipulation, muscle sculpting, body psychology, hygiene, ethics, business and legal issues.
    Level II adds clinical applications, deep tissue sculpting, oriental theory, personal assimilation.

Level III (massage therapist) adds supervised practice, anatomy and physiology, supervised clinical application, electives (such as sports massage, zone therapy, Alexander, Feldenkrais, Bartenieff fundamentals, kinesiology, dance and movement therapy), creating a professional practice.
    Level IV (Holistic Health Practitioner) adds neuromuscular therapy, supervised practice, three electives, psychotherapeutic techniques, supervised clinical application, directed study, creating your professional practice, principles of structural integration, advanced technique internship

UNIQUE ASPECTS OF SCHOOL OR CURRICULUM: The curriculum integrates the student's body/mind and supports growth and change. The school is affiliated with Reidman Center in Tel Aviv, Israel, and some IPSB classes are offered in Montana, Amsterdam, Montreal and New Orleans.

ADVANCED PROGRAMS: 600 to 1,600 additional hours are available in advanced specializations, such as Oriental massage, sports massage, Thai massage, somato-emotional integration, structural integration and neuromuscular therapy.

CONTINUING EDUCATION: contact school

#85 Mueller College of Holistic Studies
4607 Park Blvd.
San Diego, CA 92116
(619) 291-9811 or (800) 245-1976

HOURS OF TRAINING: 512

DURATION OF COURSE: 6 months to one year

DAY/EVENING/WEEKEND: day, evening and intensive programs are available

COST: $4,325 plus $340 supplies

FINANCIAL AID: work-study is available

YEAR FOUNDED: 1976

ACCREDITATIONS/APPROVALS: COMTAA

PREPARATION FOR OUT-OF-STATE LICENSING EXAM: preparation can be arranged for most states' exams; contact school for particulars

GRADUATES PER YEAR (APPROX.): 60 to 80

MODALITIES AND SUBJECTS: sports massage, trigger point, body mechanics, myo-fascial release, cranio-sacral release, hydrotherapy, cryotherapy, acupressure, principles of ayurveda, use of energy for healing, pregnancy massage, lymphatic drainage massage, palliative massage for trauma, body/mind, business procedures for private practice, entrepreneurship

UNIQUE ASPECTS OF SCHOOL OR CURRICULUM: The program can also be coordinated with community college courses, using training at Mueller for hands-on courses.

ADVANCED PROGRAMS: holistic health practitioner, 1,000 hours, adds 488 hours of instruction to massage therapist program

CONTINUING EDUCATION: Trager, foot reflexology, palpation, integrative neurology, Thai massage, introduction to ayurveda, Reiki, introduction to deep tissue massage, on-site, acupressure, jin shin, deep tissue, healing breath, fine tuning

#86 School of Healing Arts
1001 Garnet #200
San Diego, CA 92109
(619) 581-9429

HOURS OF TRAINING: 110, 500, 1,000

DURATION OF COURSE: 110 hours 2-week intensive or 11 weeks evenings/weekends; 1,000 hours approx. 2 years

COST: 110 hours $636 including books; 1,000 hours $5,200

FINANCIAL AID: payment plan

YEAR FOUNDED: 1984

ACCREDITATIONS/APPROVALS: approved for veterans benefits and vocational rehabilitation, approved for nursing CEU's

GRADUATES PER YEAR (APPROX.): 250

MODALITIES AND SUBJECTS: 110-hour massage technician certification: zen-touch, shiatsu, nutritional counseling, hypnotherapy, movement, communication, counseling, food preparation, herbology

UNIQUE ASPECTS OF SCHOOL OR CURRICULUM: flexible schedule, blending of eastern and western modalities, school's location 3 blocks from Pacific ocean

ADVANCED PROGRAMS: nutritional counselor, clinical massage therapist, fitness consultant, holistic health practitioner

CONTINUING EDUCATION: contact school

Colorado

No State licensing

Schools:

#87 Boulder School of Massage Therapy
3285 30th St.
Boulder, CO 80301
(800) 442-5131 or (303) 443-5131

HOURS OF TRAINING: 1,000

DURATION OF COURSE: days one year full-time; evenings 2 years

COST: $7,290

FINANCIAL AID: Pell grants, Stafford, loans

YEAR FOUNDED: 1975

ACCREDITATIONS/APPROVALS: COMTAA, ACCSCT

GRADUATES PER YEAR (APPROX.): 185

MODALITIES AND SUBJECTS: Required courses: movement, shiatsu, career development, communication skills, human sexuality, ethics, kinesiology, body centered therapy, integrative massage, neuromuscular therapy, myofascial release, nutrition, pathology, hydrotherapy, internship/field placement, clinic practicum. Electives include sports massage, reflexology, polarity, infant massage, herbology, yoga, intermediate shiatsu and intermediate Swedish massage

UNIQUE ASPECTS OF SCHOOL OR CURRICULUM: body/mind emphasis

ADVANCED PROGRAMS: hospital-based massage therapy

CONTINUING EDUCATION: St. John neuromuscular therapy, Feldenkrais, manual lymphatic drainage, infant massage for instructors; contact school for other courses

#88 Collinson School of Therapeutics and Massage
2596 Palmer Park Blvd.,
Colorado Springs, CO 80909
(719) 473-0145

HOURS OF TRAINING: 1,000

IN-CLASS HOURS: 160

DURATION OF COURSE: One four-hour evening class per week for 40 weeks plus 21 hours of study time each week

COST: $2,800 includes books and supplies

FINANCIAL AID: payment plan

YEAR FOUNDED: 1982

GRADUATES PER YEAR (APPROX.): 30

MODALITIES AND SUBJECTS: sports massage, stress massage, infancy and pregnancy massage, foot reflexology, acupressure therapy, shiatsu, Reiki, Trager, applied kinesiology, Touch for Health, Rolfing, herbology/nutrition, CPR, hydrotherapy, how to start a business/business law, licensing laws and regulations

#89 Colorado Institute of Massage Therapy
(formerly Stress Management Institute)
P.O. Box 1304, 934 Manitou Ave.
Manitou Springs, CO 80829
(719) 685-5431

HOURS OF TRAINING: 1,150 (including 159 hours of documented practice)

DURATION OF COURSE: one year

DAY/EVENING/WEEKEND: day and evening programs available

COST: $5,700

FINANCIAL AID: approved for V.A. benefits, Industrial Job Training and Vocational Rehabilitation, payment plan

YEAR FOUNDED: 1985

ACCREDITATIONS/APPROVALS: COMTAA, Department of Immigration

MODALITIES AND SUBJECTS: deep tissue, reflexology, neuromuscular therapy, structural kinesiology, pathology, sports massage, intuitive massage, massage for elderly, arthritic and bedridden persons, medical massage (applications to injuries and pain), psychological aspects of massage, hydrotherapy, exercise/stretching, muscle testing, nutrition, motion pressure point therapy, survey of bodywork disciplines, self-care, theory of massage and wholistic health, ethics, history, equipment, hygiene, clinical practice, business practices

UNIQUE ASPECTS OF SCHOOL OR CURRICULUM: Anatomiken models used in anatomy class, internship program in local hospital, certificate in neuromuscular therapy awarded as part of massage program

#90 Colorado School of Healing Arts
7655 West Mississippi, suite 100
Lakewood, CO 80226
(303) 986-2320

HOURS OF TRAINING: 650

IN-CLASS HOURS: 546

DURATION OF COURSE: 12 to 18 months

DAY/EVENING/WEEKEND: day, evening and weekend programs available

COST: $4,725

FINANCIAL AID: payment plans, Colorado Department of Vocational Rehabilitation, Veterans Administration Department of Rehabilitation

YEAR FOUNDED: 1988

PREPARATION FOR OUT-OF-STATE LICENSING EXAM: can prepare students for any state exam; contact school for specifics

GRADUATES PER YEAR (APPROX.): 125

MODALITIES AND SUBJECTS: Massage level I & II & III, body centered therapy, healing touch, applied kinesiology, diet & nutrition, business, sports massage I, massage clinical. Massage modalities include Swedish, deep tissue, neuromuscular, corrective soft tissue

injury intervention, hydrotherapy and emotional release facilitation.

UNIQUE ASPECTS OF SCHOOL OR CURRICULUM: The school emphasizes a sense of community, and views the field as a service to humanity, and encourages students to link the training with their spiritual and professional goals.

ADVANCED PROGRAMS: Trauma Touch Therapy, corrective tissue biomechanics, AnchorPoint system, sports massage, polarity therapy, hospital based massage, chiropractic adjunct, life credit program (350 hours of electives may be added to regular course for 1,000 hour certification)

CONTINUING EDUCATION: elective classes may be taken as continuing education

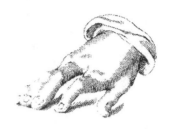

#91 Colorado Springs Academy of
Therapeutic Massage
3612 Galley Rd., suite A
Colorado Springs, CO 80909
(719) 597-3414 or (719) 597-0017

HOURS OF TRAINING: 1,100

DURATION OF COURSE: 8 months

DAY/EVENING/WEEKEND: day and evening programs available

COST: $3,000 (includes books)

FINANCIAL AID: payment plans, job training placement act

YEAR FOUNDED: 1992

GRADUATES PER YEAR (APPROX.): 65

MODALITIES AND SUBJECTS: history of massage, palpation, deep tissue, sports massage, trigger point, neuromuscular release, continuity, nutrition and weight control, hydrotherapy, lymphatic massage, stress therapy, role of massage in injury rehabilitation, building a successful business, student clinic

UNIQUE ASPECTS OF SCHOOL OR CURRICULUM: The curriculum includes 490 class hours of anatomy and physiology. The school also has a video laser-disc program with over 600 hours of human dissection that complements the anatomy class, and also uses the maniken system.

CONTINUING EDUCATION: nutrition, infant massage, geriatric massage; for other topics contact school

#92 Cottonwood School of Massage Therapy
2620 S. Parker Rd. #300
Aurora, CO 80014
(303) 745-7725

HOURS OF TRAINING: 500

DURATION OF COURSE: one year

COST: $3,000

YEAR FOUNDED: 1992

GRADUATES PER YEAR (APPROX.): 35

MODALITIES AND SUBJECTS: deep tissue massage, neuromuscular therapy

ADVANCED PROGRAMS: advanced neuromuscular technique

CONTINUING EDUCATION: therapeutic touch, Reiki, business and insurance

#93 Massage Therapy Institute of Colorado
1441 York St., suite #301
Denver, CO 80206
(303) 329-6345

HOURS OF TRAINING: 1,044

IN-CLASS HOURS: 594

DURATION OF COURSE: one year

DAY/EVENING/WEEKEND: day, evening and weekend programs available

COST: $5,645 (includes books, massage gable, supplies and insurance)

FINANCIAL AID: payment plan

YEAR FOUNDED: 1986

PREPARATION FOR OUT-OF-STATE LICENSING EXAM: Nebraska, Washington, Oregon

GRADUATES PER YEAR (APPROX.): 130

MODALITIES AND SUBJECTS: Required courses: deep tissue, neuromuscular therapy, reflexology, kinesiology, myofascial release, hydrotherapy, heliotherapy, clinical practicum, including two advanced clinics.
  Electives: polarity, Reiki, shiatsu, infant massage, geriatric massage, psychotherapy and bodywork, lomi lomi, Japanese massage, sports massage, cranio-sacral therapy, human engineering, soft tissue manipulation, Fisher method, therapeutic touch, energy work, homeopathy, acupressure, movement, chi gong, yoga

UNIQUE ASPECTS OF SCHOOL OR CURRICULUM: The program is designed for working persons, and fits their schedule. Practice-building assistance is given during the program.

ADVANCED PROGRAMS: structural integration, special programs for nurses, EMT's, respiratory therapists and physical trainers

CONTINUING EDUCATION: Elective may be taken as continuing education.

Connecticut

State Licensing 500 hours

National Certification Exam accepted

School:

#94 Connecticut Center For Massage Therapy, Inc.
75 Kitts Lane
Newington, CT 06111
(203) 667-1886
(all courses)

25 Sylvan Road South
Westport, CT 06880
(203) 221-7325
(New York licensure course only)

HOURS OF TRAINING: 600 or 635 (New York licensure program)

DURATION OF COURSE: 15 months days, 19 months evenings

COST: 600-hour course $8,325; 635-hour course $8,525

FINANCIAL AID: Pell grants, Stafford Loans, PLUS loans, approved for veterans' benefits

YEAR FOUNDED: 1982

ACCREDITATIONS/APPROVALS: COMTAA, ACCSCT

PREPARATION FOR OUT-OF-STATE LICENSING EXAM: New York

GRADUATES PER YEAR (APPROX.): 180

MODALITIES AND SUBJECTS: Massage therapist program includes acupressure, hydrotherapy, cross-fiber massage, screening clients, documenting treatment, positioning clients, athletic massage, business practices, energetic foundations, kinesiology, palpation lab, self-care, first aid/CPR, student clinic, internship.
  Shiatsu therapist program also includes alexander technique, east-west pathology, meridian theory, shiatsu.
  New York massage therapist also includes Jin Shin Do, neurology, Oriental studies, professional foundations.

UNIQUE ASPECTS OF SCHOOL OR CURRICULUM: The school offers three programs: massage therapist, shiatsu therapist, New York massage therapist. The programs include community service and outreach.

CONTINUING EDUCATION: contact school

Delaware

*State Certification: 500 hours
or 300 hours plus 2 years practice*

After several years in the works, a new massage certification law was put in place in June 1994, and the first five certified practitioners were approved in December of that year.

Delaware has long regulated massage as "adult entertainment" and has subjected the practice of massage to vice laws. This new law creates an exemption to the adult entertainment law for persons who obtain certification to practice massage or bodywork in Delaware. Certification is voluntary, but those who practice without certification fall under the adult entertainment law.

The approved curriculum for certification is 50 hours anatomy, 50 hours physiology, 300 hours technique and theory and 100 hours electives. The National Certification Exam is not accepted for Delaware certification.

For further information and for an application, call (302) 739-4522, ext. 205.

School:

#95 Owens Institute of Media, Pennsylvania
     opened a school in Wilmington in 1994.

For program information contact the Owens Institute at (800) 996-9367

District of Columbia

No local licensing

School:

#96 Potomac Massage Training Institute
     4000 Albermarle St., NW, 5th floor
     Washington, D.C. 20016
     (202) 686-7046

HOURS OF TRAINING: approx. 1,171

IN-CLASS HOURS: 500

DURATION OF COURSE: 18 months part-time

DAY/EVENING/WEEKEND: day, evening and evening/weekend programs available

COST: $4,850

FINANCIAL AID: payment plan

YEAR FOUNDED: 1976

ACCREDITATIONS/APPROVALS: COMTAA

GRADUATES PER YEAR (APPROX.): 70

MODALITIES AND SUBJECTS: kinesiology, deep tissue work, communication, business and professional skills, clinic, massage practice, study and homework, supervised fieldwork, independent fieldwork

CONTINUING EDUCATION: Touch for Health, myofascial release, sports massage, advanced sports massage, neuromuscular therapy, tui na, bodywork for the childbearing year, movement for massage therapists, lomi lomi, craniosacral therapy, visceral manipulation

Florida

State Licensing: 500 hours

National Certification Exam accepted

Approved out-of-state schools:

Alexandria School, Alexandria IN
Atlanta School, Atlanta GA
Blue Cliff School, Baton Rouge LA
Body Therapy Inst., Pittsboro NC
Massage Academy of the South, Baton Rouge LA
New Mexico Academy of Massage, Santa Fe NM
Somerset School, Somerset NJ

Schools:

#97 Academy of Healing Arts Massage & Facial
     Skin Care, Inc.
     3141 South Military Trail
     Lake Worth, FL 33463
     (407) 965-5550

HOURS OF TRAINING: 600

DURATION OF COURSE: normally seven months, can be completed in 17 weeks

COST: $3,800

ACCREDITATIONS/APPROVALS: approved for veterans' training

GRADUATES PER YEAR (APPROX.): 100

MODALITIES AND SUBJECTS: pathology, HIV/AIDS, joint movement, trigger point, hydrotherapy, statutes/rules/history, good business practices, aromatherapy, introduction to reflexology, digestive massage, neuromuscular therapy, acupressure, nutrition, soma therapy, lymphatic drainage, sports massage, Touch for Health, nutritional health management

CONTINUING EDUCATION: reflexology, lymphatic drainage methods, arthritis self-help, nature of disease, Reiki, client centered massage, shiatsu, aromatherapy, Touch for Health, embodiment workshop, facial massage techniques, connective tissue therapy, european body wraps

#98 Acupressure/Acupuncture Institute
9835 Sunset Dr., suite 206
Miami, FL 33173
(305) 595-9500

Contact the school for program information.

#99 Alpha School of Massage, Inc.
4642 San Juan Ave.
Jacksonville, FL 32210
(904) 389-9117

HOURS OF TRAINING: 500

DURATION OF COURSE: 6 months

DAY/EVENING/WEEKEND: day and evening programs available

COST: $2,500 (includes books)

YEAR FOUNDED: 1993

GRADUATES PER YEAR (APPROX.): 250

MODALITIES AND SUBJECTS: reflexology, neuromuscular therapy, structural integration, applied kinesiology, hydrotherapy, acupressure, aromatherapy, sports massage, flexibility exercise, psychology of massage, infant and pregnancy massage, HIV education

#100 America Duran Skin Care School
2100 Coral Way
Miami, FL 33145
(305) 642-4104

Contact the school for program information.

#101 American Institute of Massage Therapy, Inc.
2101 North Federal Highway
Ft. Lauderdale, FL 33305
(305) 568-6200 or (800) 752-2793

HOURS OF TRAINING: 600

DURATION OF COURSE: 6 months

DAY/EVENING/WEEKEND: day and evening programs available

COST: $3,400

FINANCIAL AID: payment plans

YEAR FOUNDED: 1983

ACCREDITATIONS/APPROVALS: ACCET

GRADUATES PER YEAR (APPROX.): 100

MODALITIES AND SUBJECTS: pathology, on-site, neuromuscular techniques, postural integration, Trager, sports massage, Rolfing, reflexology, lymphatic drainage, chiropractic modalities, infant massage, aromatherapy, hydrotherapy, cryotherapy, range of motion, colonic irrigation, natural remedies, traumatic injuries, psychology, nutrition, kinesiotherapeutic stretching, insurance billing, case assessment, goal setting, statutes and rules of massage, CPR, HIV/AIDS, field trip, practicum, communication skills, marketing and business practice

ADVANCED PROGRAMS: colonic irrigation therapy

#102 Atlantic Academy
4427 Emerson St.
Jacksonville, FL 32207
(904) 398-2359 or (800) 448-2359

HOURS OF TRAINING: 500

DAY/EVENING/WEEKEND: day and evening programs available

COST: $3,100 (includes books, supplies and instructional materials)

MODALITIES AND SUBJECTS: myology, kinesiology, massage law, hydrotherapy, AIDS, neuromuscular basics, sports massage basics, reflexology, infant massage, pregnancy massage, on-site-chair, business practices, heliotherapy.

ADVANCED PROGRAMS: advanced neuromuscular, advanced sports massage, manual lymphatic drainage, advanced reflexology, shiatsu, Bowen technique, bodywork-structural and awareness

#103 Boca Raton Institute
5499 North Federal Highway, suite A
Boca Raton, FL 33487
(407) 241-8105 or (800) 275-6764

HOURS OF TRAINING: 605

DURATION OF COURSE: 6 months days, 7½ months evenings

YEAR FOUNDED: 1983

ACCREDITATIONS/APPROVALS: National Accrediting Commission of Cosmetology Arts and Sciences

MODALITIES AND SUBJECTS: shiatsu, reflexology, sports massage, kinesiology, deep relaxation techniques, neuromuscular therapy, Rolfing, exercise physiology, stress management, somatic therapy, craniosacral techniques, hydrotherapy, business principles and Florida law, AIDS/HIV education, required clinics

UNIQUE ASPECTS OF SCHOOL OR CURRICULUM: The school offers a combined 905-hour skin care and massage program.

#104 Core Institute
      223 W. Carolina St.
      Tallahassee, FL 32301
      (904) 222-8673

HOURS OF TRAINING: 500

IN-CLASS HOURS: 500

DURATION OF COURSE: 6 months full-time, 12 months part-time

DAY/EVENING/WEEKEND: day and evening classes available

COST: $4,231.27 (includes books)

FINANCIAL AID: payment plan, VA benefits, job training program, vocational rehabilitation

YEAR FOUNDED: 1990

ACCREDITATIONS/APPROVALS: COMTAA

GRADUATES PER YEAR (APPROX.): 80

MODALITIES AND SUBJECTS: core massage, sports massage, shiatsu, polarity, Trager, trigger point, medical massage, hydrotherapy, law business, communications, wellness

UNIQUE ASPECTS OF SCHOOL OR CURRICULUM: Community service is stressed.

ADVANCED PROGRAMS: Core Body Therapy (structural integration), neuromuscular therapy certification, clinical sports massage, medical massage.

CONTINUING EDUCATION: Thai massage, seated massage experience, Trager, polarity, applied anatomy, TMJ, therapeutic touch, HIV/AIDS, feet and lower back

#105 Educating Hands School of Massage
      261 Southwest 8th St.
      Miami, FL 33130
      (305) 285-6991 or (800) 999-6991

HOURS OF TRAINING: 624

DURATION OF COURSE: 6 months days, 8 or 11 months evenings

COST: $3,645

FINANCIAL AID: payment plans

YEAR FOUNDED: 1981

ACCREDITATIONS/APPROVALS: COMTAA

GRADUATES PER YEAR (APPROX.): 104

MODALITIES AND SUBJECTS: acupressure, sports massage, polarity, lymphatic drainage, reflexology, craniosacral, shiatsu, meditation, aromatherapy, connective tissue massage, Hoshino therapy, Trager, Touch for Health, deep relaxation, guided imagery, HIV/AIDS, corrective exercise and movement, understanding the client/practitioner relationship,

relaxation techniques, pathology, kinesiology and palpation, body mechanics, student clinic, hydrotherapy, heliotherapy, business principles and development

UNIQUE ASPECTS OF SCHOOL OR CURRICULUM: Oriented toward personal growth

CONTINUING EDUCATION: connective tissue massage, on-site, infant massage, neuromuscular therapy, polarity therapy, shiatsu, sports massage, deep tissue, Hoshino, Trager, stretching

#106 Euro-Skill Therapeutic Training Center
      500 NE Spanish River Blvd., suite 25-26
      Boca Raton, FL 33431
      (407) 395-3089 or 392-5288

HOURS OF TRAINING: 600

DURATION OF COURSE: 20 weeks

DAY/EVENING/WEEKEND: day and evening programs available

COST: $3,500

FINANCIAL AID: payment plans

YEAR FOUNDED: 1989

ACCREDITATIONS/APPROVALS: Southern Association of Colleges and Schools Commission on Occupational Educational Institutions, approved for veterans' benefits

MODALITIES AND SUBJECTS: shiatsu, sports massage, kinesiology, deep tissue, neuromuscular, chair massage, reflexology Trager, trigger point, connective tissue, lymphatic drainage, pathology, dietetics and nutrition, hydrotherapy, HIV/AIDS course, remedial exercises, self-care and communication, business management, Florida rules and regulations, hygiene, public health, first aid/CPR, heliotherapy, clinical lab practice

UNIQUE ASPECTS OF SCHOOL OR CURRICULUM: Transfer credit may be arranged for courses taken at another educational institution. The school also offers a 100-hour colon therapy course.

#107 Fabulous Fingers Academy
      209 Dunlawton
      Port Orange 32119
      (904) 788-5550

HOURS OF TRAINING: 510

DURATION OF COURSE: 6 months

DAY/EVENING/WEEKEND: day and evening programs available

COST: $3,200 (plus lab fee of approx. $20)

FINANCIAL AID: payment plans

YEAR FOUNDED: 1985

GRADUATES PER YEAR (APPROX.): 80 to 100

MODALITIES AND SUBJECTS: sports massage, polarity therapy, animal massage, reflexology, neuromuscular therapy, trigger point, meditation/relaxation, touch therapy, shiatsu, hydrotherapy, osteology, kinesiology, state laws, business course, HIV/AIDS/CPR and vitals

UNIQUE ASPECTS OF SCHOOL OR CURRICULUM: Class size is kept small for individualized attention.

CONTINUING EDUCATION: kinesiology, reflexology, polarity therapy

#108 Florida Academy of Massage
      8695 College Parkway suite 110
      Ft. Myers, FL 33919
      (813) 489-2282

Contact the school for program information.

#109 Florida Institute of Massage Therapy and
      Esthetics
      5453 N. University Dr.
      Lauderhill, FL 33351
      (305) 742-8399 or (800) 541-9299

      7925 NW 12th St., Suite 201
      Miami, FL 33126
      (305) 597-9599 or (800) 599-9599

HOURS OF TRAINING: 624

DURATION OF COURSE: 5 to 7 months

DAY/EVENING/WEEKEND: day and evening programs available

COST: $4,215 (includes books)

FINANCIAL AID: federal Pell grants, supplemental educational opportunity grant, work-study, Stafford loans, PLUS loans

YEAR FOUNDED: 1986

ACCREDITATIONS/APPROVALS: ACCSCT, COMTAA

GRADUATES PER YEAR (APPROX.): 250

MODALITIES AND SUBJECTS: hydrotherapy, shiatsu, reflexology, sports massage, kinesiology, deep relaxation techniques, neuromuscular therapy, Trager, Rolfing, exercise physiology, CPR, stress management, infant massage, craniosacral therapy, HIV/AIDS, state law, business principles and development

UNIQUE ASPECTS OF SCHOOL OR CURRICULUM: The school's courses in skin care or sports massage can be combined with the massage program.

ADVANCED PROGRAMS: Skin care/esthetics, Advanced sports massage

CONTINUING EDUCATION: infant massage, practice building, aromatherapy, seated massage, spa therapy, acupressure, equine massage, Oriental massage

#110 Florida School of Massage
      6421 SW 13th Street
      Gainesville, FL 32608
      (904) 378-7891

HOURS OF TRAINING: 1,000

IN-CLASS HOURS: 650

DURATION OF COURSE: approx. 5½ months

COST: $4,250

YEAR FOUNDED: 1973

ACCREDITATIONS/APPROVALS: COMTAA, Department of Vocational Rehabilitation, Bureau of Blind Services, Office for Social Security, approved for veterans' training, approved by national YMCA Health Service Director's Society

PREPARATION FOR OUT-OF-STATE LICENSING EXAM: New York (additional training required)

GRADUATES PER YEAR (APPROX.): 150

MODALITIES AND SUBJECTS: reflexology, neuromuscular therapy, sports massage, polarity, connective tissue massage, massage for infants, pregnant, elderly, or arthritic persons, five element theory, treatments for specific pathologies, clinic internship, hydrotherapy, pathology, awareness and communication skills, stress awareness and movement, massage law and business practices, first aid/CPR, living with AIDS, directed independent study project

UNIQUE ASPECTS OF SCHOOL OR CURRICULUM: Credit may be given for study completed elsewhere.

ADVANCED PROGRAMS: polarity certification program, sports massage certification program, structural bodywork and awareness program, teacher's assistant program

CONTINUING EDUCATION: living with AIDS, arthritis massage, colonic irrigation certification workshop, connective tissue therapy, evaluation and treatment of shoulder injuries, advanced neuromuscular therapy, ortho-bionomy, shiatsu, pregnancy massage, present centered awareness therapy, reflexology, soft tissue injuries in athletics, soft tissue injury assessment and therapeutic techniques

#111 Florida's Therapeutic Massage School
      1300 East Gadsden St.
      Pensacola, FL 32501
      (904) 433-8212

HOURS OF TRAINING: 600 including 100 hours clinic internship

DURATION OF COURSE: 6 months

DAY/EVENING/WEEKEND: day and evening programs available

COST: $3,400 including required textbooks

FINANCIAL AID: payment plan

MODALITIES AND SUBJECTS: reflexology, sports massage, neuromuscular therapy, deep tissue massage, polarity, kinesiology, pathology, hydrotherapy, massage laws, AIDS/HIV education, communication skills, business ethics and practices, movement, nutrition, herbology, CPR, clinic internship

UNIQUE ASPECTS OF SCHOOL OR CURRICULUM: Class size is limited to 22 to allow for individualized instruction. Transfer credit may be allowed for work completed at other schools.

ADVANCED PROGRAMS: polarity certification

CONTINUING EDUCATION: neuromuscular therapy, Touch for Health, advanced sports massage, introduction to herbal medicine, AIDS awareness for LMT's, Trager

#112 Humanities Center School of Massage
4045 Park Blvd.
Pinellas Park, FL 34665
(813) 541-5200

HOURS OF TRAINING: 625

DURATION OF COURSE: 8 months days, 9 months evenings

COST: $5,230 (includes books)

FINANCIAL AID: Stafford loans, Pell grants

YEAR FOUNDED: 1981

ACCREDITATIONS/APPROVALS: COMTAA, ACCSCT

GRADUATES PER YEAR (APPROX.): 160

MODALITIES AND SUBJECTS: maniken anatomy, Esalen, sexual ethics, body mechanics, range of motion, sports therapy, Rolfing, polarity, reflexology, business practices, shiatsu, clinic internship, massage law, hydrotherapy, HIV/AIDS education, neuromuscular therapies (trigger point, strain-counterstrain, muscle energy technique, myofascial release, shiatsu, postural analysis, clinic)

UNIQUE ASPECTS OF SCHOOL OR CURRICULUM: small classes, emphasis on neuromuscular therapies

ADVANCED PROGRAMS: myofascial release

CONTINUING EDUCATION: contact school

#113 International Unisex Academy
529-537 East 9 Street
Hialeah, FL 33010
(305) 884-2499

Contact the school for program information.

#114 Jacksonville School of Massage Therapy
6524 San Juan Ave.
Jacksonville, FL 32210
(904) 781-3153

HOURS OF TRAINING: 510

DURATION OF COURSE: six months, evenings

COST: $2,215 including books and supplies

YEAR FOUNDED: 1980

MODALITIES AND SUBJECTS: joint movements, case studies, pathology, hydrotherapy, heliotherapy, neuromuscular therapy, structural integration, reflexology, applied kinesiology, aromatherapy, acupressure, exercise, sports massage, nutrition, psychology of massage, florida laws, rules, history of massage, HIV/AIDS

UNIQUE ASPECTS OF SCHOOL OR CURRICULUM: Transfer credits from another school may be recognized.

CONTINUING EDUCATION: back pain chair and beyond, massage as a help for arthritis and strokes, colon hygiene course

#115 Lindsey Hopkins Technical Education Center
750 Northwest 20th St.
Miami, FL 33127
(305) 324-6070

HOURS OF TRAINING: 720

DURATION OF COURSE: 8 months

DAY/EVENING/WEEKEND: day and evening programs available

COST: $350

FINANCIAL AID: approved for veterans, JTPA, and other agencies. Call for specific information.

YEAR FOUNDED: around 1960

ACCREDITATIONS/APPROVALS: Southern University System

MODALITIES AND SUBJECTS: theory of massage, professionalism, client/therapist relationship, joint movement and range of motion, Florida law and rules, hydrotherapy, survey of allied modalities, AIDS education

#116 Mandarin School of Chinese Medicine
11018 Old St. Augustine Rd. #136
Jacksonville, FL 32257
(904) 292-0009

HOURS OF TRAINING: 530

DURATION OF COURSE: 9 months

DAY/EVENING/WEEKEND: day and evening programs available

COST: $3.075

YEAR FOUNDED: 1986

GRADUATES PER YEAR (APPROX.): 30

MODALITIES AND SUBJECTS: hydrotherapy, rules and regulations, AIDS education, reflexology, therapeutic touch, neuromuscular therapy, shiatsu, polarity, Reiki, massage for elderly, disabled, pregnant, athletes, AIDS patients, body mechanics, body/mind, self care, business and marketing, professional development, supervised student clinic, CPR

ADVANCED PROGRAMS: The school also offers a 3-year acupuncture training.

CONTINUING EDUCATION: contact school

#117 Orlando Institute School of Massage
      Therapy, Inc.
      Casselberry Collection
      3385 S. Hwy 17-92, suite 221
      Casselberry, FL 32707
      (407) 331-1101

HOURS OF TRAINING: 500

DURATION OF COURSE: Students can proceed at their own pace.

DAY/EVENING/WEEKEND: day and evening programs available

COST: $3,000 (includes books)

FINANCIAL AID: payment plan

YEAR FOUNDED: 1989

MODALITIES AND SUBJECTS: hydrotherapy, acupressure, polarity, lymphatic drainage, muscle testing, connective tissue massage, deep relaxation techniques, business principles and development, HIV/AIDS

CONTINUING EDUCATION: 12 hours advanced massage

#118 Port Charlotte School of Massage Therapy
      1057 Colllingswood Blvd., Unit A
      Port Charlotte, FL 33953
      (813) 255-1966

Contact the school for program information.

#119 Reese Institute, Inc.
      School of Massage Therapy
      425 Geneva Drive
      Oviedo, FL 32765
      (407) 365-9283

HOURS OF TRAINING: 600

DURATION OF COURSE: days 6 months, evenings one year

COST: $4,465 (includes books)

FINANCIAL AID: payment plan

YEAR FOUNDED: 1983

ACCREDITATIONS/APPROVALS: COMTAA

MODALITIES AND SUBJECTS: hydrotherapy, reflexology, integrative massage, deep tissue massage, business practices, high-level wellness, allied modalities, practicum/professional issues, first aid & CPR, HIV/AIDS, statutes, rules and history of massage, therapeutic stretching, pathology, sports massage, shiatsu, assisted flexibility stretching

UNIQUE ASPECTS OF SCHOOL OR CURRICULUM: The school is on a 6½ acre campus with landscaped gardens, pool and sauna.

ADVANCED PROGRAMS: 100-hour clinical internship, 300-hour program in pain and stress management

CONTINUING EDUCATION: numerous programs offered; contact school

#120 Ridge Technical Center
      7700 State Road 544
      Winter Haven, FL 33881
      (813) 422-6402 or (813) 299-2512

HOURS OF TRAINING: 518

DURATION OF COURSE: approx. six months

DAY/EVENING/WEEKEND: day and evening programs available

COST: $329 evenings, $536 days

FINANCIAL AID: veterans administration, vocational rehabilitation, Pell grants, JTPA, Single Parent/Displaced Homemaker, farm-worker, scholarships, workers compensation, social security

ACCREDITATIONS/APPROVALS: Southern Association of Colleges and Schools

MODALITIES AND SUBJECTS: hydrotherapy, hygiene, legal aspects of massage practice, allied modalities, leadership, leadership, human relations skills, health and safety, CPR and employability skills

#121 Sarasota School of Massage Therapy
      1970 Main St.
      Sarasota, FL 34236
      (813) 957-0577

HOURS OF TRAINING: 540

DURATION OF COURSE: 25 weeks

DAY/EVENING/WEEKEND: day and evening programs available

COST: $3,075

YEAR FOUNDED: 1991

GRADUATES PER YEAR (APPROX.): 90

MODALITIES AND SUBJECTS: hydrotherapy, Florida law, HIV/AIDS education, introduction to instrumentation, client rapport, business management and marketing, movement physiology, nutrition, pathology, CPR, sports massage, neuromuscular therapy, medical terminology, zen shiatsu, polarity, Rolfing, Jin Shin Do, reflexology, positional release, infant massage, animal massage, spinal touch

UNIQUE ASPECTS OF SCHOOL OR CURRICULUM: internship with Florida Marlins, hospital internship

CONTINUING EDUCATION: contact school

#126 Suncoast School
4910 Cypress St.
Tampa, FL 33607
(813) 287-1099 or (813) 287-1050

HOURS OF TRAINING: 500 or 600

DURATION OF COURSE: 6 months

COST: 500 hours $3,575; 600 hours $4,275

FINANCIAL AID: Pell grants, Stafford Loans, SLS/Plus loans

YEAR FOUNDED: 1982

Accreditations/Approvals: COMTAA, ACCSCT, approved for full veterans' benefits, approved for nursing CEU's, vocational rehabilitation

Preparation for out-of-State licensing exam: New York (by arrangement)

GRADUATES PER YEAR (APPROX.): 160

MODALITIES AND SUBJECTS: 500-hour program includes history and theory of massage, hygiene, Esalen, creative and intuitive massage, sports massage, myofascial release, hydrotherapy, Florida massage law, HIV/AIDS, introduction to instrumentation, helping relationship, health care practice building, exercise physiology, musculo-skeletal pathology, CPR. The 600-hour program adds a specialization in one of the following: Oriental modalities, basic sports massage, coremassage.

ADVANCED PROGRAMS: 300-hour core bodywork practitioner program, acupuncture and traditional Chinese medicine program

#127 Venice School of Massage Therapy, Inc.
10915 Bonita Beach Rd., S.E. #212-1
Bonita Springs, FL 33923
(813) 495-0714

HOURS OF TRAINING: 500

DURATION OF COURSE: 24 weeks full-time, 36 or 48 weeks part-time

DAY/EVENING/WEEKEND: day and evening programs available

COST: $2,700

FINANCIAL AID: payment plans, loans, job training partnership act grants

YEAR FOUNDED: 1988

GRADUATES PER YEAR (APPROX.): 120

MODALITIES AND SUBJECTS: history of massage, stress reduction, pain management, health assessment skills, pathology, sports massage conditioning, myofascial release, lymphology, flexibility exercise, neuromuscular therapy, rehabilitative exercise, hydrotherapy, massage law, nutritional counseling, HIV/AIDS

UNIQUE ASPECTS OF SCHOOL OR CURRICULUM: Students attend class in white clothing.

ADVANCED PROGRAMS: colon hydrotherapy, advanced neuromuscular therapy, exercise for rehabilitation

#128 Wood Hygienic Inst., Inc.
2220 East Irlo Bronson Hwy. #11
Kissimmee, FL 34744
(407) 933-0009

HOURS OF TRAINING: 500

DURATION OF COURSE: 5 to 6 months days, 9 months evenings

COST: $3,000

FINANCIAL AID: veterans' benefits, payment plan

MODALITIES AND SUBJECTS: neuromuscular therapy, positional release, sports massage, treatments for TMJ, bronchial drainage, joint injury and mobilization, myofascial approaches, clinical terms and pathology, palpation, postural evaluation, hydrotherapy, statutes and rules, HIV/AIDS, CPR/first aid, business marketing and management, field trips

UNIQUE ASPECTS OF SCHOOL OR CURRICULUM: Credit may be arranged for prior coursework completed elsewhere.

ADVANCED PROGRAMS: colonic irrigation course

CONTINUING EDUCATION: pre- and post-surgical breastwork, on-site, pathology and trauma treatment, TMJ dysfunction and treatment, aromatherapy, equine myofascial treatment

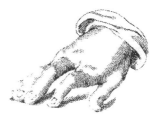

Georgia

No State licensing

Schools:

#129 Academy of Somatic Healing Arts
1924 Cliff Valley Way
Atlanta, GA 30329
(404) 315-0394

HOURS OF TRAINING: 660

DURATION OF COURSE: 8 months days, one year evenings or weekends

COST: $5,675

FINANCIAL AID: payment plans

YEAR FOUNDED: 1991

PREPARATION FOR OUT-OF-STATE LICENSING EXAM: Florida

GRADUATES PER YEAR (APPROX.): 60

MODALITIES AND SUBJECTS: kinesiology, pathology, maniken: sculpting anatomy, palpation, assessment skills, hygiene, first aid/CPR, neuromuscular therapy, clinical sports massage, hydrotherapy, heliotherapy, somatic nutrition, body mechanics/passive stretching, business, ethics, law

UNIQUE ASPECTS OF SCHOOL OR CURRICULUM: The school's focus is on clinical/rehabilitation massage. Graduates earn three-fold certifications in massage, neuromuscular therapy and clinical sports massage

CONTINUING EDUCATION: Paul St. John, Dallas Hancock and others; contact school for current schedule.

#130 Atlanta School of Massage
2300 Peachford Rd., suite 3200
Atlanta, GA 30338
(404) 454-7167

HOURS OF TRAINING: 620

DURATION OF COURSE: days 6 months or evenings for one year

COST: $6,575

FINANCIAL AID: payment plans and financial aid are available; contact school for details

YEAR FOUNDED: 1980

ACCREDITATIONS/APPROVALS: COMTAA, VA approved, ACCSCT

PREPARATION FOR OUT-OF-STATE LICENSING EXAM: Florida

GRADUATES PER YEAR (APPROX.): 200

MODALITIES AND SUBJECTS: hydrotherapy, electrical and thermal modalities, sports massage, deep tissue, energy and the body, injury assessment, trigger point, cross-fiber friction, reflexology, polarity, shiatsu, therapeutic touch, joint movements, movement skills, on-site, pregnancy massage, postural analysis, altered states of consciousness and massage, bodywork and awareness, communication skills, focusing, imagination, intuition, emotions and massage, AIDS awareness, ethics, massage theory and history, law, research and study skills, personal success, business aspects of massage, professional preparation, stretching, biomechanics, CPR/first aid, exercise physiology, hygiene, research presentations, case study, client evaluation and assessment, community events, student clinic

UNIQUE ASPECTS OF SCHOOL OR CURRICULUM: The school also offers a 620-hour massage therapist/clinical sports massage course

ADVANCED PROGRAMS: clinical sports massage, energy healing, bodywork for the childbearing year, infant massage instructor training, manual lymphatic drainage, spa training seminar, polarity certification

CONTINUING EDUCATION: HIV/AIDS, Feldenkrais, new paradigm anatomy for the bodyworker, pathophysiology, reflexology, myofascial manipulation of the neck and back, TMJ seminar

Hawaii

State licensing: 570 hours

Schools:

#131 Aisen Shiatsu School
1314 South King St., suite 601
Honolulu, HI 96814
(808) 596-7354

The school trains students in Shiatsu as preparation for licensure as Massage Therapists by the Hawaii Board of Massage. For program information, contact the school.

#132 All Hawaiian School of Massage
1750 Kalakaua Ave., suite 512
Honolulu, HI 96826
(808) 941-8101

Contact the school for program information.

#133 Aloha Kauai Massage Workshop
Devaki and Kevin Holman
Box 622, Hanalei
Kauai, HI 96714
(808) 826-9990

No catalogue

HOURS OF TRAINING: 570 (150 workshop, 420 apprenticeship)

In-class hours: 370 (150-hr workshop plus 220 in-class hours during apprenticeship)

Duration of course: one year, evenings and weekends

Cost: approximately $3,000

Year founded: 1985

Graduates per year (approx.): 10 to 16

Modalities and subjects: Esalen, Hawaiian Lomi lomi, sports massage, deep tissue, shiatsu

Unique aspects of school or curriculum: Class size is kept small for individual attention. All classes are taught by directors Devaki and Kevin.

Advanced programs: contact school

#134 Big Island Academy of Massage
197 Kino'ole St.
Hilo, HI 96720
(808) 935-1405

Hours of training: 150, 600

Duration of course: 150 hours 3 months, 600 hours 9 to 12 months

Cost: 150 hours $1,295

Financial aid: $500 to part-Hawaiians or American Indians, payment plans

Year founded: 1992

Graduates per year (approx.): 20

Modalities and subjects: sports massage, Masunaga shiatsu, advanced injury care, CST, polarity, reflexology, deep tissue, lomi-lomi, business matters

Unique aspects of school or curriculum: After the initial 150 hours, students receive partial tuition waivers in return for work done in the clinic.

Advanced programs: injury care, sports massage, clinical anatomy and physiology

Continuing education: Thai medical massage, injury care

#135 Hawaiian Islands School of Body Therapies
P.O. Box 390188
Kailua-Kona, HI 96739
(808) 322-0048

Hours of training: 160, 640, 1,000

Duration of course: 160 hours 3 months, 640 hours one year, 1,000 hours 15 months

Cost: 160 hours $1,520, 640 hours $5,024, 1,000 hours $6,950 (all plus tax)

Financial aid: payment plans

Year founded: 1984

Accreditations/approvals: State of Florida continuing education provider

Graduates per year (approx.): 25

Modalities and subjects: aromatherapy, lomi lomi, brain gym, shiatsu, geriatric massage lymphatic drainage, reflexology, polarity, sports massage, pathology, exercise therapy, kinesiology and clinical anatomy, principles of assessment and treatment, business, clinical practicum

Unique aspects of school or curriculum: The school teaches the Knight-Wind Method of restorative treatment therapies.

Advanced programs: Knight-Wind method of medical massage, offered in several levels that each explore anatomy and treatment of a portion of the body; 150-hour and 200-hour alchemical hpynotherapy trainings

Continuing education: All programs at the school may be taken by individually as continuing education. In addition, numerous workshops are offered throughout the year. Examples include sports massage, cranial-sacral therapy, neuromuscular therapy, joint play, Thai massage, Reiki, Touch for Health, polarity, zero balancing, yoga, t'ai chi.

#136 Honolulu School of Massage, Inc.
1123 11th Ave., #301
Honolulu, HI 96816
(808) 733-0000

Hours of training: basic 150; professional 450 (total 600)

Duration of course: basic 3 months; professional 7 months (combined program one year)

Day/evening/weekend: day and evening programs are available

Cost: basic $1,700; professional $4,400

Financial aid: payment plan

Year founded: 1981

Accreditations/approvals: COMTAA

Graduates per year (approx.): 100

Modalities and subjects: reflexology, kinesiology, pregnancy massage, senior citizen massage, CPR, first aid, hydrotherapy, professionalism, myology, neuroanatomy, deep tissue, applied kinesiology, pathology, shiatsu, cranial sacral technique, sports massage, energy work, lymphatic massage, student clinic

Unique aspects of school or curriculum: Students can begin the curriculum at any of four entry points each year.

ADVANCED PROGRAMS: 450-hour program may be taken as advanced training.

CONTINUING EDUCATION: Individual courses in the 450-hour program may be taken as continuing education.

#137 Institute of Body Therapeutics
P.O. Box 11634
Lahaina, HI 96761
(808) 667-5058

No Catalogue

HOURS OF TRAINING: 600

DURATION OF COURSE: 6 months

COST: $2,500

YEAR FOUNDED: 1978

GRADUATES PER YEAR (APPROX.): 20

MODALITIES AND SUBJECTS: structural kinesiology, sports massage, shiatsu, medical massage, integrated body therapies, energy balancing

UNIQUE ASPECTS OF SCHOOL OR CURRICULUM: The school can assist out-of-State trained therapists toward Hawaii licensure, and can tailor its program to the needs of individuals or small groups.

#138 Maui Academy of the Healing Arts
Administrative Office
1993 South Kihei Rd., suite 210
Kihei, HI 96753
(808) 879-4266

Classroom
1325 L. Main St. #201
Wailuhi, HI 96793
(808) 244-3440

HOURS OF TRAINING: 600

IN-CLASS HOURS: 450

DURATION OF COURSE: 11 months, two evenings per weeks plus half-day Saturday

COST: $3,965

YEAR FOUNDED: 1988

GRADUATES PER YEAR (APPROX.): 30

MODALITIES AND SUBJECTS: structural kinesiology, body mechanics, Esalen, lomi lomi, acupressure, reflexology, polarity therapy, treatment of injury, lymphatic drainage massage, basic counseling and communication skills, integrative body/mind therapies,

trigger point, Jin Shin Do, business practices, laws & ethics, health and sanitation, Thai massage, zen shiatsu, somatic exercise

CONTINUING EDUCATION: contact school

#139 The Pacific Center for Bodywork and Awareness
P.O. Box 672
Kilauea, Kauai, HI 96754
(808) 828-6797

The Body Suite - satellite classroom
3501 Rice St, unit 115
Lihue, HI 96766
(808) 245-2413

HOURS OF TRAINING: 150 and 600

YEAR FOUNDED: 1991

MODALITIES AND SUBJECTS: reflexology, neuromuscular therapy, connective tissue massage, structural integration, gestalt therapy, polarity, hypnosis, body-centered psychotherapy, meditation, sports massage, pregnancy massage, arthritis, rehabilitation

ADVANCED PROGRAMS: awareness oriented structural therapy, counseling trainings for psychotherapists, meditation retreats

CONTINUING EDUCATION: connective tissue massage, present centered awareness therapy, hypnotherapy, polarity

Please note: Programs at the school were undergoing revision at the time of publication. The school anticipates opening a branch on Maui. Please contact the school for specifics of programs offered.

Non-Licensure Program:

#140 American Institute of Massage Therapy, Inc.
407 Uluniu St.
Kailua, HI 96734
(808) 266-2468

HOURS OF TRAINING: 160

DURATION OF COURSE: 3 months, two evenings per week plus Sundays

COST: $1,600, $100 registration fee

FINANCIAL AID: scholarships, payment plans

YEAR FOUNDED: 1985

CONTINUING EDUCATION: Intensives and electives are scheduled throughout the year; contact school for current listings.

Idaho

No State licensing

School:

#141 The Idaho School of Massage Therapy
        5353 Franklin Rd.
        Boise, ID 83705
        (208) 343-1847

Contact the school for program information.

Illinois

No State licensing

Schools:

#142 Academy of Massage Therapy
        (Formerly Shock's Educational Center)
        1518 5th Avenue, suite 201
        Moline, IL 61265
        (309) 762-8231

HOURS OF TRAINING: 720 to 900

DURATION OF COURSE: 6 months

MODALITIES AND SUBJECTS: pathology, holistic health, acupuncture/acupressure, Touch for Health, psychology, sociology, sexuality and spirituality, t'ai chi, CPR/first aid, small business practices, documented clinic

CONTINUING EDUCATION: reflexology, shiatsu, sports massage, tui na, qi gong

#143 Chicago School of Massage Therapy
        2918 North Lincoln Ave.
        Chicago, IL 60657
        (312) 477-9444

HOURS OF TRAINING: 650

IN-CLASS HOURS: 525

DURATION OF COURSE: 12 months or 14 months

DAY/EVENING/WEEKEND: day and evening/weekend programs available

COST: $6,700 includes books and professional treatments

FINANCIAL AID: payment plans

YEAR FOUNDED: 1981

ACCREDITATIONS/APPROVALS: COMTAA

GRADUATES PER YEAR (APPROX.): 150

MODALITIES AND SUBJECTS: body mechanics and self-care, palpation, maniken or cadaver intensive, body mobilization techniques, hydrotherapy, cryotherapy, stretching, sports massage, sports injuries, kinesiology, pathology, trigger point, client management, myofascial therapy, Oriental medicine, acupressure/shiatsu, energy approaches, reflexology, stress management, hospice work, on-site, pregnancy massage, zen shiatsu stretches, history of massage, current trends and issues, professional ethics and credentialing, communication skills, starting a practice, clinical and community internship, directed independent study, hygiene, first aid

UNIQUE ASPECTS OF SCHOOL OR CURRICULUM: Community outreach has students doing massage with homeless, hospice clients, drug-exposed infants, domestic violence sufferers and AIDS patients.

ADVANCED PROGRAMS: neuromuscular therapy certification, myofascial therapy certification, sports massage certification

CONTINUING EDUCATION: infant massage, bodywork for the childbearing year, maniken workshop, aromatherapy, cadaver workshop, bodymind renewal in Jamaica, qi gong

#144 LifePath School of Massage Therapy
        7820 N. University, suite 110
        Peoria, IL 61614
        (309) 693-7284

HOURS OF TRAINING: 660

DURATION OF COURSE: 9 months, evenings and weekends

COST: $5,275 ($200 discount for payment in full)

YEAR FOUNDED: 1992

GRADUATES PER YEAR (APPROX.): 12 to 16

MODALITIES AND SUBJECTS: kinesiology, nutrition, reflexology, lymphatic drainage massage, connective tissue massage, cross-fiber, deep tissue, trigger point, sports massage, joint mobilization and stretching, hydrotherapy, polarity, neuromuscular principles in deep tissue bodywork, business ethics and professional practice, psychology for the bodyworker, wellness concepts, clinical experience

CONTINUING EDUCATION: contact school

#145 Redfern Training Systems School of
        Massage
        9 S. 531 Wilmette Ave.,
        Darien, IL 60561
        (708) 960-5636

HOURS OF TRAINING: 690

IN-CLASS HOURS: 150

DURATION OF COURSE: 30 weeks

DAY/EVENING/WEEKEND: day and evening programs available

COST: $3,600 (includes books and supplies)

YEAR FOUNDED: 1990

GRADUATES PER YEAR (APPROX.): 36

MODALITIES AND SUBJECTS: history of massage, acupressure, reflexology, sports massage, deep tissue, myo-fascial release, cranial therapy, day spa treatments

UNIQUE ASPECTS OF SCHOOL OR CURRICULUM: Classes are kept small for individual attention.

ADVANCED PROGRAMS: sports massage, reflexology

**#146 Wellness & Massage Training Institute
614 Executive Dr.
Willowbrook, IL 60521
(708) 325-3773**

HOURS OF TRAINING: 700

DURATION OF COURSE: minimum of one year

DAY/EVENING/WEEKEND: day, evening and weekend programs available

COST: approximately $7,000 (varies with electives chosen)

YEAR FOUNDED: 1989

ACCREDITATIONS/APPROVALS: (curriculum approval by AMTA pending)

GRADUATES PER YEAR (APPROX.): 60

MODALITIES AND SUBJECTS: Required subjects (583 hours) are kinesiology, wellness concepts, anatomy and physiology for bodyworkers, joint mobilization, hydrotherapy, deep tissue, trigger point, professional practice and business of massage therapy, integrative studies, massage clinic, community outreach.

Electives (117 hours) include seated massage, sports massage, positional release, active assisted stretching, Esalen, principles of structural massage, clinical symposia, advanced sports massage, Touch for Health, ortho-bionomy, Jin Shin Do acupressure, shiatsu, bodywork and the adult child, bodywork for survivors of sex abuse, introduction to nutrition, communication skills, boundary issues for massage therapists, t'ai chi, creative success through productive thinking, stress management.

ADVANCED PROGRAMS: ortho-bionomy

CONTINUING EDUCATION: first aid/CPR, how to study effectively, medical terminology, introduction to prescription medications, introduction to skin disease, how to market your work, marketing on-site massage, self-massage, techniques for the back, techniques for the feet, techniques for the neck and shoulders, massage for couples, pressure sensitivity techniques, infant and toddler massage, geriatric massage, trigger point, on-site, prenatal massage, manual lymphatic drainage, reflexology, aromatherapy, cranial sacral,

Touch for Health, Feldenkrais, somatic re-education, readings in bodywork theory, presence, energy and intention, t'ai chi, shiatsu

Indiana

No State licensing

Schools:

**#147 Alexandria School of Scientific Therapeutics
809 S. Harrison, P.O. Box 287
Alexandria, IN 46001
(317) 724-7745**

Contact the school for program information.

**#148 Health Enrichment Center, Inc.
Indiana Branch
6801 Lake Plaza Drive, Suite A102
Indianapolis, IN 46220
(317) 841-1414**

See Listing for Health Enrichment Center, Inc. in Michigan

**#149 Lewis School & Clinic of Massage Therapy
3400 Michigan St.
Hobart, IN 46342
(219) 962-9640**

Contact the school for program information.

Iowa

State Licensure: 500 hours

National Certification Exam not accepted

Approved out-of-state schools:

Boulder School of Massage, Boulder CO
Academy of Massage Therapy, Moline IL
Chicago School of Massage, Chicago IL
Deep Muscle Therapy Inst., King of Prussia PA
Desert Institute, Tucson, AZ
Dr. Welbe's College, Omaha NE
Heartwood Institute, Garberville CA
Mueller College, San Diego CA
New Mexico School, Albuquerque NM
Pennsylvania School, King of Prussia PA
Swedish Institute, New York NY

Schools:

**#150 Capri College of Massage Therapy
315 2nd Ave. SE
Cedar Rapids, IA 52401
(319) 354-1541**

1815 E. Kimberly Rd.
Davenport, IA 52807
(319) 359-1306 or (800) 728-1336

395 Main St.
P.O. Box 873
Dubuque, IA 52004
(319) 588-2379 or (800) 728-0712

HOURS OF TRAINING: 650

IN-CLASS HOURS: 510

DURATION OF COURSE: 19 weeks

COST: $4,686.50 (includes massage table and accessories, uniforms and textbooks)

FINANCIAL AID: Pell grants, Stafford loans, PLUS loans, supplement education opportunity grants, work-study, scholarships

YEAR FOUNDED: school 1977; massage program 1994

ACCREDITATIONS/APPROVALS: ACCSCT

PREPARATION FOR OUT-OF-STATE LICENSING EXAM: may be available; contact school for specifics

MODALITIES AND SUBJECTS: history, laws and licensing, health and sanitary practices, business ethics, hygiene, professionalism, kinesiology, pathology, first aid/CPR, consultation and preparation, body mechanics, hydrotherapy, heat and light, sports massage, rehabilitation massage, prenatal massage, infant massage, lymph massage, deep tissue, acupressure, shiatsu, reflexology, nutrition, therapeutic exercise, building a successful business

UNIQUE ASPECTS OF SCHOOL OR CURRICULUM: The school also offers cosmetology and esthetics curricula.

CONTINUING EDUCATION: contact school

Capri College has branches in Davenport, Daybook, and Madison, WI. Programs vary slightly from the above description. Contact each school for specifics about their program.

#151 Carlson College of Massage Therapy
      11809 County Rd. x-28
      Anamosa, IA 52205
      (319) 462-3402

HOURS OF TRAINING: 625

DURATION OF COURSE: 5 months

COST: $4,000

YEAR FOUNDED: 1984

ACCREDITATIONS/APPROVALS: COMTAA

GRADUATES PER YEAR (APPROX.): 50-60

MODALITIES AND SUBJECTS: polarity, stretches, deep tissue, connective tissue, reflexology, sports massage,

hydrotherapy, musculoskeletal pathology, aromatherapy, nutrition and diet, herbs, t'ai chi/body movement, on-site, CPR/first aid, professional ethics, business practices, outreach, clinic

UNIQUE ASPECTS OF SCHOOL OR CURRICULUM: The school recently moved to a rural setting offering peaceful surroundings and outdoor activities.

#152 Dr. Welbe's College of Massage Therapy
      17½ N. Federal, Apt. 2
      Hampton, IA 50441
      (515) 456-4528

HOURS OF TRAINING: 500

IN-CLASS HOURS: 400 plus 100 hours externship

DURATION OF COURSE: 30 weeks

DAY/EVENING/WEEKEND: classes meet Saturday/Sunday or Tuesday/Wednesday

COST: $3,550 plus uniform and books

FINANCIAL AID: educational loans and payment plans are available

YEAR FOUNDED: 1993

MODALITIES AND SUBJECTS: deep tissue massage, infant massage, reflexology, stress management techniques, ethics, legalities and business basics, clinical externship, CPR/first aid

UNIQUE ASPECTS OF SCHOOL OR CURRICULUM: class size is between 6 and 12

#153 Dr. Welbe's College of Massage Therapy
      4242 Gordon Drive
      Sioux City, IA 51106
      (712) 274-8696

Contact the school for program information.

#154 Iowa School of Natural Therapeutics and
      Clinic
      2733 Douglas Ave.
      Des Moines, IA 50310
      (515) 277-2126

HOURS OF TRAINING: 1,000

IN-CLASS HOURS: 500

DURATION OF COURSE: 6 months, evenings and Saturdays

COST: $3,775 (includes books)

FINANCIAL AID: payment plan

YEAR FOUNDED: 1986

GRADUATES PER YEAR (APPROX.): 30

MODALITIES AND SUBJECTS: sports massage, deep muscle therapy, postural and breathing techniques, nutrition, foot reflexology, on-site, polarity, shiatsu, business, ethics, CPR/first aid

UNIQUE ASPECTS OF SCHOOL OR CURRICULUM: Proximity to Drake University provides housing within walking distance.

CONTINUING EDUCATION: contact school

#155 Millennium College of Massage Therapy
      and Reflexology
      1605 First Ave. North
      Fort Dodge, IA 50501
      (515) 955-2296

HOURS OF TRAINING: 1,200 including internship hours and 200 hours of reflexology

DURATION OF COURSE: 6 months

COST: $5,000

MODALITIES AND SUBJECTS: history of massage, Touch for Health, musculoskeletal pathology, reflexology, pregnancy massage, infant massage, acupressure, stress reduction, hydrotherapy, exercise and movement, professional ethics, business practices, first aid/CPR

Kansas

No State licensing

Certified Instructors:

Maggie Kelley   June M. Jones
707 SE Quincy   4348 SW Wanamaker
Topeka, KS 66603   Topeka, KS 66610
(913) 233-7073   (913) 478-9643

Please contact Maggie or June for details about their instructional programs.

Kentucky

No State Licensing

#156 The Louisville School of Massage
      Therapeutics
      7410 New LaGrange Road, #320
      Louisville, KY 40222
      (502) 429-5765

HOURS OF TRAINING: 150 or 300

DURATION OF COURSE: 150 hours 6 months, 300 hours 12 months

DAY/EVENING/WEEKEND: day and evening programs available

Cost: 150 hour course $1,165 plus books and supplies

FINANCIAL AID: payment plans

YEAR FOUNDED: 1986

GRADUATES PER YEAR (APPROX.): 150

MODALITIES AND SUBJECTS: deep tissue, trigger point, polarity, Jin Shin Do acupressure, yoga, t'ai chi, healing touch, infant massage and additional modalities

UNIQUE ASPECTS OF SCHOOL OR CURRICULUM: Housed in Stillpoint Center, the school is part of a wellness center that includes an in-house M.D., a research library, food co-op, and a gift shop/supply center.

ADVANCED PROGRAMS: The basic 150 hour course is a prerequisite for the 150-hour advanced training.

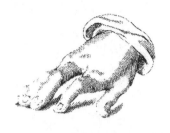

Louisiana

State Licensing: 500 hours

National Certification Exam accepted

Schools:

#157 Blue Cliff School of Therapeutic Massage
      1919 Veterans Blvd., suite 310
      Kenner, LA 70062
      (504) 471-0294

HOURS OF TRAINING: 600

DURATION OF COURSE: days 6½ months, evenings 13 months, weekends 15 months

COST: $4,299.50 (includes books)

FINANCIAL AID: payment plan

YEAR FOUNDED: 1987

ACCREDITATIONS/APPROVALS: COMTAA

PREPARATION FOR OUT-OF-STATE LICENSING EXAM: Florida

GRADUATES PER YEAR (APPROX.): 60

MODALITIES AND SUBJECTS: body systems balancing, cranio-sacral therapy, neuromuscular therapy, subtle body energetics, shiatsu, deep tissue massage, hydrotherapy, pathology, reflexology, sports kinesiology, sports massage, sports shiatsu, supervised clinical practice, t'ai chi, CPR/first aid/HIV, laws and legislation, marketing, therapeutic communication, business practices and professionalism

UNIQUE ASPECTS OF SCHOOL OR CURRICULUM: All students take a 460 hour core curriculum and choose one of two 140-hour specialty tracks to complete their training.

ADVANCED PROGRAMS: 140-hour specialty in Oriental bodywork, 140-hour specialty in western bodywork

CONTINUING EDUCATION: traditional Chinese medicine, neuromuscular therapy

#158 In-Touch Bodyworks
11715 Bricksome Ave., suite B-4
Baton Rouge, LA 70816
(504) 293-8555

HOURS OF TRAINING: 520

DURATION OF COURSE: Classes meet two nights per week and alternate weekends for 7½ months

COST: $3,650 including books and supplies

FINANCIAL AID: Student loans are available at a nearby bank for those who qualify.

YEAR FOUNDED: 1992

GRADUATES PER YEAR (APPROX.): 25

MODALITIES AND SUBJECTS: Sports massage, reflexology, polarity, nutrition, deep tissue, connective tissue, business, therapeutic communication, CPR/first aid, t'ai chi, meditation

UNIQUE ASPECTS OF SCHOOL OR CURRICULUM: The school is small and selective and maintains a very personal approach.

CONTINUING EDUCATION: shiatsu, Reiki

#159 Louisiana Institute of Massage Therapy
1108 Lafitte St.
Lake Charles, LA 70601
(318) 474-9435
(Classroom: 401 W. 18th St)

HOURS OF TRAINING: 300, 325, 500

COST: 300 hours $2,500 (Texas), 325 hours $2,450, 500 hours $3,200

FINANCIAL AID: payment plan

YEAR FOUNDED: 1990

PREPARATION FOR OUT-OF-STATE LICENSING EXAM: Texas, other states by arrangement

GRADUATES PER YEAR (APPROX.): 25-30

MODALITIES AND SUBJECTS: deep tissue, neuromuscular therapy, pregnancy massage, infant massage, sports massage, reflexology, hydrotherapy, polarity, on-site, body mechanics

UNIQUE ASPECTS OF SCHOOL OR CURRICULUM: In-hospital internship program, Maniken Muscle sculpting system, all classes are taught on weekends.

CONTINUING EDUCATION: contact school

#160 Massage Academy of the South
4939 Jamestown Ave., suite 201
Baton Rouge, LA 70808
(504) 926-5820

HOURS OF TRAINING: 650

IN-CLASS HOURS: 610

DURATION OF COURSE: 5½ months days, 7½ months evenings/weekends

COST: $4,200

FINANCIAL AID: Vocational rehabilitation, Veterans' Administration, bank financing

YEAR FOUNDED: 1992

PREPARATION FOR OUT-OF-STATE LICENSING EXAM: Florida

GRADUATES PER YEAR (APPROX.): 35

MODALITIES AND SUBJECTS: neuromuscular therapy, sports massage, connective tissue, shiatsu, reflexology, polarity, pregnancy and infant massage, hydrotherapy, nutrition, business, law, CPR/first aid, psychology and communications, herbology, kinesiology, HIV/AIDS

UNIQUE ASPECTS OF SCHOOL OR CURRICULUM: Focus is on health care and community involvement.

Maine

State Certification/registration

National Certification Exam accepted

Schools:

#161 Downeast School of Massage
P.O. Box 24, 99 Moose Meadow Lane
Waldoboro, ME 04572
(207) 832-5531

HOURS OF TRAINING:
Program I: Swedish and sports massage 608
Program II: Swedish and shiatsu 689
Program III: Swedish and body/mind 600

DURATION OF COURSE: 10 months or 2 years

DAY/EVENING/WEEKEND: day and evening programs available

COST: Program I $5,100; Program II $5,700; Program III $5,100

FINANCIAL AID: payment plans

YEAR FOUNDED: 1980

ACCREDITATIONS/APPROVALS: COMTAA, military and veterans approved, approved for vocational rehabilitation

GRADUATES PER YEAR (APPROX.): 80

MODALITIES AND SUBJECTS: t'ai chi, shiatsu, body/mind, pregnancy massage, reflexology, body mechanics, seated massage, nutrition, neuromuscular therapy, hydrotherapy, pathology, kinesiology, movement analysis, ethics, maniken muscles, chronic pain, the art of practice design, integrating business, first aid/CPR, polarity, sports massage, energy field healing, psychological aspects of massage therapy, working with incest and trauma survivors, clinic program

CONTINUING EDUCATION: neuromuscular therapy, herbology, craniosacral therapy, spa training seminar, family massage, seated massage

#162 Polarity Realization Institute
        Portland, ME
        (800) 497-2908 or (508) 356-0980

600-hour massage and bodywork training

See listing for Polarity Realization Institute, Ipswich, MA

Maryland

No State licensing

School:

#163 Baltimore School of Massage
        6401 Dogwood Rd.
        Baltimore, MD 21207
        (410) 944-8855

HOURS OF TRAINING: 500

DURATION OF COURSE: 60 weeks

DAY/EVENING/WEEKEND: day and evening programs available

COST: $4,675 (includes books)

FINANCIAL AID: contact school

YEAR FOUNDED: 1981

ACCREDITATIONS/APPROVALS: COMTAA, Maryland Higher Education Council

GRADUATES PER YEAR (APPROX.): 200

MODALITIES AND SUBJECTS: deep tissue work, deep muscle release work, myofascial release, energy work, sensitivity training, psycho-emotional release work, contraindications, how to make a living successfully doing massage therapy

UNIQUE ASPECTS OF SCHOOL OR CURRICULUM: The same founding director, faculty and administrative staff have been at the school since its inception in 1981. The program focuses on sensitivity and inner training.

ADVANCED PROGRAMS: contact school

CONTINUING EDUCATION: acupressure, sports massage, craniosacral therapy, zero balancing

Massachusetts

No State licensing

Schools:

#164 Bancroft School of Massage Therapy
        50 Franklin St., suite 370
        Worcester, MA 01608
        (508) 757-7923

HOURS OF TRAINING: 750

DURATION OF COURSE: 17 months days or 22 months evenings

COST: $8,500

FINANCIAL AID: Stafford Loans, PLUS loans, payment plans

YEAR FOUNDED: 1950

ACCREDITATIONS/APPROVALS: COMTAA, Accrediting Commission of Career Schools/Colleges of Technology

PREPARATION FOR OUT-OF-STATE LICENSING EXAM: Florida, Washington, New Hampshire, Rhode Island, New York (Oriental massage application II required for New York)

GRADUATES PER YEAR (APPROX.): 115-120

MODALITIES AND SUBJECTS: movement and palpation, reflexology, Oriental massage applications, hydrotherapy, sports massage, on-site, first aid/CPR, business practices/life skills, clinical massage applications, internship

UNIQUE ASPECTS OF SCHOOL OR CURRICULUM: The Maniken system is used in anatomy and physiology class.

ADVANCED PROGRAMS: myology, neurology and Oriental massage applications II

CONTINUING EDUCATION: Variety of programs offered; contact school.

#165 The Central Mass. School of Massage and Therapy
318 N. Main St.
North Brookfield, MA 01535
(508) 867-7951

HOURS OF TRAINING: 500

IN-CLASS HOURS: 325

COST: $5,000

FINANCIAL AID: payment plan

YEAR FOUNDED: 1970

MODALITIES AND SUBJECTS: general health, hypnosis, foot care, body balancing, reflexology, muscle therapy

#166 Healing Touch Institute, Inc. School of Muscle Therapy
27 Water Street, suite 405
Wakefield, MA 01880
(617) 246-2449

HOURS OF TRAINING: 500

IN-CLASS HOURS: 160

DURATION OF COURSE: one evening per week for 40 weeks

YEAR FOUNDED: 1992

UNIQUE ASPECTS OF SCHOOL OR CURRICULUM: The institute is a non-profit corporation. Class size is limited to six and classes begin on an on-going basis throughout the year.

#167 Kripalu Center
P.O. Box 793
Lenox, MA 01240
(413) 448-3400

HOURS OF TRAINING: 150

DURATION OF COURSE: 27 days (residential)

COST: $1,944 (dormitory accommodation) includes room and board and use of the facilities; room with half-bath $2,214, semi-private room $3,105, private room $4,050

FINANCIAL AID: partial scholarships available; call (800) 967-3577

YEAR FOUNDED: 1982

GRADUATES PER YEAR (APPROX.): 100 to 150

MODALITIES AND SUBJECTS: body dynamics, grounding exercises, yoga postures, energy balancing, meditation, breath awareness

UNIQUE ASPECTS OF SCHOOL OR CURRICULUM: Meditative approach and emphasis on personal growth promote bodymind integration for both practitioner and client. Facilitated group process and yoga curriculum help practitioners develop body awareness, strength and stamina. The program includes daily yoga, dance class, vegetarian cuisine, hot tub and sauna, wooded grounds in the Berkshire mountains.

ADVANCED PROGRAMS: 7-day energy balancing training

#168 Massage Institute of New England, Inc.
439 Cambridge St.
Cambridge, MA 02141
(617) 547-6554

HOURS OF TRAINING: 1,028 (including 300 supervised clinic)

IN-CLASS HOURS: 728

DURATION OF COURSE: 12 to 36 months

DAY/EVENING/WEEKEND: day and evening programs available

COST: $8,500

FINANCIAL AID: payment plan

YEAR FOUNDED: 1982

ACCREDITATIONS/APPROVALS: COMTAA

PREPARATION FOR OUT-OF-STATE LICENSING EXAM: The curriculum meets most states' criteria for licensing; contact school for information about individual states.

GRADUATES PER YEAR (APPROX.): 48

MODALITIES AND SUBJECTS: trigger point, craniosacral, zero balancing, clinical modalities, pathology, business, marketing and placement, electives, t'ai chi

UNIQUE ASPECTS OF SCHOOL OR CURRICULUM: The school offers flexible scheduling and allow students to develop their own technique, from light energy work to deep, sports massage therapy.

CONTINUING EDUCATION: zero balancing, sports massage, deep structural technique

#169 Muscular Therapy Institute
122 Rindge Ave.
Cambridge, MA 02140-2527
(617) 576-1300

HOURS OF TRAINING: 51.9 credit hours

IN-CLASS HOURS: 900

DURATION OF COURSE: 1½ years (3 semester format) or 2 years (4 semesters)

DAY/EVENING/WEEKEND: weekend programs available

COST: $10,833 including fees (3 semester) or $10,868 including fees (4 semester)

FINANCIAL AID: financial aid available if qualified

YEAR FOUNDED: 1974

ACCREDITATIONS/APPROVALS: COMTAA, ACCET

GRADUATES PER YEAR (APPROX.): 80

MODALITIES AND SUBJECTS: Benjamin system of muscle therapy, pathology, sports massage, skills and dynamics of therapeutic relationship, practice development, alternative approaches to holistic therapies, foundations of professional massage, professional development

UNIQUE ASPECTS OF SCHOOL OR CURRICULUM: Individual coaching sessions with faculty, extensive communications curriculum, class advisors system

ADVANCED PROGRAMS: Benjamin system training in injury work

CONTINUING EDUCATION: contact school

#170 Polarity Realization Institute
126 High St.,
Ipswich, MA 01938
(800) 497-2908 or (508) 356-0980

HOURS OF TRAINING: 180 or 600

IN-CLASS HOURS: 144 or 529

DURATION OF COURSE: 180 hours 6 months; 600 hours 12 to 24 months

COST: 180 hours $1,640; 600 hours $4,754 (plus insurance and required outside sessions)

FINANCIAL AID: payment plans

YEAR FOUNDED: 1981

ACCREDITATIONS/APPROVALS: program approved by American Polarity Therapy Association, approved for nursing CEU's in Massachusetts and Maine

MODALITIES AND SUBJECTS: Basic course includes body mechanics, communication skills, business skills, self-care and stretching, ice and heat, clinics.
For contents of polarity certification, contact school. Additional electives include reflexology, sports massage, craniosacral therapy, advanced vitality balancing, color and light, sacral and sacroiliac, advanced chakra and energetic anatomy, advanced spinal and client evaluation, sound therapy, advanced aura and energetic anatomy, distance healing, hips and pelvic alignment, intuitive symbolic interpretation, psychosynthesis and body awareness, eating disorders, additions, sexual abuse and transitions, polarity nutrition and yoga, running your subtle energies, business skills

UNIQUE ASPECTS OF SCHOOL OR CURRICULUM: The combination of physical work and energetic work promotes a deeper level of understanding of the whole being and the healing process. The modular structure of the program allows the student to begin a professional practice after completing the first 180 hours.

ADVANCED PROGRAMS: The five modules offered may be taken individually. Module 1 is Swedish massage, 180 hours; module 2 is polarity therapy certification, 160 hours; module 3 is advanced anatomy and physiology, 56 hours; module 4 is advanced massage and polarity electives, 148 hours; module 5 is advanced integration and evaluation, 56 hours.

The school also offers this program in Portland, ME

#171 Stillpoint Center
P.O. Box 15
60 Main St.
Hatfield, MA 01038
(413) 247-9322

HOURS OF TRAINING: 878

DURATION OF COURSE: 10 months full-time, two years part-time. Also offered is an evening program with occasional weekends.

COST: $6,000 including insurance

FINANCIAL AID: payment plan

YEAR FOUNDED: 1980

ACCREDITATIONS/APPROVALS: COMTAA

PREPARATION FOR OUT-OF-STATE LICENSING EXAM: New York (additional coursework required)

MODALITIES AND SUBJECTS: deep compression massage, trigger point therapy, connective tissue massage, skin rolling, foot reflexology, polarity therapy, shiatsu, on-site, massage for the elderly, neurology, myology, Feldenkrais/body mechanics, council, kinesiology, pathology, hydrotherapy, massage clinic, community service/field placement, professional worklife/professional development, first aid/CPR, final project, supervised practice

UNIQUE ASPECTS OF SCHOOL OR CURRICULUM: The school is located in picturesque rural setting in Western Massachusetts, and is a non-profit corporation. Vocational training is combined with opportunities for personal growth and spiritual awareness. The program emphasizes holism, massage with awareness and compassionate action.

Michigan

No State licensing

Schools:

#172 Health Enrichment Center, Inc.
1820 N. Lapeer Road
Lapeer, MI 48446
(810) 667-9453

HOURS OF TRAINING: 1,000

IN-CLASS HOURS: 500

DURATION OF COURSE: 6 months or 10 months

DAY/EVENING/WEEKEND: day, evening and weekend programs are available

COST: $3,750 (includes books and supplies)

FINANCIAL AID: limited scholarships available

YEAR FOUNDED: 1985

ACCREDITATIONS/APPROVALS: COMTAA

PREPARATION FOR OUT-OF-STATE LICENSING EXAM: Washington, Oregon, Texas, Ohio, Province of Ontario

GRADUATES PER YEAR (APPROX.): 250

MODALITIES AND SUBJECTS: pathology, nutrition, body mechanics, connective tissue therapy, integration of eastern and western bodywork styles, sports massage, movement re-education, proprioceptive integration, applied kinesiology, hydrotherapy, supervised work experience, law, history, ethics, business practices, communication, client/practitioner dynamics

UNIQUE ASPECTS OF SCHOOL OR CURRICULUM: Coursework may be taken at the school in Lapeer, or in Adrian, Grand Rapids, Livonia, Warren, Traverse City, or Indianapolis, IN.

ADVANCED PROGRAMS: School of Clinical Approaches (designed to interface with medical practitioners); School of Shiatsu and Oriental Approaches; School of Subtle Energy Therapies; Massage Practitioner (advanced courses for graduates of the 1000-hour program); Advanced Practitioner (2000-hour diploma); Master Bodywork Therapist (5000-hour diploma)

CONTINUING EDUCATION: The school also offers a modified correspondence course.

Weekend workshops include chronic pain, chronic fatigue, Three in One Concepts Brain Integration Programs, manual medicine technician, Russian medical massage, triune polarity, massage and mental health, chiropractic massage assistant, reflexology, bodywork for pregnancy, labor and delivery, equine massage, sports massage, structural dynamics, activated neuromuscular correction, advanced techniques, bio-energy, art of knowing, body mechanics, clinical evaluation and correction, communication skills, on-site, discover the emotional you, homeopathy, integrated energy series, interpersonal skills, magnets, maniken, muscle testing, professionalism, TMJ, vibration

#173 Irene's Myomassology Institute
      18911 Ten Mile Rd. #200
      Southfield, MI 48075
      (313) 569-HAND/4263

HOURS OF TRAINING: 500

IN-CLASS HOURS: 382

DURATION OF COURSE: 46 weeks, one day per week, plus self-scheduled electives

DAY/EVENING/WEEKEND: some weekend classes available

COST: $2,332 (includes some books)

FINANCIAL AID: payment plans

YEAR FOUNDED: 1987

GRADUATES PER YEAR (APPROX.): 150

MODALITIES AND SUBJECTS: Required classes are reflexology, craniology, energy balancing, body mechanics, hydrotherapy, paraffin therapy, side-lying massage, leg exercises, sanitary practices, ethics, business procedures, research thesis, journal/summary, clinical experience, anatomy coloring book, special credit.

Electives include sports massage, shiatsu, polarity, Touch for Health, structural and postural evaluation and treatment, Hellerwork, on-site, trigger points, prenatal and infant massage, labor massage, therapeutic touch, aromatherapy, herbology, nutrition, macrobiotics, carpal tunnel, iridology, spiritual development, crystal healing, biomagnets, response to emotional release, qi gong, bach flower remedies, neuro-linguistic programming, Feldenkrais, reflexology in depth, colon health, CPR, skin care, chakra basics, first aid, exercise, stress management, meditation, spinal subluxation, three in one concepts series

ADVANCED PROGRAMS: contact school

CONTINUING EDUCATION: Electives may be taken as continuing education.

#174 Kalamazoo Center for the Healing Arts
      3715 West Main, suite 3
      Kalamazoo, MI 49006
      (616) 373-1000

HOURS OF TRAINING: 120, 520

DURATION OF COURSE: 520-hour course 1½ to 2 years

DAY/EVENING/WEEKEND: Classes meet primarily evenings and weekends

COST: 120-hour program $1,100; 520-hour program $3,890

YEAR FOUNDED: 1986

MODALITIES AND SUBJECTS: myofascial release, craniosacral therapy, polarity, t'ai chi and yoga for bodyworkers, acupressure, five element theory, advanced anatomy, body reading, posturing, emotional anatomy, community service, professional seminars, business issues, professional issues

UNIQUE ASPECTS OF SCHOOL OR CURRICULUM: Introductory 20-hour seminar is a prerequisite for the 100-hour basic training. 100-hour basic training is a prerequisite for 400-hour professional level training. The program is oriented toward personal growth.

#175 Lansing Community College
P.O. Box 40010
Lansing, MI 48901
(517) 483-1410 or 483-1455

HOURS OF TRAINING: 26 credit hours, or 400 class hours

YEAR FOUNDED: 1977

ACCREDITATIONS/APPROVALS: North Central Association of Colleges and Schools

MODALITIES AND SUBJECTS: healthy lifestyles, stress management, massage practicum, Touch for Health, polarity, business, clinical approach to massage, sports massage, self-awareness/wellness, consumer/health issues, nutrition-critical issues

#176 Michigan Institute of Myomassology
25711 Southfield Rd., ste. 101
Southfield, MI 48075
(810) 443-1669

HOURS OF TRAINING: 500

IN-CLASS HOURS: 332

DURATION OF COURSE: 41 weeks, one class per week

DAY/EVENING/WEEKEND: day or evening program available

COST: $2,290 to $2,385 (depending on electives chosen)

YEAR FOUNDED: 1992

MODALITIES AND SUBJECTS: Required courses include craniosacral therapy, resistive movements, strain/counterstrain, reflexology, energy balancing, deep tissue massage, compression, face massage, paraffin therapy, hydrotherapy, modified massage, business procedures, sanitary procedures, massage ethics, review, research thesis, journal, clinical experience, anatomy coloring book, special credit.

Students also take 168 hours of elective subjects including sports massage, shiatsu, polarity, Touch for Health, one brain, under the code, louder than words, physical therapy techniques, prenatal and infant massage, myofascial release, herbs, nutrition, iridology, labor massage, beyond on-site, physiology, CPR, therapeutic touch, colon health, neurolinguistic programming, Alexander technique, pathology

UNIQUE ASPECTS OF SCHOOL OR CURRICULUM: Satellite classes are also available in Richmond and East Pointe

CONTINUING EDUCATION: See electives, listed above. These may be taken individually as continuing education.

#177 Wellspring Institute School of Therapeutic Bodywork
20312 Chalon
St. Clair Shores, MI 48080
(810) 772-8520

HOURS OF TRAINING: 100, 300, 500

Cost: 100 hours $1,200, 300 hours $2,500, 500 hours $4,000

MODALITIES AND SUBJECTS: The 100-hour accelerated training program includes gentle deep tissue massage, reflexology, trigger point, chair massage, hot herbal wraps, hygiene, and practice management. The 300-hour course adds exposure to other types of bodywork and massage, such as cranial massage, energy balancing, five element theory, acupressure, shiatsu, therapeutic touch, polarity, cranio-sacral therapy, massaging the elderly, sports massage, emotional self-influencing and elective workshops.

UNIQUE ASPECTS OF SCHOOL OR CURRICULUM: A unique offering is "Radical Energy Balancing," a high-trust approach to polarity and hypnosis. The massage school is part of Wellspring Institute, a growth center that offers a variety of programs. Transfer credit can be arranged for coursework taken at other schools or with recognized teachers.

ADVANCED PROGRAMS: A 200-hour advanced program, when combined with the 300-hour training, completes a 500-hour course. This advanced program includes advanced massage practicum, practical anatomy, modern medical massage, radical energy balancing and independent study.

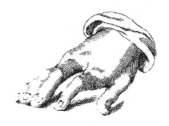

Minnesota

No State licensing

Schools:

#178 Minneapolis School of Massage and Bodywork, Inc.
220 Lowry Ave. NE
Minneapolis, MN 55418
(612) 788-8907

HOURS OF TRAINING: Course I Massage Practitioner 174 hours (136 in-class); course II Sports Massage

Practitioner 410 hours (270 in-class); course III Comprehensive Massage Therapy 630 hours (440 in-class)

DURATION OF COURSE: Course I: 4 months full-time, 5 months part-time; course II: 8 months full-time, 10 months part-time; course III: 10 months full-time or 13 months part-time (or students may proceed at their own pace)

DAY/EVENING/WEEKEND: day and evening programs available

COST: course I $1,546.25 including books, course II $3,480.25 including books, course III $5,212.25 including books (plus cost of electives)

FINANCIAL AID: Minnesota State grants, VA benefits, DRS funding, other sources, payment plans

YEAR FOUNDED: 1975

ACCREDITATIONS/APPROVALS: ACCSCT

MODALITIES AND SUBJECTS: Course I: Esalen massage, pressure and release points, communications and boundaries, business, critiques. Course II adds joint massage, connective tissue, body wellness strokes and sports anatomy, body wellness testing, movements and sports balance. Course III adds CPR, pre/post natal and infant massage, intuitive awareness and self body care, structural alignment and the nervous system, electives, history of massage.

UNIQUE ASPECTS OF SCHOOL OR CURRICULUM: Credit may be arranged for coursework previously taken elsewhere.

ADVANCED PROGRAMS: The five phase way of shiatsu training program (10 months), day-break geriatrics training program (3 months)

CONTINUING EDUCATION: CPR, head/neck/back, nutrition, seated chair massage, t'ai chi, "energy" the heart and soul of bodywork, celebrating and healing the feminine, exploring/creating/healing the inner self, reflexology, lymphatic massage, infant massage instructor training workshop, the radiance technique, yoga. Program classes may also be taken as individual workshops.

#179 Northern Lights School of Massage Therapy
1313 S.E. Fifth St., ste. 202
Minneapolis, MN 55414
(612) 379-3822

HOURS OF TRAINING: 600

DURATION OF COURSE: one year (classes meet two weekdays from 1:30 p.m. to 9:00 p.m., and some Saturdays)

COST: $4,550

FINANCIAL AID: payment plans

YEAR FOUNDED: 1985

ACCREDITATIONS/APPROVALS: COMTAA

GRADUATES PER YEAR (APPROX.): 60

MODALITIES AND SUBJECTS: deep tissue, on-site, sports massage, cross-fiber friction, trigger points, communication and client management, clinical applications and pathology, business and practice management, first aid/CPR

CONTINUING EDUCATION: contact school

#180 Sister Rosalind Gefre's School of
Professional Massage
400 Selby Ave., suite G
St. Paul, MN 55102
(612) 228-0960 or (612) 698-9123

HOURS OF TRAINING: 550

DURATION OF COURSE: one year to two years

DAY/EVENING/WEEKEND: day and evening programs available

COST: $3,700

FINANCIAL AID: payment plans

MODALITIES AND SUBJECTS: kinesiology, reflexology, on-site, nutrition, ethical issues, massage & disabilities, massage & the elderly, business practices & communication, anatomy & the physiology of aging, Chinese acupressure, charting, muscular therapy, sports massage, CPR/first aid, spirituality & massage, student practicum

UNIQUE ASPECTS OF SCHOOL OR CURRICULUM: The school is based on Christian principles.

Missouri

No State licensing

Schools:

#181 Heartland School of Massage
1719½ W. 39th St.
Kansas City, MO 64111
(816) 753-8566

HOURS OF TRAINING: 250

IN-CLASS HOURS: 160

DURATION OF COURSE: 8 weeks in class plus four months student clinic (90 hours)

DAY/EVENING/WEEKEND: day, evening and weekend programs available

COST: $2,100 including book fee (10% discount for pre-payment)

FINANCIAL AID: payment plans

YEAR FOUNDED: 1988

GRADUATES PER YEAR (APPROX.): 20 to 30

MODALITIES AND SUBJECTS: ethics, marketing, business practices, personal integration, student clinic

UNIQUE ASPECTS OF SCHOOL OR CURRICULUM: Multi-level teaching accommodates different learning styles of students in class.

#182 National Institute for Muscle Therapy
      777 S. New Ballas Rd., suite 230E
      St. Louis, MO 63141
      (314) 993-9083

HOURS OF TRAINING: 100

IN-CLASS HOURS: approximately 65

DURATION OF COURSE: nine one-day workshops over a four-month period

COST: $850

YEAR FOUNDED: 1977

GRADUATES PER YEAR (APPROX.): 12 to 18

MODALITIES AND SUBJECTS: Esalen, muscle stretching, establishing your business, sports massage, sports injury techniques

UNIQUE ASPECTS OF SCHOOL OR CURRICULUM: Class size is kept small for individual attention to each student.

#183 The Oasis School of Massage Therapy
      519 S. Fifth
      St. Charles, MO 63301
      (314) 949-0232 or 949-0448

No Catalogue

HOURS OF TRAINING: 100

DURATION OF COURSE: 3 months, evenings and weekends

COST: $800

YEAR FOUNDED: 1991

GRADUATES PER YEAR (APPROX.): 35

MODALITIES AND SUBJECTS: foot reflexology, trigger point, chair massage, marketing

CONTINUING EDUCATION: sports massage, Touch for Health, polarity

#184 Ozark Institute of Natural Therapies
      1271 E. Montclair
      Springfield, MO 65804
      (417) 883-0300

HOURS OF TRAINING: 600

DURATION OF COURSE: nine months

YEAR FOUNDED: 1989

MODALITIES AND SUBJECTS: medical terminology, pathological conditions, range of motion, palpation, prenatal massage, sports massage, reflexology, hydrotherapy, hygiene, business practices, ethical guidelines

ADVANCED PROGRAMS: contact school

CONTINUING EDUCATION: contact school

Nebraska

State Licensing: 1,000 hours

National Certification Exam accepted

Approved out-of-state schools:

   Collinson School, Colorado Springs CO
   Massage Therapy Institute, Denver CO
   New Mexico Academy, Santa Fe NM

Schools:

#185 Dr. Welbe's College of Massage Therapy
      2602 J. Street
      Omaha, NE 68107
      (402) 731-6768

Contact the school for program information.

#186 Myotherapy Institute
      6001 South 58th Street, Bldg. D, Box 16
      Lincoln, NE 68516
      (402) 421-7410

No Catalogue

HOURS OF TRAINING: 1,000 to 1,500

DURATION OF COURSE: nine months or longer

DAY/EVENING/WEEKEND: day or evening programs available

YEAR FOUNDED: 1993

GRADUATES PER YEAR (APPROX.): 30

MODALITIES AND SUBJECTS: applied anatomy, pathology, kinesiology, massage practicum, massage clinic, hydrotherapy, business, hygiene, Eastern techniques, kinetics seminar

CONTINUING EDUCATION: sports massage certification, medical massage certification, spa treatment certification

#187 Omaha School of Massage Therapy
      7905 "L" St., suite 230
      Omaha, NE 68127
      (402) 331-3694

HOURS OF TRAINING: 1,000 (500 in-class)

DURATION OF COURSE: 9 months

DAY/EVENING/WEEKEND: day and evening/weekend programs are available

COST: $4,150 (includes books)

FINANCIAL AID: arrangements pending at time of publication; contact school

YEAR FOUNDED: 1991

GRADUATES PER YEAR (APPROX.): 30 to 40

MODALITIES AND SUBJECTS: nutrition, kinesiology, exercise training, sports massage, executive massage, deep tissue, pregnancy massage, hydrotherapy, business and health service management, stress management, pathology

UNIQUE ASPECTS OF SCHOOL OR CURRICULUM: Students work in the student clinic and donate 20 hours of community service massage.

CONTINUING EDUCATION: contact school

New Hampshire

State Licensing: 750 hours

National Certification Exam not accepted

Schools:

#188 Dovestar Alchemian Institute
50 Whitehall Road
Hooksett, NH 03106-2104
(603) 669-9497 or (603) 669-5104

HOURS OF TRAINING: 750

DURATION OF COURSE: average 10 months; varies with individual students' schedules

DAY/EVENING/WEEKEND: day, evening and weekend programs available

COST: $4,500

FINANCIAL AID: work-study available

YEAR FOUNDED: 1979

ACCREDITATIONS/APPROVALS: transformational hypnotherapists Assoc., American council of hypnotist examiners

GRADUATES PER YEAR (APPROX.): 50

MODALITIES AND SUBJECTS: kriya massage, trigger point, Reiki, myofascial therapy, neuromuscular therapy, strain/conterstrain, pathology, hygiene, sports massage, acupressure, applied kinesiology, reflexology, hydrotherapy, CPR, client analysis, practicum, clinical, business and marketing

UNIQUE ASPECTS OF SCHOOL OR CURRICULUM: Students may begin the program at any time during the year and go at their own pace. The focus is on sensitivity, and credit can be arranged for prior training and experience.

ADVANCED PROGRAMS: Reiki-alchemia, alchemical synergy, alchemia heart breath, therapeutic massage advanced study, sports massage, Oriental bodywork, jin shin acupressure, alchemical hypnotherapy, equine massage, holistic health practitioner

CONTINUING EDUCATION: contact school

#189 New England Academy of Therapeutic Sciences
402 Amherst St.
Nashua, NH 03063
(603) 886-8433

HOURS OF TRAINING: 950

IN-CLASS HOURS: 800

DURATION OF COURSE: nine months, 3 evenings per week plus Saturdays (day program to be added in 1995)

COST: $5,600

FINANCIAL AID: payment plans

MODALITIES AND SUBJECTS: polarity, reflexology, reflex point therapy, lymphatic drainage massage, sports massage, circulatory massage, pathology, biomechanics, exercise physiology, hydrotherapy, nutrition, homeopathy, first aid/CPR, public health and hygiene, business practices, ethics, practicum

CONTINUING EDUCATION: medical massage, sports massage; contact school for additional offerings.

#190 New Hampshire Institute for Therapeutic Arts
School of Massage Therapy
153 Lowell Rd.
Hudson, NH 03051
(603) 882-3022

HOURS OF TRAINING: 1,500

IN-CLASS HOURS: 750

DURATION OF COURSE: 9 months, two evenings per week plus Saturdays

COST: $4,825

YEAR FOUNDED: 1983

ACCREDITATIONS/APPROVALS: COMTAA

MODALITIES AND SUBJECTS: embryology, first aid/CPR, ethics and professionalism, business and legal issues, reflexology, pressure point therapies, health and hygiene, pathology, hydrotherapy, neuromuscular technique, human sexuality, nutrition, neurology, circulatory massage, lymphatic drainage massage, sports massage, polarity, acupressure, shiatsu, five element theory, research and report, massage practicum

ADVANCED PROGRAMS: polarity certification course, Russian energy techniques

CONTINUING EDUCATION: otology, iridology, advanced reflexology, hydrotherapy, homeopathy, a day for therapists, bach remedies, awakening your light body, speech and sound therapy, art therapy, introduction to radionics, herbology

#191 North Eastern Institute of Whole Health, Inc.
      School of Massage Therapy
      22 Bridge St.
      Manchester, NH 03101
      (603) 623-5018

HOURS OF TRAINING: 750

DURATION OF COURSE: one year

DAY/EVENING/WEEKEND: day, evening and Saturday programs available

COST: $4,725

FINANCIAL AID: payment plan

YEAR FOUNDED: 1993

MODALITIES AND SUBJECTS: history and theory of massage, rules/professionalism/ethics, sports massage, seated massage, reflexology, acupressure, shiatsu, cranio-sacral therapy, neuromuscular technique, hygiene, business practices and marketing, hydrotherapy, CPR, massage practicum, electives

CONTINUING EDUCATION: aromatherapy, cranio-sacral therapy, Esalen massage, lymphatic drainage massage, NLP, physical and emotional rebalancing, polarity, trigger point and pressure point therapy, equine massage, geriatric massage

New Jersey

No State licensing

Schools:

#192 The Center for Transpersonal Body/Mind
      Studies
      51 Upland Ave.
      Metuchen, NJ 08840
      (908) 548-8579

HOURS OF TRAINING: 225

IN-CLASS HOURS: 175

DURATION OF COURSE: 6 months, evenings and weekends

COST: $1,890

YEAR FOUNDED: 1990

ACCREDITATIONS/APPROVALS: approved for independent college credit

GRADUATES PER YEAR (APPROX.): 40

MODALITIES AND SUBJECTS: Polarity, myofascial techniques, Trager, shiatsu, cross-cultural massage and healing methods, medical intuitiveness, gestalt therapy, bioenergetics, transpersonal bodywork and psychology

UNIQUE ASPECTS OF SCHOOL OR CURRICULUM: Faculty has a mental health and bodywork background, and has studied with shamans and healers in other countries. The school emphasizes psycho-physical aspects of bodywork and energetic and shamanic approaches to healing.

ADVANCED PROGRAMS: The program may be taken as advanced training for bodyworkers who wish to learn or deepen counseling skills.

#193 Healing Hands Institute for Massage
      Therapy
      63 Franklin Court
      Emerson, NJ 07630
      (201) 265-6970

HOURS OF TRAINING: 500

DURATION OF COURSE: 11 months

DAY/EVENING/WEEKEND: day and evening programs available

COST: $5,060 (includes books)

FINANCIAL AID: various forms available, contact school

YEAR FOUNDED: 1990

ACCREDITATIONS/APPROVALS: NJ Dept. of Education

GRADUATES PER YEAR (APPROX.): 50

MODALITIES AND SUBJECTS: pathology, art of touch and biomechanics, professional ethics, deep tissue, hydrotherapy, business management, sports massage, pre and postnatal massage, practicum, body integration, reflexology, shiatsu

ADVANCED PROGRAMS: chinese massage, advanced reflexology

CONTINUING EDUCATION: on-site, sports massage

#194 Health Choices Center for the Healing Arts
      166 Bunn Drive
      Princeton, NJ 08540
      (609) 252-0895

HOURS OF TRAINING: 550

IN-CLASS HOURS: 475

DURATION OF COURSE: one year

DAY/EVENING/WEEKEND: day and evening/weekend programs available

COST: $5,675 including books

FINANCIAL AID: payment plan

YEAR FOUNDED: 1978

GRADUATES PER YEAR (APPROX.): 40

MODALITIES AND SUBJECTS: shiatsu, neuromuscular therapy, polarity, aromatherapy, Trager, reflexology, clinical application, field work, metaphysics, body mechanics, intuition development, self-care, stress management, business practice

UNIQUE ASPECTS OF SCHOOL OR CURRICULUM: The school maintains an informal atmosphere and emphasizes the body/mind/spirit connection.

CONTINUING EDUCATION: on-site, couples massage, Gateway training (spiritual transformational bodywork), aromatherapy, shiatsu

#195 Helma Corp. Institute of Massage Therapy
853 Garrison Ave.
Teaneck, NJ 07666
(201) 836-8176

HOURS OF TRAINING: 500 (includes 220 hours of supervised clinic practice)

DURATION OF COURSE: 6 to 7 months, 3 evening per week plus half-day Sunday

COST: $3,025 (includes required texts)

FINANCIAL AID: payment plan

YEAR FOUNDED: 1984

GRADUATES PER YEAR (APPROX.): 45 to 50

MODALITIES AND SUBJECTS: pathology, kinesiology, CPR, shiatsu, on-site, prenatal massage, hydrotherapy, sports massage, reflexology, geriatric massage, business and marketing, clinic practicum

CONTINUING EDUCATION: contact school

#196 Ingeborg Schlobohm
Certified Instructor
177 Weston Ave.
Chatham, NJ 07928
(201) 635-4655

250-hour curriculum with 8-student maximum. Please contact Ms. Schlobohm for complete program information.

#197 Kinley Institute for Massage and Related Studies
668 Raritan Road
Clark, NJ 07066
(908) 382-2434

HOURS OF TRAINING: 100

DURATION OF COURSE: 4½ months

DAY/EVENING/WEEKEND: day, evening and Saturday programs available

COST: $1,695

YEAR FOUNDED: 1963

UNIQUE ASPECTS OF SCHOOL OR CURRICULUM: flexible scheduling and individualized instruction

ADVANCED PROGRAMS: shiatsu

CONTINUING EDUCATION: reflexology, Touch for Health, scalp massage, vibro-percussive techniques, chairside massage, relaxation training

#198 Morris Institute of Natural Therapeutics
3108 Rt. 10 West
Denville, NJ 07834
(800) 360-MINT or (201) 989-8939

HOURS OF TRAINING: 520

DURATION OF COURSE: 25 weeks

DAY/EVENING/WEEKEND: day and evening programs available

COST: $2,395

YEAR FOUNDED: 1963

GRADUATES PER YEAR (APPROX.): 60

MODALITIES AND SUBJECTS: professional ethics, hygiene, legislation and insurance, business skills

UNIQUE ASPECTS OF SCHOOL OR CURRICULUM: Class size is limited for individual instruction.

ADVANCED PROGRAMS: shiatsu certification course

CONTINUING EDUCATION: sports massage, reflexology, aromatherapy, Touch for Health, on-site, neuromuscular therapy, facelift massage system, craniosacral therapy, zero balancing

#199 New Jersey School of Massage
3699 Rt. 46
Parsippany, NJ 07054
(201) 263-2229

The school teaches shiatsu combined with Western bodywork disciplines. The student-teacher ratio is 2:1. Please contact the school for complete program information.

#200 Ocean Massage Institute
3321 Doris Ave., Bldg. B
Ocean, NJ 07712
(908) 531-3059

HOURS OF TRAINING: 520

DURATION OF COURSE: two to three evenings per week plus some weekends for one year

COST: $4,995

FINANCIAL AID: payment plan

YEAR FOUNDED: 1985

MODALITIES AND SUBJECTS: history of massage, self-care, hygiene, client/therapist relationship, professional ethics, body mechanics, medical terminology, CPR/first aid, business and career guidance, deep tissue, sidelying techniques, joint structure techniques, chiropractic adjunct massage, pathology, hydrotherapy, HIV, reflexology, sports massage, shiatsu, myofascial techniques, medical massage, 5-element theory, Touch for Health,

UNIQUE ASPECTS OF SCHOOL OR CURRICULUM: Advanced standing may be granted based on completion of prior massage training at another school.

ADVANCED PROGRAMS: 100-hour medical externship

CONTINUING EDUCATION: craniosacral therapy, sports massage, shiatsu, on-site, reflexology, Touch for Health, infant massage, yoga

---

#201 Somerset School of Massage Therapy
      7 Cedar Grove Lane
      Somerset, NJ 08873
      (908) 356-0787

HOURS OF TRAINING: 564

DURATION OF COURSE: 12 months

DAY/EVENING/WEEKEND: day and evening programs available

COST: $4,795 (includes books)

FINANCIAL AID: approved for veterans' benefits, some state funding programs

YEAR FOUNDED: 1987

ACCREDITATIONS/APPROVALS: COMTAA, NJ Dept. of Ed.

PREPARATION FOR OUT-OF-STATE LICENSING EXAM: Florida

MODALITIES AND SUBJECTS: sports massage, on-site, reflexology, myofascial and deep tissue massage, prenatal massage, neuromuscular therapy, CPR/first aid, t'ai chi, hydrotherapy, clinic, HIV/AIDS, business and ethics

CONTINUING EDUCATION: advanced myofascial therapy, pre-natal certification, lymphatic drainage certification, sports massage certification, neuromuscular certification, spa workshop, therapeutic touch, massage for survivors of abuse

---

#202 Time-Out Professional Massage School
      285 Parker Rd.
      Eatontown, NJ 07724
      (908) 229-8300

HOURS OF TRAINING: 112

IN-CLASS HOURS: 100

Duration of course: 4 months

DAY/EVENING/WEEKEND: day and evening program available

COST: $1,160 (includes textbook)

YEAR FOUNDED: 1991

GRADUATES PER YEAR (APPROX.): 60

UNIQUE ASPECTS OF SCHOOL OR CURRICULUM: The director is a registered nurse and massage therapist, and the program is geared toward those in the medical field. Prior experience as a physical trainer, physical therapy assistant, medical technician, nurse or other health or human services position is a prerequisite for enrollment.

Continuing education: reflexology, aromatherapy, sports massage, chair massage, chiropractic and massage, creative marketing

---

New Mexico

State Licensing: 650 hours

National Certification Exam accepted

Schools:

#203 Crystal Mountain Apprenticeship in the
      Healing Arts
      118 Dartmouth SE
      Albuquerque, NM 87106
      (505) 268-4411

HOURS OF TRAINING: 675

DURATION OF COURSE: 6 months

Day/evening/weekend: day and evening programs are available

COST: $3,250 (includes books)

FINANCIAL AID: payment plans, work-study, loans

YEAR FOUNDED: 1988

ACCREDITATIONS/APPROVALS: New Mexico Commission on Higher Education, Division of Vocational Rehabilitation

GRADUATES PER YEAR (APPROX.): 85

MODALITIES AND SUBJECTS: sports massage, therapeutic exercise, Esalen, neuromuscular therapy, polarity, polar-reflexology, movement re-education, deep tissue massage, body reading/postural analysis, cranio-sacral therapy, emotional release and clearing work, process work, abuse issues, business skills, pregnancy massage, interviewing techniques, hydrotherapy, CPR/first aid, nutrition, morality/ethics, herbology, pathology, business internship and 150 hours of clinical internship

CONTINUING EDUCATION: Programs are offered regularly; contact school for current offerings.

#204 Dr. Jay Scherer's Academy of Natural Healing
1443 S. St. Francis Dr.
Santa Fe, NM 87505
(505) 982-8398

HOURS OF TRAINING: 670 plus 120-hour practicum and internship

DURATION OF COURSE: 6 months full-time in Santa Fe, 12 months evening/weekend program available in Taos, NM

COST: $4,500

FINANCIAL AID: work-study positions, payment plans

YEAR FOUNDED: 1979

ACCREDITATIONS/APPROVALS: COMTAA

PREPARATION FOR OUT-OF-STATE LICENSING EXAM: program meets most states' requirements — contact school with specific inquiries

GRADUATES PER YEAR (APPROX.): 50

MODALITIES AND SUBJECTS: self-awareness for massage professionals, kinesiology, sensitivity training, business practice, ethics, hygiene, connective tissue massage, pathology, Oriental self-help techniques, stretches for postural alignment, foot reflexology, naturopathic uses of herbs and folk remedies, Touch for Health, applied kinesiology, homeopathic theory, massage therapy for specific conditions, first aid, CPR, shiatsu, financial management, movement, chair massage

UNIQUE ASPECTS OF SCHOOL OR CURRICULUM: small classes, holistic focus, volunteer outreach program

ADVANCED PROGRAMS: Life Impression Bodywork

CONTINUING EDUCATION: polarity, shiatsu, trigger point, massage for the child-bearing year, herbology, infant massage instructor training

#205 Higher Knead
3107 Eubank N.E. suite 1
Albuquerque, NM 87111
(505) 275-2100

HOURS OF TRAINING: 650

DURATION OF COURSE: 8 months

DAY/EVENING/WEEKEND: day and evening programs available (plus one weekend per month)

COST: $3,500

MODALITIES AND SUBJECTS: acupressure, Alexander technique, applied kinesiology, ayurveda, business, centering, chair massage, chakra balancing, emotional release and facilitation, deep tissue massage, dry massage, Feldenkrais method, first aid/CPR, herbs, hydrotherapy, iridology, nutrition, professional ethics, reflexology, running a practice, shiatsu, skin cancer identification, t'ai chi, Thai massage, massage for animals and plants, use of machines in massage therapy

#206 Inochi Institute
330 Garfield St., #201
Santa Fe, NM 87501
(505) 986-0638

No Catalogue available

HOURS OF TRAINING: 660

DURATION OF COURSE: one year

DAY/EVENING/WEEKEND: evening program available

COST: $8,000

YEAR FOUNDED: 1985

GRADUATES PER YEAR (APPROX.): 2-4

MODALITIES AND SUBJECTS: Japanese systems; shiatsu, amma, sotai, sakai hon li, te a te, self-health care, first aid.

UNIQUE ASPECTS OF SCHOOL OR CURRICULUM: The curriculum is coordinated with the first year of the Inochi acupuncture training. 100 hours of anatomy and physiology is required for admission. Swedish massage is a survey course and the training emphasizes Oriental styles of therapy.

CONTINUING EDUCATION: contact school

#207 The Medicine Wheel
1243 B West Apache
Farmington, NM 87401
(505) 327-1914

HOURS OF TRAINING: 650-hour massage therapist, 1,000-hour holistic health practitioner

DURATION OF COURSE: (650-hour course) classes meet evenings and weekends for one year

COST: $4,555.32 (includes required coursebooks) The 1,000-hour program tuition is $6,885.95. Electives make be taken for $9 per class hour with payment two weeks in advance.

FINANCIAL AID: payment plan

YEAR FOUNDED: 1992

ACCREDITATIONS/APPROVALS: approved for veterans

GRADUATES PER YEAR (APPROX.): 12

MODALITIES AND SUBJECTS: chinese massage, deep tissue, infant massage, integrative massage, jin shin ki, lymphatic massage, neuromuscular therapy, on-site, polarity, pre-natal, reflexology, shiatsu, sports massage, supervised clinic, business practicum, client relationship & stress management, mind-body connection, first aid & CPR, hydrotherapy, legal guidelines, ethical issues

UNIQUE ASPECTS OF SCHOOL OR CURRICULUM: The school offers life experience credit and allows transfer of credit from other schools. Students may begin the program at any time, and choose between Swedish, Oriental and energy classes offered in weekend intensives.

ADVANCED PROGRAMS: 1,000-hour holistic health practitioner program. Courses include aromatherapy, bach flower remedies, body reading, chakra, color & crystal healing, cranio-sacral, diet and nutrition, herbology, bio-feedback, personal growth, Reiki, t'ai chi, therapeutic touch, tibetan healing sounds, TMJ workshop, yoga for specifics.

CONTINUING EDUCATION: Some of the advanced courses are offered as continuing education.

#208 Mesilla Valley School of Therapeutic Arts
1803 W. Union Ave.
Las Crusas, NM 88005
(505) 527-1239

Contact the school for program information.

#209 New Mexico Academy of Healing Arts
P.O. Box 932
Santa Fe, NM 87504
(505) 982-6271

HOURS OF TRAINING: 650

DURATION OF COURSE: 650-hour course six months days or twelve months evenings; 1000-hour course nine months; 1200-hour course 11 months

COST: 650-hours $4,600; 1,000 hours $6,500; 1,200 hours $7,000

FINANCIAL AID: Job Training Partnership Act, vocational rehabilitation, veterans' benefits, payment plans

YEAR FOUNDED: 1981

ACCREDITATIONS/APPROVALS: COMTAA, approved for nursing CEU's

UNIQUE ASPECTS OF SCHOOL OR CURRICULUM: Community service, meditation and commitment to holistic healing are key concepts at the Academy.

ADVANCED PROGRAMS: Associate Polarity Practitioner, Registered Polarity Practitioner, shiatsu, advanced sports/clinical massage

CONTINUING EDUCATION: sports massage, shiatsu, recovering from grief, anatomy and physiology with Manikens, aromatherapy, bodyreading, ortho-bionomy, polarity, cranial work, ayurvedic medicine, medicinal herbs, deep tissue/trigger point therapy

#210 New Mexico School of Natural Therapeutics
117 Richmond NE
Albuquerque, NM 87106
(505) 268-6870

HOURS OF TRAINING: 750

DURATION OF COURSE: 6 months day, one year evenings and Saturdays

COST: $5,000 including supplies

YEAR FOUNDED: 1974

ACCREDITATIONS/APPROVALS: COMTAA, NM Division of vocational rehabilitation

PREPARATION FOR OUT-OF-STATE LICENSING EXAM: can be arranged; contact school for specifics

GRADUATES PER YEAR (APPROX.): 100

MODALITIES AND SUBJECTS: sports massage, Swedish gymnastics, polarity therapy, herbology, bach flowers, homeopathic first aid, shiatsu, reflexology, body/mind counseling techniques, hydrotherapy, philosophy of natural therapeutics, business procedures and professional ethics, nutrition, first aid/CPR, hygiene, AIDS education, internship/clinical practice

UNIQUE ASPECTS OF SCHOOL OR CURRICULUM: The school emphasizes energy work and holistic approaches. Core faculty have 10 to 18 years teaching experience at this school.

CONTINUING EDUCATION: cranio-sacral, sports massage, colonic irrigation, advanced polarity, myofascial technique and others—contact school for current offerings

#211 Somatic Therapy Institute
546 Harkle Road, suite B
Santa Fe, NM 87501
(505) 983-9695

At the time of publication (1/1/95), the school's massage training program was in a process of revision and final information was not available.

In addition to its state-approved massage training program, Somatic Therapy Institute is creating a new program in conjunction with Southwestern College to offer a Masters in Counseling that will qualify graduates for dual licensure as mental health counselor and massage therapist.

Once the masters program is implemented, the revised massage program will be resumed. Please contact the school for current program information.

#212 Universal Therapeutic Massage Institute, Inc.
3410 Aztec Rd. NE
Albuquerque, NM 87107
(505) 888-0020 or (800) 557-0020

HOURS OF TRAINING: 670

IN-CLASS HOURS: 520

DURATION OF COURSE: 6 months

DAY/EVENING/WEEKEND: day and evening programs available

COST: $3,450 plus tax (includes books)

FINANCIAL AID: payment plan

YEAR FOUNDED: 1993

GRADUATES PER YEAR (APPROX.): 80

MODALITIES AND SUBJECTS: pathology, interview techniques, range of motion, palpation, massage theory and history, joint mobilization, stretches, exercise, relaxation, stress management, sports massage, shiatsu, reflexology, body reading deep tissue therapy, chair massage, body mechanics, clinic internship, business and professional ethics

UNIQUE ASPECTS OF SCHOOL OR CURRICULUM: small class size for personal attention

ADVANCED PROGRAMS: contact school

CONTINUING EDUCATION: contact school

New York

State Licensing: 605 hours

National Certification Exam not accepted

Schools:

#213 Finger Lakes School of Massage
1251 Trumansburg Road
Ithaca, NY 14850
(607) 272-9024

A Branch of the Florida School of Massage

HOURS OF TRAINING: 850

DURATION OF COURSE: 5½ months full-time, 1½ to 2 years weekends

COST: $5,800

YEAR FOUNDED: 1993

PREPARATION FOR OUT-OF-STATE LICENSING EXAM: Florida

GRADUATES PER YEAR (APPROX.): 135

MODALITIES AND SUBJECTS: connective tissue massage, neuromuscular therapy, polarity, sports massage, reflexology, shiatsu and Oriental theory, massage for infants, pregnant women and the elderly, awareness and communication skills, massage practicum, hydrotherapy, kinesiology, massage law and business practices, AIDS education, directed independent study

UNIQUE ASPECTS OF SCHOOL OR CURRICULUM: student internship with developmentally disabled adults, children who are physically handicapped, senior citizens and people with AIDS; opportunity for directed independent study

ADVANCED PROGRAMS: neuromuscular therapy, structural integration, sports massage, homeopathy, polarity, reflexology

CONTINUING EDUCATION: contact school

#214 The New Center For Wholistic Health Education & Research
6801 Jericho Tpke
Syosset, NY 11791
(516) 364-0808

HOURS OF TRAINING: 1,072

DURATION OF COURSE: normally 18 months, can be completed in 12 months or up to 27 months

COST: $9,504

FINANCIAL AID: Federal Pell grants, Stafford Loans, SLS/Plus, veterans benefits, vocational rehabilitation

YEAR FOUNDED: 1981

ACCREDITATIONS/APPROVALS: New York State Board of Regents, ACCET, COMTAA

GRADUATES PER YEAR (APPROX.): 75 to 100

MODALITIES AND SUBJECTS: AMMA therapy, Oriental anatomy and physiology, t'ai chi, ethics, sexuality and emotional functioning, myology, trigger point therapy, deep tissue, active and passive exercises, treatments for pathological conditions, professional business practice and management, Oriental clinic assessment, massage therapy clinic, neurology, pathology, first aid/CPR

ADVANCED PROGRAMS: Advanced AMMA therapy program

CONTINUING EDUCATION: A variety of continuing education programs are regularly offered. Contact school for current listing.

#215 New York Institute of Massage
P.O. Box 645
Buffalo, NY 14231
(716) 633-0355

HOURS OF TRAINING: 735

IN-CLASS HOURS: 675

DURATION OF COURSE: 30 weeks

DAY/EVENING/WEEKEND: day and evening programs available

COST: $6,325 (includes books and supplies)

YEAR FOUNDED: 1994

GRADUATES PER YEAR (APPROX.): 200

MODALITIES AND SUBJECTS: spa therapies, sports massage, polarity, neuromuscular therapy, pathology, myology, Oriental massage, CPR & first aid, neurology, hydrotherapy, exercise physiology, business management, health and hygiene, infection control, student clinic (40 hours), community service (20 hours)

Unique aspects of school or curriculum: cooperative training with chiropractic and physical therapy colleges

ADVANCED PROGRAMS: contact school

CONTINUING EDUCATION: contact school

#216 Swedish Institute, Inc.
226 West 26th St., Fifth Floor
New York, NY 10001
(212) 924-5900

HOURS OF TRAINING: 692

DURATION OF COURSE: 12 months

DAY/EVENING/WEEKEND: day and evening programs available

COST: $6,535 plus approximately $400 for books and uniforms

FINANCIAL AID: Stafford Loans, Unsubsidized Stafford Loans, Parent Plus Loans, Pell grants; contact school financial aid officer for information regarding eligibility

YEAR FOUNDED: 1916

ACCREDITATIONS/APPROVALS: COMTAA, Career College Association, New York Bureau of Veterans Education, Commission for the Blind and Visually Handicapped, New York Department of Vocational Education for Individuals with Disabilities, Department of Immigration and Naturalization

PREPARATION FOR OUT-OF-STATE LICENSING EXAM: can be arranged — contact school

MODALITIES AND SUBJECTS: arthrology, kinesiology, pathology, joint manipulation, deep tissue, medical massage, clinical internship program, shiatsu, business practices seminar, first aid, CPR

UNIQUE ASPECTS OF SCHOOL OR CURRICULUM: Students work in a medically-oriented clinic, treating patients referred by their doctors.

CONTINUING EDUCATION: A wide range of continuing education programs are offered — contact the Director of Continuing Education for information or a brochure.

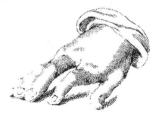

North Carolina

No State licensing

Schools:

#217 Body Therapy Institute
South Wind Farm
P.O. Box 1
Pittsboro, NC 27312
(919) 663-3111

HOURS OF TRAINING: 600

IN-CLASS HOURS: 527

DURATION OF COURSE: 7 months days or 11 months evenings and weekends

COST: $5,770 (includes books)

FINANCIAL AID: payment plan, work study

YEAR FOUNDED: 1983

ACCREDITATIONS/APPROVALS: COMTAA

PREPARATION FOR OUT-OF-STATE LICENSING EXAM: Florida

GRADUATES PER YEAR (APPROX.): 40

MODALITIES AND SUBJECTS: deep tissue, polarity, shiatsu, body psychology, hydrotherapy, business and marketing, body mechanics

UNIQUE ASPECTS OF SCHOOL OR CURRICULUM: wholistic/transformational model

ADVANCED PROGRAMS: somatic therapy

CONTINUING EDUCATION: contact school

#218 Carolina School of Massage Therapy
103 W. Weaver St
Carrboro, NC 27510
(919) 933-2212

HOURS OF TRAINING: 525

DURATION OF COURSE: days 6 months; weekends, alternate weekends for one year

DAY/EVENING/WEEKEND: weekend program available

COST: $4,620

FINANCIAL AID: payment plan

YEAR FOUNDED: 1987

ACCREDITATIONS/APPROVALS: COMTAA

GRADUATES PER YEAR (APPROX.): 60

MODALITIES AND SUBJECTS: deep tissue, sports massage, polarity, hydrotherapy, business practices, communications, somatics, case studies

UNIQUE ASPECTS OF SCHOOL OR CURRICULUM: The school is a program of the non-profit Community

Wholistic Health Center which offers a variety of continuing education classes. Its location near Chapel Hill provides a wide range of cultural and educational activities.

CONTINUING EDUCATION: contact school

#219 The Southeastern School of Neuromuscular and Massage Therapy of Charlotte, Inc.
4 Woodlawn Green, suite 200
Charlotte, NC 28217
1-800-420-HAND or (704) 527-4979

HOURS OF TRAINING: 500

IN-CLASS HOURS: 500

DURATION OF COURSE: 6 months full-time or one year part-time

DAY/EVENING/WEEKEND: morning and evening programs available

COST: $5,300

FINANCIAL AID: Contact school for information

YEAR FOUNDED: 1994

PREPARATION FOR OUT-OF-STATE LICENSING EXAM: Florida

GRADUATES PER YEAR (APPROX.): (anticipated) 50-120

MODALITIES AND SUBJECTS: neuromuscular and structural bodywork, hydrotherapy, ethics, laws and rules

UNIQUE ASPECTS OF SCHOOL OR CURRICULUM: Certification in neuromuscular and structural bodywork is built into 500 hour course. A 200-hour certification in NMT and structural bodywork is also available.

ADVANCED PROGRAMS: Advanced trainings in neuromuscular and structural integration by Kyle Wright, L.M.T.

CONTINUING EDUCATION: contact school

Ohio

State Licensing: 600 hours

National Certification Exam not accepted

Approved Out-of-State Schools

Boulder School of Massage Therapy, Boulder, CO
Brenneke School of Massage, Seattle, WA
Chicago School of Massage Therapy, Chicago, IL
Desert Institute of the Healing Arts, Tucson, AZ
Health Enrichment Center, Lapeer, MI
New Mexico Academy of Healing Arts, Santa Fe, NM
Reese Institute, Ovieda, FL
Swedish Institute, New York, NY

Schools:

#220 American Institute of Massotherapy, Inc.
212 Jefferson
Tiffin, OH 44883
(419) 448-1355

Contact the school for program information.

#221 Central Ohio School of Massage
1120 Morse Rd., suite 250
Columbus, OH 43229
(614) 841-1122 or (800) 466-5676

HOURS OF TRAINING: 670

DURATION OF COURSE: 18 months

DAY/EVENING/WEEKEND: day and evening programs available

COST: $5,850 plus application fee

FINANCIAL AID: payment plan

YEAR FOUNDED: 1964

ACCREDITATIONS/APPROVALS: COMTAA

MODALITIES AND SUBJECTS: pathology, ethics, business practices, patient approach, uses of heat and cold, restorative exercises

ADVANCED PROGRAMS: 170-hour MyoFascial Therapist program

#222 Hocking College
3301 Hocking Parkway
Nelsonville, OH 45764
(614) 753-3591 or (800) 282-4163

HOURS OF TRAINING: 33 credit hours (approximately 600 classroom hours)

DURATION OF COURSE: six quarters (two academic years)

COST: Ohio residents $55 per credit hour ($1,815 total), non-residents $110 per credit hour ($3,630 total)

FINANCIAL AID: Contact school for financial aid information.

MODALITIES AND SUBJECTS: fascia and joint release, healing through the human energy field, massage techniques, massage theory, the human organism, professionalism and ethics, movement analysis, craniosacral release

#223 Midwestern College of Massotherapy
Office: 3857 East Broad St.
Classroom: 3589 E. Main St.
Columbus, OH 43213
(614) 231-1973

HOURS OF TRAINING: 600 or 630

DURATION OF COURSE: evening program one year; Thursday/Saturday program 19 months

Cost: $6,157 (includes books, insurance and two re-quired seminars)

Financial aid: payment plan

Year founded: 1989

Accreditations/approvals: Veterans' Administration Rehabilitation Division

Modalities and subjects: Rolfing, strain-counter-strain, neuromuscular therapy, Nimmo technique, craniosacral technique, musculoskeletal pathology, medical clinical skills, physiotherapy modalities, hygiene, ethics, on-site clinic, massage practicum, business practice, first aid/CPR

#224 National Institute of Massotherapy
2110 Copley Rd.
Akron, OH 44320
(216) 867-1996

Hours of training: 600

Duration of course: 12 months or 18 months

Day/evening/weekend: day and evening programs available, and both meet some weekends

Cost: $6,335

Financial aid: payment plan, veterans benefits, Title IV monies

Year founded: 1991

Graduates per year (approx.): 40

Modalities and subjects: shiatsu, Touch for Health, movement, ethics, kinesiology, massage clinic, CPR

Advanced programs: myofascial therapy, conscious touch, manual lymphatic drainage, craniosacral therapy, Feldenkrais, Alexander, advanced shiatsu, therapeutic touch, polarity, advanced Touch for Health, professional kinesiology practitioner, maximum athletic performance system, stress management, consultation, taijiquan, psychotherapeutic issues in massotherapy

Continuing education: contact school

#225 Ohio College of Massotherapy, Inc.
1014-16-18 Kenmore Blvd.
Akron, OH 44314
(216) 745-6170

Hours of training: 602 including 50 hours clinic

Duration of course: 18 months, one day per week (Wed., Th., Fri. or Sat.)

Cost: $6,774 including books and insurance

Financial aid: payment plans

Year founded: 1973

Accreditations/approvals: ACCSCT

Modalities and subjects: joint mobilization, TMJ treatment, hydrotherapy, structural analysis, posture and body mechanics, neurologic and orthopedic screening, pathology, palpation, communicable diseases, sexuality, ethics and spirituality, business and law, insurance and record-keeping, SOAP charting

Unique aspects of school or curriculum: Class size is limited to 25 for individual attention.

Continuing education: neuromuscular therapy, myofascial release, craniosacral technique, on-site, Touch for Health

#226 Ohio College of Medical Arts
School of Massotherapy
10605 Chester Ave.
Cleveland, OH 44106
(216) 791-1150

Hours of training: 670

Duration of course: 21 months (Saturdays or two mornings per week)

Cost: $7,575

Financial aid: veterans' benefits, payment plans

Year founded: 1989

Modalities and subjects: pathology, joint movements, heat, cold and electrical modalities, flexibility and stretching, outpatient clinical practice, CPR and emergency care, seminar, autopsy

#227 Self-Health, Inc. School of Medical Massage
P.O. Box 474
130 Cook Road
Lebanon, OH 45036
(513) 932-8712

Hours of training: 600

Duration of course: 18 months evenings or 12 months Honors program days

Cost: 18-months $5,200; 12-months $5,500 (includes books; $400 discount for prepayment)

Financial aid: payment plan

Year founded: 1980

Accreditations/approvals: COMTAA

Graduates per year (approx.): 90

Modalities and subjects: cranio-sacral, myofascial release, joint mobilization, seated massage, sports massage

Unique aspects of school or curriculum: The school has a holistic emphasis and offers students community outreach with social services agencies

Continuing education: joint mobilization, cranio-sacral, acupressure, myofascial therapy

Oklahoma

No State licensing

Schools:

#228 Massage Therapy Institute of Oklahoma
9433 East 51st St., suite H
Tulsa, OK 74145
(918) 622-6644

HOURS OF TRAINING: 250 or 500

DURATION OF COURSE: 16 weeks for each 250-hour program

DAY/EVENING/WEEKEND: day and evening programs available

COST: $1,500 per 250-hour program (10% discount for prepayment)

FINANCIAL AID: payment plans, work study programs available

YEAR FOUNDED: 1992

GRADUATES PER YEAR (APPROX.): 40

MODALITIES AND SUBJECTS: 250-hour program includes on-site, shiatsu, acupressure, passive joint movement, reflex/zone therapy, hydrotherapy, spa standards, first aid/CPR, hygiene, business and ethics, clinical practicum. The 500-hour program adds pathology, massage for specific conditions, body psychology, neuromuscular re-education, range of motion, passive stretching, subtle bodywork, connective tissue and deep tissue techniques, Jyn Shyn Jytsu, tui na, practice management, medical and clinical terminology, clinical practicum II.

UNIQUE ASPECTS OF SCHOOL OR CURRICULUM: maximum class size is limited to 20 students.

CONTINUING EDUCATION: geriatric massage, prenatal massage, infant massage, chronic pain workshop, body mind workshop, shiatsu-Oriental therapies, reflexology

#229 The Oklahoma School of Natural Healing
1660 E. 71st St., suite 2-0
Tulsa, OK 74136
(918) 496-9401 or (800) 496-9401

HOURS OF TRAINING: technician 250, therapist 650

IN-CLASS HOURS: technician 140; therapist 420

DURATION OF COURSE: technician one month days or three months weekends (plus practicum); therapist 2½ months days or 10 months weekends (plus practicum)

COST: technician $1,743 including books and massage table ($1,495 if prepaid); therapist $4,338 including books and massage table ($3,695 if prepaid)

FINANCIAL AID: job training partnership act, vocational rehabilitation

YEAR FOUNDED: 1980

GRADUATES PER YEAR (APPROX.): 20

MODALITIES AND SUBJECTS: polarity, reflexology, sports massage, deep tissue, myofascial release, hydrotherapy, heliotherapy, body mobilization, on-site, business skills, acupressure, craniosacral therapy, manual lymphatic drainage, geriatric massage, nutrition, herbology, counseling skills, attitudinal healing, neurolinguistic programming

UNIQUE ASPECTS OF SCHOOL OR CURRICULUM: All coursework can be applied to a Doctor of Naturopathic Medicine program at select universities. The programs include clinical practicum, which may be taken at the school, and/or with physicians, counselors and graduate massage therapists.

ADVANCED PROGRAMS: masters (1,000 hours) and instructor of massage (1,290 hours)

CONTINUING EDUCATION: All courses are in workshop format and can be taken as continuing education.

#230 Praxis College
P.O. Box 75507
Oklahoma City, OK 73107
(405) 949-2244

HOURS OF TRAINING: 500 or 1,100

IN-CLASS HOURS: 500 or 1,100

DURATION OF COURSE: 500 hours 90 days; 1,100 hours two years

DAY/EVENING/WEEKEND: evening and weekend programs are available

COST: 500 hours $500, including books and supplies; 1,100 hours $2,800, books and supplies approximately $822 additional

FINANCIAL AID: scholarships, loans, grants, work-study

YEAR FOUNDED: founded 1976, state licensed 1987

PREPARATION FOR OUT-OF-STATE LICENSING EXAM: contact school

GRADUATES PER YEAR (APPROX.): 51

MODALITIES AND SUBJECTS: 500-hour course includes sports massage, reflexology, massage for the childbearing year, on-site, origins of the profession, ethics, business, techniques of healthy living, supervised practice and apprenticeship.

The 1,100 program also includes skilled touch, nutrition, human relations, additional anatomy training, hydrotherapy, pain control, non-traditional medicine, physical assessment, pharmacology and pathology, psychotherapeutic massage, Oriental massage, energy field massage, life power, externship.

UNIQUE ASPECTS OF SCHOOL OR CURRICULUM: The program is taught in part at medical school, with clinical rotation at major hospitals

ADVANCED PROGRAMS: Masters program available, and reflexology certification.

CONTINUING EDUCATION: pregnancy, infant and geriatric massage, aromatherapy, Knieppism, hydrotherapy, bath attendant

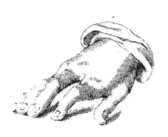

Oregon

State Licensing: 330 hours

National Certification Exam not accepted

Approved out-of-state schools:

Brenneke School, Seattle WA
Brian Utting School, Seattle WA
Dr. Jay Scherer's, Santa Fe NM
Hawaiian Islands School, Kailua-Kona HI
Health Enrichment Center, Lapeer MI
Heartwood Institute, Garberville CA
Massage Therapy Institute, Denver CO
Mueller College, San Diego CA
New Hampshire Institute, Hudson NH
New Mexico Academy, Santa Fe NM
New Mexico School, Albuquerque NM
Richmond Academy of Massage, Richmond VA
Seattle Massage School, Seattle WA
S.W. Washington Massage Th. Sch., Vancouver WA

Schools:

#231 Ashland Massage Institute
P.O. Box 1233
Ashland, OR 97520
(503) 482-5134

HOURS OF TRAINING: 375

DURATION OF COURSE: evenings and some weekends for nine months

COST: $2,720

YEAR FOUNDED: 1988

GRADUATES PER YEAR (APPROX.): 30

MODALITIES AND SUBJECTS: hydrotherapy, business and ethics, ortho-bionomy, survey of soft tissue tech-

niques, Jin Shin Do, release point therapy, board orientation, supervised clinic, kinesiology, pathology

CONTINUING EDUCATION: shiatsu, ortho-bionomy, intuitive bodywork, soft tissue techniques, Jin Shin Do, release point therapy, movement awareness

#232 Cascade Institute of Massage & Body Therapies
1250 Charnelton St.
Eugene, OR 97401
(503) 687-8101

HOURS OF TRAINING: 565

DURATION OF COURSE: one year, three or four evenings per week plus occasional Saturdays

COST: $3,985 ($200 discount for pre-payment)

FINANCIAL AID: payment plan

YEAR FOUNDED: 1989

PREPARATION FOR OUT-OF-STATE LICENSING EXAM: approval in Washington State is pending.

GRADUATES PER YEAR (APPROX.): 30

MODALITIES AND SUBJECTS: kinesiology, acupressure, deep tissue, onsen technique, myofascial release, trigger point therapy, body reading, pathology, hydrotherapy, first aid/CPR, business management, ethics, massage clinic, community outreach

UNIQUE ASPECTS OF SCHOOL OR CURRICULUM: small class size, and emphasis on proper body mechanics

CONTINUING EDUCATION: muscle sculpting bodywork, human cadaver lab, sports massage onsen technique, on-site, business mastery (for additional offerings contact school)

#233 East-West College of the Healing Arts
4531 S.E. Belmont St.
Portland, OR 97215
(503) 231-1500 or (800) 635-9141

HOURS OF TRAINING: Oregon licensure program 405; intermediate (AMTA-approved) program 536; see also advanced trainings, below

DURATION OF COURSE: 405 hours 9 months; 536 hours 11 months

DAY/EVENING/WEEKEND: day and evening programs are available

COST: 405 hours $4,115; 536 hours $5,404 (costs include required books)

FINANCIAL AID: payment plan

YEAR FOUNDED: 1972 (Midway School); 1981 East-West College

ACCREDITATIONS/APPROVALS: COMTAA, Veterans Administration, U.S. Dept. of Immigration and Naturalization, Oregon State Vocational Rehabilitation Division, Oregon Commission for the Blind, Job Training Partnership Act.

PREPARATION FOR OUT-OF-STATE LICENSING EXAM: Washington (school can create a program to meet the licensing requirement of any state)

GRADUATES PER YEAR (APPROX.): 130

MODALITIES AND SUBJECTS: kinesiology, pathology, self-care, client confidentiality and vulnerability, deep tissue, trigger point, myofascial release, cross-fiber friction, hydrotherapy, clinical practice, first aid, CPR, business practices, bodymind therapy, externship, movement therapy, neuro-humeral massage, polarity, shiatsu, sports massage, transformational hypnotherapy

ADVANCED PROGRAMS: Students who complete the intermediate program may take any of four advanced trainings, composed of subjects in the above list. Advanced training options range from 132 additional hours to 528 additional hours.

CONTINUING EDUCATION: contact school

#234 The Ewing Institute of Therapeutic Massage
3800 SW Cedar Hills Blvd., suite 195
Beaverton, OR 97005
(503) 644-1307

HOURS OF TRAINING: 544

DURATION OF COURSE: 8 to 12 months

DAY/EVENING/WEEKEND: day and evening programs available

COST: $3,850

FINANCIAL AID: payment plans

YEAR FOUNDED: 1993

MODALITIES AND SUBJECTS: Pregnancy massage, deep tissue, trigger point, kinesiology, pathology, business practices and preparation, clinic/supervised practicum, first aid/CPR, HIV/AIDS education, ethics, hygiene. Electives include on-site, manual lymphatic drainage, geriatric massage, infant massage, pregnancy massage, marketing strategies, Russian massage, sports massage and injury management, supervised clinic, advanced massage techniques, business mastery, student assistant, special studies, hydrotherapy, myofascial awareness, movement dynamics, issues of abuse

ADVANCED PROGRAMS: 750 and 1,500-hour advanced diploma courses

CONTINUING EDUCATION: introduction to aromatherapy, polarity therapy, manual lymphatic drainage, sports massage—contact school for current listings

#235 Lane Community College
1059 Willamette St.
Eugene, OR 97401
(503) 747-4501

Contact the school for program information.

#236 National Health Care Institute
1445 State St.
Salem, OR 97301
(503) 585-8912

HOURS OF TRAINING: 392

DURATION OF COURSE: 8 months, evenings

COST: $4,260

FINANCIAL AID: payment plan

YEAR FOUNDED: 1990

GRADUATES PER YEAR (APPROX.): 40

MODALITIES AND SUBJECTS: kinesiology, hydrotherapy, introduction to other modalities (see continuing education programs), pathology, professional development, student practicum clinic

UNIQUE ASPECTS OF SCHOOL OR CURRICULUM: School emphasizes holistic perspective and preventative health maintenance.

ADVANCED PROGRAMS: certified nutrition program (home study)

CONTINUING EDUCATION: herbology, aromatherapy, infant massage, manual lymphatic drainage, Touch for Health, myofascial release, polarity, reflexology, shiatsu, sohtai, sports massage

#237 Oregon School of Massage
9500 SW Barbur Blvd., suite 100
Portland, OR 97219
(503) 244-3420 or (800) 844-3420

HOURS OF TRAINING: 360 or 525

DURATION OF COURSE: minimum of one year; students proceed at their own pace.

COST: 360-hour program $3,245; 525-hour program $4,790 (discounts for early payment)

YEAR FOUNDED: 1984

PREPARATION FOR OUT-OF-STATE LICENSING EXAM: Washington (525-hour program)

GRADUATES PER YEAR (APPROX.): 140

MODALITIES AND SUBJECTS: foot reflexology, shiatsu, Hakomi integrative somatics, deep tissue massage, side-lying massage, sports massage, Reiki, polarity the psychology of touch, pathology, kinesiology, nutrition, hydrotherapy, clinic-student practicum clinic, professional development

UNIQUE ASPECTS OF SCHOOL OR CURRICULUM: The emphasis is on psycho-spiritual and communication dimensions of bodywork.

ADVANCED PROGRAMS: shiatsu certification, deep tissue massage

CONTINUING EDUCATION: ABC's of Chinese medicine, belly work, body rock massage, compassionate touch, deep tissue massage, EDGU, first aid/CPR, foot reflexology, hakomi integrative somatics, lifelong career options, massage-clinical applications, nutrition, on-site, polarity, pregnancy massage, psychology of touch, shiatsu, side-lying massage, sports massage

---

#238 Rogue Community College
3345 Redwood Highway
Grants Pass, OR 97527
College: (503) 471-3500
Massage Program: (503) 471-3519

HOURS OF TRAINING: 46 credits

COST: $882 to $4,738 depending on residency

FINANCIAL AID: grants, loans, scholarships and part-time work

MODALITIES AND SUBJECTS: business math, reading, chemistry, medical terminology, first aid/CPR, business english, acupressure, Esalen, hydrotherapy, reflexology, stress reduction techniques, kinesiology, pathology, psychology of human relations, plus electives, such as small business management, personal health, algebra, nutrition, physical conditioning, basic communication.

#239 South Coast School of Healing Arts
Rt. 4 Box 30
Bandon, OR 97411
(503) 347-4124 or 347-9877

HOURS OF TRAINING: 330

DURATION OF COURSE: 8 months, three evenings per week plus Saturdays

COST: $2,535

YEAR FOUNDED: 1988

GRADUATES PER YEAR (APPROX.): 10 to 14

MODALITIES AND SUBJECTS: pathology, kinesiology, survey of bodywork techniques, hydrotherapy, business development, ethics, laws, hygiene

CONTINUING EDUCATION: contact school

Pennsylvania

No State licensing

Schools:

#240 Career Training Academy
Main Campus
703 Fifth Ave.
New Kensington, PA 15068
(412) 337-1000 or (800) 660-3470

Branch Campus
244 Center Road
Monroeville, PA 15146
(412) 372-3900 or (800) 491-3470

HOURS OF TRAINING: 300 and 600-hour massage programs, 300 and 600-hour shiatsu programs

DURATION OF COURSE: Courses meet Mon-Thurs, 6:00 pm to 10:00 pm. 300-hour program meets for 4.7 months, 600-hour program for 9.5 months

COST: 300-hour program $1,950; 600-hour program $3,660

FINANCIAL AID: Federal grants are available for the 600-hour program

YEAR FOUNDED: 1986

ACCREDITATIONS/APPROVALS: ACCSCT

GRADUATES PER YEAR (APPROX.): 75

MODALITIES AND SUBJECTS: aromatherapy, homeopathic remedies, career development, kinesiology, healing power of magnets, clinical evaluation, client interaction, first aid, CPR, practicum, acupressure, shiatsu, reflexology, sports massage, stretching, alexander, chiropractic assistance, Touch for Health, myotherapy, hydrotherapy

UNIQUE ASPECTS OF SCHOOL OR CURRICULUM: The school trains students for a variety of careers in medical Allied Health. In addition to massage and shiatsu, the school offers programs in dental assistant and medical assistant.

CONTINUING EDUCATION: contact school

#241 Health Options Institute
1410 Main St.
Northampton, PA 18067
(610) 261-0680

HOURS OF TRAINING: 120 (increasing to 200 during 1995)

DURATION OF COURSE: 36 weeks

DAY/EVENING/WEEKEND: day and evening classes available

COST: $1,974

YEAR FOUNDED: 1984

GRADUATES PER YEAR (APPROX.): 70

MODALITIES AND SUBJECTS: deep muscle massage, sports massage, nutrition, herbology

UNIQUE ASPECTS OF SCHOOL OR CURRICULUM: Students learn anatomy with the Anatomiken system

CONTINUING EDUCATION: St. John neuromuscular therapy, nutrition and holistic health

#242 International Academy of Massage Sciences
The Well-Person Place
P.O. Box 277
Park Mount & Lungren Roads
Glen Riddle, PA 19037
(215) 558-3140

HOURS OF TRAINING: 500 hours

IN-CLASS HOURS: 128

DURATION OF COURSE: 17 Sundays

YEAR FOUNDED: 1977

ACCREDITATIONS/APPROVALS: Susan B. Anthony University, Montreal

School programs are described in a catalogue for which the school charges $5.00.

#243 Lancaster School of Massage
323 N. Queen St.
Lancaster, PA 17603
(717) 293-9698

HOURS OF TRAINING: 500

DURATION OF COURSE: approx. 5½ months

COST: $3,950

MODALITIES AND SUBJECTS: reflexology, polarity therapy, neuromuscular therapy, connective tissue massage, cranio-sacral, sports massage, pathology, nutrition, hydrotherapy, heliotherapy and instrumentation, CPR/first aid, business practices

#244 Lehigh Valley Healing Arts Center
School of Bodywork
5677 Greens Dr.
Wescosville, PA 18106
(610) 398-9642

HOURS OF TRAINING: 230

IN-CLASS HOURS: 101

DURATION OF COURSE: 12 Sundays

COST: $1,250 includes books

FINANCIAL AID: Monroe County Job Partnership Training, Private Industry Council, payment plans

MODALITIES AND SUBJECTS: healing philosophy, pathology, applied exercises, business procedures, documented fieldwork

ADVANCED PROGRAMS: 50-hour advanced trainings available on topics including cranial-sacral, body-mind, Trager, sports massage, PNF, energy balancing, five element theory, aromatherapy, deep connective tissue strokes, trigger point. Advanced trainings can be combined to acquire a total of 500 hours training.

CONTINUING EDUCATION: Touch for Health, polarity, shiatsu, Trager, Yoga, Reiki, reflexology

#245 Massage Arts and Sciences Center of Philadelphia
1625 Spruce St.
Philadelphia, PA 19103
(215) 985-0674

HOURS OF TRAINING: 120 (school plans to increase hours in 1995)

DURATION OF COURSE: 5 months, 2 evenings per week or one day and one evening per week)

COST: $2,035

YEAR FOUNDED: 1984

GRADUATES PER YEAR (APPROX.): 40

MODALITIES AND SUBJECTS: body mechanics, joint movements and stretches, business seminar, tutorial

CONTINUING EDUCATION: reflexology, pathology, aromatherapy, medical massage, myofascial technique, sports massage

#246 Owens Institute of Massage & Wholistic Sciences, Inc.
Regional Administrative Office
P.O. Box 1812
Media, PA 19063
1-800-99-OWENS 1-800-996-9367

HOURS OF TRAINING: 500

IN-CLASS HOURS: 100 to 500

DURATION OF COURSE: 6 months, 9 months or 12 months

DAY/EVENING/WEEKEND: day, evening, weekend or combination

COST: $3,045 (includes books)

FINANCIAL AID: $600 scholarship available to most students

YEAR FOUNDED: 1986

PREPARATION FOR OUT-OF-STATE LICENSING EXAM: Delaware

GRADUATES PER YEAR (APPROX.): 200

MODALITIES AND SUBJECTS: business practice and management, psychological-mental-spiritual success integration

UNIQUE ASPECTS OF SCHOOL OR CURRICULUM: The student personally tailors a schedule to meet his or her needs. Curriculum is approved for credit toward Westbrook University's wholistic health arts and sciences certification and degree programs.

CONTINUING EDUCATION: reflexology, on-site, aromatherapy, Reiki, Touch for Health, therapeutic touch

#247 Pennsylvania School of Muscle Therapy
      651 South Gulph Road
      King of Prussia, PA 19406
      (610) 265-7939

HOURS OF TRAINING: 521

DURATION OF COURSE: 9 months

DAY/EVENING/WEEKEND: day, evening and weekend programs are available

COST: $4,850

YEAR FOUNDED: 1980

ACCREDITATIONS/APPROVALS: COMTAA, International assoc. of Pfrimmer deep muscle therapists

GRADUATES PER YEAR (APPROX.): 100

MODALITIES AND SUBJECTS: COMTAA-approved program: sports massage, pathology, hydrotherapy, business and professional ethics, CPR/first aid

ADVANCED PROGRAMS: Pfrimmer deep muscle therapy, evaluation and correction of the muscular system through advanced techniques, advanced anatomy and physiology, myofascial release, structural evaluation, palpation, digestive and circulatory system massage

CONTINUING EDUCATION: Pfrimmer deep muscle therapy, reflexology, on-site, mother massage, advanced techniques, sports massage, shiatsu

#248 Pittsburgh School of Massage Therapy
      10989 Frankstown Ave.
      Penn Hills, PA 15235
      (800) 860-1114

HOURS OF TRAINING: 247 (longer program in development)

DURATION OF COURSE: 19 weeks or 38 weeks

DAY/EVENING/WEEKEND: day and evening programs are available

COST: $1,930 (includes books)

FINANCIAL AID: loans and partial scholarships are available

YEAR FOUNDED: 1986

GRADUATES PER YEAR (APPROX.): 85

MODALITIES AND SUBJECTS: Required courses include pathology, business, client interaction. Students also choose electives, such as reflexology, sports massage, shiatsu, Russian sports massage, joint mobilization, Alexander, bioenergetics, working with a chiropractor.

UNIQUE ASPECTS OF SCHOOL OR CURRICULUM: School donates 1% of corporate gross revenue to local and national charities.

CONTINUING EDUCATION: on-site, trigger point, cranio-sacral therapy, advanced sports massage, geriatric massage, bodywork for the childbearing year, body sculpting, chua-ka, spa techniques, counterstrain techniques

#249 Rose Meta-Therapy
      1317 Markley St.
      Norristown, PA 19401
      (610) 272-6585

HOURS OF TRAINING: 25

DURATION OF COURSE: five weeks

COST: $300 ($60 per class session)

YEAR FOUNDED: 1985

MODALITIES AND SUBJECTS: Edgar Cayce lymphatic massage, Reiki, deep tissue, chakra balancing, Oriental theory, reflexology, intuitive and energy theory, on-site, sports massage.

UNIQUE ASPECTS OF SCHOOL OR CURRICULUM: The program is flexible and can be tailored to individual needs and interests. Students may pay one class at a time and may also continue open-ended training after completing the five week course.

South Dakota

No State licensing

Schools:

#250 Carrie's Kadesh
      School of Massage Theory and Practice
      104 W. 4th Ave.
      Mitchell, SD 57301
      (605) 996-3916

HOURS OF TRAINING: 1,100

IN-CLASS HOURS: 900

DURATION OF COURSE: 5 months

COST: $2,550

YEAR FOUNDED: 1982

GRADUATES PER YEAR (APPROX.): 3 to 12

MODALITIES AND SUBJECTS: sports massage, infant massage, deep tissue, acupressure, reflexes, zone therapy, kinesiology, craniology, iridology, yoga, magnet therapy, light therapy, color therapy, hydrotherapy, nutrition, exercise, health and hygiene, business, professionalism, ethics, first aid/CPR, Heimlich maneuver, social studies, medical terminology, field trips, documented independent work

UNIQUE ASPECTS OF SCHOOL OR CURRICULUM: Class size is kept small, allowing one-on-one attention.

#251 South Dakota School of Massage Therapy
P.O. Box 96
Sioux Falls, SD 57101
(605) 335-8736

HOURS OF TRAINING: 500 plus clinical practice

DURATION OF COURSE: 6 months

COST: $4,500

FINANCIAL AID: approved for veterans' benefits

YEAR FOUNDED: 1987

PREPARATION FOR OUT-OF-STATE LICENSING EXAM: contact school

GRADUATES PER YEAR (APPROX.): 25

MODALITIES AND SUBJECTS: deep tissue, acupressure, reflexology, hydrotherapy, business, TMJ, sports massage, on-site, emotional release and breathwork, personal growth and enrichment, yoga, CPR/first aid, clinical practice

UNIQUE ASPECTS OF SCHOOL OR CURRICULUM: The focus is on personal growth.

ADVANCED PROGRAMS: contact school

CONTINUING EDUCATION: contact school

Tennessee

No State licensing

Schools:

#252 Cumberland Institute for Wellness Education
500 Wilson Pike Circle, suite 121
Brentwood, TN 37027
(615) 370-9794

HOURS OF TRAINING: Holistic Massage Practitioner 412, Holistic Massage Therapist 743

DURATION OF COURSE: Students proceed at their own pace

DAY/EVENING/WEEKEND: 412-hour course evenings or weekends, 743-hour course days or weekends

COST: 412 hours course $6,305 including books; 743-hour course $10,005 including books

FINANCIAL AID: Two school-sponsored scholarships ($5,000 and $3,000), State Vocational Rehabilitation grants, Veterans Administration loans, payment plans, 10% discount to ABMP members

YEAR FOUNDED: 1987

MODALITIES AND SUBJECTS: 412-hour course includes introduction to massage, touch dynamics, therapist-client interdynamics, bodywork ethics, applied anatomy, kinesiology, nutrition concepts, CPR, Esalen, structural observation and assessment, posture dynamics, lymphatic massage, reflexology, business and marketing, internship.

The 743-hour course adds neuromuscular-somatic therapy, cranio-sacral therapy, Touch for Health, aromatherapy, polarity therapy, touch therapy for abuse survivors, transformational hypnotherapy, internship.

#253 The Massage Institute of Memphis
804-806 S. Cooper
Memphis, TN 38104
(901) 725-7355

HOURS OF TRAINING: 500

DURATION OF COURSE: days 6 months, evenings 10 months

COST: $3,950 (includes books and supplies)

FINANCIAL AID: payment plan

YEAR FOUNDED: 1987

PREPARATION FOR OUT-OF-STATE LICENSING EXAM: Arkansas

GRADUATES PER YEAR (APPROX.): 6

MODALITIES AND SUBJECTS: foot reflexology, remedial exercises, traction, meditation, communication with clients, body reading, law and ethics, first aid/CPR/AIDS awareness, health and hygiene, health services management, hydrotherapy, electrotherapy, heliotherapy, student clinic, research paper

UNIQUE ASPECTS OF SCHOOL OR CURRICULUM: Meditation and wholistic philosophy are incorporated in the curriculum. Class size is kept small for individual attention.

ADVANCED PROGRAMS: contact school

CONTINUING EDUCATION: contact school

#254 Tennessee Institute of Healing Arts, Inc.
5779 Brainerd Road
Chattanooga, TN 37411
(800) 735-1910 or (615) 892-9882

HOURS OF TRAINING: 1,000

IN-CLASS HOURS: 920

DURATION OF COURSE: one year

COST: $6,000

FINANCIAL AID: payment plan

YEAR FOUNDED: 1989

ACCREDITATIONS/APPROVALS: authorized by Tennessee Department of Higher Education, ACCSCT application pending

Preparation for out-of-State licensing exam: Florida

GRADUATES PER YEAR (APPROX.): 40

MODALITIES AND SUBJECTS: deep tissue massage, neuromuscular therapy, russian massage technique, sports massage, transformational bodywork, Oriental therapies, reflexology, polarity, pregnancy massage, on-site, hydrotherapy, geriatric massage, illness care massage, pathology, professional ethics, communication skills, marketing and business, movement integration, nutrition, CPR and first aid, self-care, statutes, rules and history of massage, HIV/AIDS, documented practice, student clinic, research project, community outreach

UNIQUE ASPECTS OF SCHOOL OR CURRICULUM: special emphasis on anatomy and physiology, neuromuscular therapy and transformational bodywork

CONTINUING EDUCATION: craniosacral, partner massage, functional assessment, transformational bodywork

#255 Tennessee School of Massage
4726 Poplar, #4
Memphis, TN 38117
(901) 767-8484 or (901) 360-8866

HOURS OF TRAINING: 500

DURATION OF COURSE: 9 months

DAY/EVENING/WEEKEND: day and evening programs available

COST: $3,360 (includes printed materials)

FINANCIAL AID: payment plan

YEAR FOUNDED: 1988

ACCREDITATIONS/APPROVALS: approved by Tennessee Higher Education Association

GRADUATES PER YEAR (APPROX.): 16-20

MODALITIES AND SUBJECTS: Required courses include sports massage, pathology, nutrition, polarity, business career development, human sexuality and ethical massage, hydrotherapy, personal support, basic counseling, CPR, clinic.

Students also choose electives, such as reflexology, hypnosis, maternity and infant massage, aromatherapy, abnormal psychology, homeopathic approaches, trigger points and on-site.

UNIQUE ASPECTS OF SCHOOL OR CURRICULUM: The school is located in Wilson World hotel, and students are offered full-time employment in its day spa while in school and afterward.

ADVANCED PROGRAMS: Electives may be taken as advanced programs.

CONTINUING EDUCATION: contact school

Texas

State Licensing/registration: 300 hours

National Certification Exam not accepted

Schools:

#256 Asten Center of Natural Therapeutics
797 Grove Rd., suite 101
Richardson, TX 75081
(214) 669-3245

HOURS OF TRAINING: basic 300, advanced 250

DURATION OF COURSE: basic 5 to 12 months; advanced 5 to 12 months

DAY/EVENING/WEEKEND: day, evening and Sunday programs available

COST: basic $2,980, advanced $2,395 (includes textbooks and massage table)(5% discount for payment in full)

FINANCIAL AID: contact school

YEAR FOUNDED: 1983

ACCREDITATIONS/APPROVALS: COMTAA

GRADUATES PER YEAR (APPROX.): 65-100

MODALITIES AND SUBJECTS: The basic course includes health and hygiene, hydrotherapy, cryotherapy, business practices and ethics, internship.

The advanced course includes sports massage, trigger point, reflexology, clinical treatment for 12 specific injuries, and electives such as infant massage, elderly and pregnancy massage, chair massage, lymphatic massage, polarity.

ADVANCED PROGRAMS: advanced program described above

CONTINUING EDUCATION: All courses may be taken individually as continuing education.

#257 Austin School of Massage Therapy (ASMT)
2600 W. Stassney Ln.
Austin, TX 78745
(512) 462-3005

HOURS OF TRAINING: 300

DURATION OF COURSE: 6 months or 3-month summer intensive

DAY/EVENING/WEEKEND: evening and weekend programs are available

COST: $2,200

FINANCIAL AID: partial scholarship to one student per class

YEAR FOUNDED: 1985

GRADUATES PER YEAR (APPROX.): 250

MODALITIES AND SUBJECTS: stretching, range of motion, awareness of energetics, sports massage, trigger points, special applications, on-site massage, kinesiology, postural analysis, hydrotherapy, health and hygiene, business practices and professional ethics, practice massages, internship

UNIQUE ASPECTS OF SCHOOL OR CURRICULUM: The school provides a focus on business goals and self-awareness.

ADVANCED PROGRAMS: The school offers a 300-hour training in neuromuscular therapy, as well as internships and teacher training.

CONTINUING EDUCATION: myofascial release, trigger point therapy, reflexology, rhythmic massage, energetic techniques

The Austin school training is offered in other cities in the weekend format, on alternating weekends for a total of fifteen class weekends. Cities in which the program is offered are (as of 1/1/95):

Amarillo	Dallas	El Paso
Fort Worth	Houston	Lubbock
Midland/Odessa	San Angelo	San Antonio
Waco	Wichita Falls	

#258 Christian Associates
25030 I-45 N
Spring, TX 77386
(713) 367-6515

HOURS OF TRAINING: 300

DURATION OF COURSE: days 3 to 4 months, evenings 6 months

COST: $2,725 (includes books)

FINANCIAL AID: payment plan, work exchange

YEAR FOUNDED: 1990

ACCREDITATIONS/APPROVALS: veterans administration, Texas rehabilitation commission, Texas commission for the blind

GRADUATES PER YEAR (APPROX.): 24

MODALITIES AND SUBJECTS: hydrotherapy, health and hygiene, business practices and ethics and internship

UNIQUE ASPECTS OF SCHOOL OR CURRICULUM: Small class size allows individual attention, and the school maintains a Christian environment.

ADVANCED PROGRAMS: contact school

CONTINUING EDUCATION: sports massage, muscle balancing, nutrition, healthy cooking, vitamin supplements

#259 European Health and Science Institute
1201 Airway, suite A-2
El Paso, TX 79925
(915) 772-4243

Contact the school for program information.

#260 European Institute
33 East Shady Lane
Houston, TX 77063
(713) 783-1446

Contact the school for program information.

#261 European Massage Therapy Institute
7220 Louis Pasteur, suite 140
San Antonio, TX 78229
(210) 615-8207 or (800) 458-5440

HOURS OF TRAINING: 300

DURATION OF COURSE: 9 months

DAY/EVENING/WEEKEND: day and evening programs available

COST: $2,075

FINANCIAL AID: payment plan

YEAR FOUNDED: 1988

MODALITIES AND SUBJECTS: hydrotherapy, health and hygiene, ethics and business practices, internship

#262 Hands-On Therapy School of Massage
625 Gatewood
Garland, TX 75043
(214) 240-9288

HOURS OF TRAINING: 300 (State requirement) or 500

DURATION OF COURSE: 6 months

DAY/EVENING/WEEKEND: day and evening programs available

COST: 300 hours $2,250; 500 hours $3,550

FINANCIAL AID: contact school

YEAR FOUNDED: 1991

GRADUATES PER YEAR (APPROX.): 100

MODALITIES AND SUBJECTS: hydrotherapy, health and hygiene, business practices, internship

UNIQUE ASPECTS OF SCHOOL OR CURRICULUM: The school emphasizes personal growth and the psychological aspects of bodywork.

CONTINUING EDUCATION: contact school

#263 Harmony Massage Institute
2547 S. Austin
Pearland, TX 77584
(713) 485-2177

Contact the school for program information.

#264 Health Masters
9928 Fulton
Houston, TX 77076
(713) 529-3296

Contact the school for program information.

#265 HealthTouch
1409 Kingwood Dr.
Kingwood, TX 77339
(713) 358-0600

HOURS OF TRAINING: 300

DURATION OF COURSE: day class 4 months plus internship, evening class 6 months plus internship

COST: $2,600

FINANCIAL AID: payment plan

MODALITIES AND SUBJECTS: hydrotherapy, business practices and professional ethics, health and hygiene, internship

UNIQUE ASPECTS OF SCHOOL OR CURRICULUM: The school may grant credit for previous education.

#266 Houston Massage Center Massage School
2611 Stanford
Houston, TX 77006
(713) 520-0177

HOURS OF TRAINING: 300

DURATION OF COURSE: courses are taken individually; average course time 10 months

DAY/EVENING/WEEKEND: day and evening classes are available

COST: $2,100 (includes most textbooks)

FINANCIAL AID: payment plan

YEAR FOUNDED: 1980

GRADUATES PER YEAR (APPROX.): 20

MODALITIES AND SUBJECTS: history of massage, hydrotherapy, business practices and professional ethics, health and hygiene

UNIQUE ASPECTS OF SCHOOL OR CURRICULUM: Students can take courses in any order and can enter the program at any time during the year.

#267 Institute of Cosmetic Arts
1105 Airline
Corpus Christi, TX 78412
(512) 991-8868

No Catalogue

HOURS OF TRAINING: 300

DURATION OF COURSE: 10 weeks

COST: $3,058

FINANCIAL AID: Texas rehabilitation — Commission for the Blind

YEAR FOUNDED: 1982

GRADUATES PER YEAR (APPROX.): 30

MODALITIES AND SUBJECTS: hydrotherapy, business, hygiene

#268 The Institute of Natural Healing Sciences
4100 Felps Drive, suite E
Colleyville, TX 76034
(817) 498-0716

HOURS OF TRAINING: 300

DURATION OF COURSE: day program four months, evening program 8½ months

COST: $1,950

FINANCIAL AID: payment plan

YEAR FOUNDED: 1985

ACCREDITATIONS/APPROVALS: COMTAA

GRADUATES PER YEAR (APPROX.): 60

MODALITIES AND SUBJECTS: joint mobilization, health and hygiene, business practices and ethics, hydrotherapy, internship

UNIQUE ASPECTS OF SCHOOL OR CURRICULUM: Student-teacher ratio of 10:1 assures personal supervision

ADVANCED PROGRAMS: The programs listed below, taken together, comprise an advanced program, offered in the evenings.

CONTINUING EDUCATION: reflexology, sports massage, shiatsu, chair massage, polarity, craniosacral and myofascial release, clinical applications

#269 In-Touch School of Massage
770 S. Post Oak Ln. suite 610
Houston, TX 77056
(713) 961-1669

Contact the school for program information.

#270 The Lauterstein-Conway Massage School and Clinic
213 South Lamar, Suite 101
Austin, TX 78704
(512) 474-1852

HOURS OF TRAINING: 300 (one semester) to 800 (three semesters)

IN-CLASS HOURS: 300 to 800

DURATION OF COURSE: 3½ to 21 months

DAY/EVENING/WEEKEND: semester 1 can be taken days or evenings; semester 2 combines days and evenings; semester 3 is days only.

COST: $2,200 per semester plus required texts

FINANCIAL AID: payment plans, partial scholarships

YEAR FOUNDED: 1989

GRADUATES PER YEAR (APPROX.): sem. 1: 118; sem. 2: 42; sem. 3: 12

MODALITIES AND SUBJECTS:
Semester 1 is the basic Texas 300 hour curriculum. Semester 2 adds sports massage, advanced anatomy, injury assessment and theory, zen shiatsu, deep massage, psychosomatic theory and application, integrative bodywork, business practice, CPR and first aid. Semester 3 includes basic and advanced structural bodywork, emotional growth work, cranio-sacral, advanced session design, zero balancing and integrative bodywork.

ADVANCED PROGRAMS: See semester 2 and semester 3

CONTINUING EDUCATION: deep massage certification, sports massage certification, zero balancing, craniosacral work, advanced structural bodywork, other workshops as scheduled

#271 Massage Education Institute
3195 Calder
Beaumont, TX 77702
(409) 832-3020

HOURS OF TRAINING: 300

DURATION OF COURSE: alternate weekends for eight months

COST: $2,500 plus books and supplies

YEAR FOUNDED: 1988

GRADUATES PER YEAR (APPROX.): 12 to 14

MODALITIES AND SUBJECTS: reflexology, deep tissue, business, hydrotherapy, health and hygiene, herbal nutrition, internship

CONTINUING EDUCATION: t'ai chi, reflexology, herbal nutrition, aromatherapy, personal massage, sports massage, infant and pregnancy massage, deep tissue, on site, CPR, stress management

#272 Massage Resources, Inc.
2880 LBJ Freeway #501
Dallas, TX 75234
(214) 484-8180

HOURS OF TRAINING: basic 300, advanced up to 250 additional

IN-CLASS HOURS: basic 250

DURATION OF COURSE: basic 6 months (4 months in-class, 2 months internship)

DAY/EVENING/WEEKEND: basic training may be taken days or evenings; advanced training may be taken days or weekends

COST: basic $2,100 (includes books), advanced $10 per hour per course or $2,250 if taken as a series

YEAR FOUNDED: 1994

ACCREDITATIONS/APPROVALS: Texas Rehab. Comm.

GRADUATES PER YEAR (APPROX.): 25 to 30

MODALITIES AND SUBJECTS: business practices, professional ethics, health and hygiene, hydrotherapy

UNIQUE ASPECTS OF SCHOOL OR CURRICULUM: emphasis on efficient body mechanics; personalized table-side attention

ADVANCED PROGRAMS: reflexology, trigger point, myofascial tension reduction, sports massage, injuries and special conditions

#273 Massage Therapy Clinic & School
400 Medical Center Blvd., suite 211
Webster, TX 77598
(713) 332-3994

HOURS OF TRAINING: 300

DURATION OF COURSE: 3 months days, 5½ months evenings. Weekend program also available

COST: $2,662 includes textbooks, sheets, towels and oil

FINANCIAL AID: payment plan

YEAR FOUNDED: 1990

ACCREDITATIONS/APPROVALS: Texas Rehabilitation Commission, Texas Commission for the Blind, Department of Veterans Affairs

MODALITIES AND SUBJECTS: hydrotherapy, business practices and ethics, human health and hygiene, internship

UNIQUE ASPECTS OF SCHOOL OR CURRICULUM: Credit may be arranged for coursework previously completed.

ADVANCED PROGRAMS: 300- and 700-hour advanced training programs were pending approval at the time for publication.

CONTINUING EDUCATION: Touch for Health, Sports massage I and II, myofascial release, neuromuscular therapy I, II, III and IV, reflexology, marketing

#274 MRC School of Massage
2990 Richmond, suite 142
Houston, TX 77098
(713) 522-1423

HOURS OF TRAINING: 300

DURATION OF COURSE: 5 months days, 6½ months evenings

COST: $2,500 including most books and all supplies; discounts for pre-payment and for morning class

FINANCIAL AID: payment plans

YEAR FOUNDED: 1989

GRADUATES PER YEAR (APPROX.): 100

MODALITIES AND SUBJECTS: health and hygiene, hydrotherapy, business practices, professional ethics, internship

CONTINUING EDUCATION: reflexology, deep tissue, carpal tunnel, pregnancy massage, infant massage

#275 Neuromuscular Concepts Massage Therapy School
8607 Wurzbach Road, Bldg. R, suite 150
San Antonio, TX 78240
(210) 558-3112

HOURS OF TRAINING: 300

IN-CLASS HOURS: 250

DURATION OF COURSE: 3 evenings per week for 5½ months

COST: $2,102

YEAR FOUNDED: 1989

GRADUATES PER YEAR (APPROX.): 30

MODALITIES AND SUBJECTS: hydrotherapy, health and hygiene, business practice, business ethics, internship

ADVANCED PROGRAMS: spinal touch, soft-tissue manipulation, palpatory literacy, spa work, chi-gong, zen bodywork, acupuncture, nutrition, shamanic healing, awareness through movement

#276 North Texas School of Swedish Massage
2335 Green Oaks Blvd. West
Arlington, TX 76016
(817) 446-6629

HOURS OF TRAINING: 300

DURATION OF COURSE: 3 months or 6 months

DAY/EVENING/WEEKEND: day and evening programs available, plus some Saturdays

COST: $2,648 (includes books) ($250 discount for payment in full at start of class)

YEAR FOUNDED: 1994

GRADUATES PER YEAR (APPROX.): 120

MODALITIES AND SUBJECTS: hydrotherapy, business and ethics, health and hygiene, internship

ADVANCED PROGRAMS: contact school

CONTINUING EDUCATION: contact school

#277 Phoenix School of Wholistic Health
6610 Harwin #256
Houston, TX 77036
(713) 974-5976

Contact the school for program information.

#278 School of Natural Therapy
4309-B N. 10th
McAllen, TX 78504
(210) 630-0928 or (800) 870-0670

HOURS OF TRAINING: 300

DURATION OF COURSE: 6 months

DAY/EVENING/WEEKEND: day and evening programs available

COST: approx $3,075 including supplies

FINANCIAL AID: payment plan, C.C., JTPA

YEAR FOUNDED: 1989

ACCREDITATIONS/APPROVALS: Texas Rehab. Comm., Commission for Blind, JTPA

GRADUATES PER YEAR (APPROX.): 50

MODALITIES AND SUBJECTS: health and hygiene, hydrotherapy, business practices, professional ethics, internship

UNIQUE ASPECTS OF SCHOOL OR CURRICULUM: Extra tutoring is offered as needed.

ADVANCED PROGRAMS: contact school

CONTINUING EDUCATION: contact school

#279 S.T.A.R.
School of Therapeutically Advanced Relaxation
2204 NW Loop 410
San Antonio, TX 78230
(210) 342-7444

HOURS OF TRAINING: 300

DURATION OF COURSE: four months or eight months

DAY/EVENING/WEEKEND: evening and weekend programs available

COST: $2,000 including books and supplies

YEAR FOUNDED: 1991

GRADUATES PER YEAR (APPROX.): 8 to 12

UNIQUE ASPECTS OF SCHOOL OR CURRICULUM: A therapy center on the premises provides internship opportunity.

ADVANCED PROGRAMS: colon hydrotherapy, sports massage

#280 Texas Massage Institute
      1750 Blalock
      Houston, TX 77080
      (713) 973-9345

Contact the school for program information.

#281 Texas Massage Therapy Corp.
      3617 Red Bluff
      Pasadena, TX 77503
      (713) 472-0383

Contact the school for program information.

#282 Third Coast Center
      3425 Bee Cave Rd.
      Austin TX 78756
      (512) 458-8435

HOURS OF TRAINING: 300

DURATION OF COURSE: 3 months days, 7 to 8 months evenings

COST: $2,150

MODALITIES AND SUBJECTS: aromatherapy, reflexology, health and hygiene, hydrotherapy, business practices and ethics, clinical internship

ADVANCED PROGRAMS: shiatsu, polarity

CONTINUING EDUCATION: Reiki

#283 Wellness Skills, Inc.
      6102 E. Mockingbird Lane, suite 401
      Dallas, TX 75214
      (214) 828-4000

Classes also offered at:

      Wellness Center
      6301 Airport Freeway
      Fort Worth, TX 76117
      (817) 838-3800

HOURS OF TRAINING: 300 (semester I); 650 (semester I + II)

DURATION OF COURSE: Semester I: 4-months, 7 months part-time, or one course at a time; Semester II: approx. 9 months

DAY/EVENING/WEEKEND: day program and evening/weekend program available

COST: Semester I: $2,185 (discounts up to $285 are available); Semester I + II: $4,370

FINANCIAL AID: payment plans, job training partnership act, private industry commission, barter

YEAR FOUNDED: 1985

ACCREDITATIONS/APPROVALS: Texas rehabilitation commission, Texas commission for the blind

GRADUATES PER YEAR (APPROX.): 250

MODALITIES AND SUBJECTS: Semester I includes health and hygiene, hydrotherapy, business practices and ethics, clinical internship.
Semester II includes sports massage, manual lymphatic drainage, therapeutic touch, polarity, bodymind, on-site, reflexology, applied kinesiology, aromatherapy, hydrotherapy, nutrition, movement, adjunctive therapies, massage for the medical setting

ADVANCED PROGRAMS: somatic practitioner 350 hours; partial semester 200 hours; polarity therapy 155 hours; seven-fold process (bodymind) 175 hours

CONTINUING EDUCATION: contact school

#284 Williams Institute School of Massage
      810 S. Mason Rd., suite 290
      Katy, TX 77450
      (713) 392-9212

HOURS OF TRAINING: 300

COST: $2,499

MODALITIES AND SUBJECTS: history of massage, personal development, guided relaxation techniques, medical terminology, hydrotherapy, business practices and professional ethics, human health and hygiene, internship

UNIQUE ASPECTS OF SCHOOL OR CURRICULUM: Credit may be arranged for coursework previously completed elsewhere.

#285 The Winters School
      3333 Eastside, suite 265
      Houston, TX 77098
      (713) 523-1023

HOURS OF TRAINING: 300

DURATION OF COURSE: 4 months days, 8 months evenings

COST: $2,400

FINANCIAL AID: payment plans

YEAR FOUNDED: 1984

ACCREDITATIONS/APPROVALS: Texas Rehabilitation Commission, Texas Commission for the Blind

GRADUATES PER YEAR (APPROX.): 40

MODALITIES AND SUBJECTS: hydrotherapy, human health and hygiene, business practices and ethics, internship

Non-School Instructors

In addition to certifying massage schools, the State of Texas also certifies instructors who may teach independent of a school. The following certified non-school instructors provided their program information for publication:

#286 Paul Frizzell
8607 Wurzbach Road, Bldg. R, suite 150
San Antonio, TX 78240
(210) 558-3112

HOURS OF TRAINING: 300

IN-CLASS HOURS: 250

DURATION OF COURSE: 3 evenings per week for 5½ months

COST: $2,102

YEAR FOUNDED: 1989

MODALITIES AND SUBJECTS: hydrotherapy, health and hygiene, business practice, business ethics, internship

ADVANCED PROGRAMS: spinal touch, soft-tissue manipulation, palpatory literacy, spa work, chi-gong, zen bodywork, acupuncture, nutrition, shamanic healing, awareness through movement

#287 Wanda Yvonne Loggins
Conroe, TX
(409) 441-3139

HOURS OF TRAINING: 300

DURATION OF COURSE: 7 to 8 months, Friday evenings and Saturdays

COST: $2,470 (includes books and supplies)

FINANCIAL AID: payment plans

YEAR FOUNDED: 1989

MODALITIES AND SUBJECTS: hydrotherapy, business practices, professional ethics, human health and hygiene

UNIQUE ASPECTS OF SCHOOL OR CURRICULUM: Focus is on developing an awareness of the human energy field.

ADVANCED PROGRAMS: business and personal development

#288 Dan Martin
1200 North Louise
Atlanta, TX
(501) 772-8622

HOURS OF TRAINING: 300

COST: $3,000

YEAR FOUNDED: Registered as instructor since 1991

MODALITIES AND SUBJECTS: history of massage, joint mobilization, exercise therapy, hydrotherapy, clinical massage, trigger point, business practices and ethics, human health and hygiene, AIDS, psychology and sexuality, internship

UNIQUE ASPECTS OF SCHOOL OR CURRICULUM: Two classrooms are available; one in Atlanta, one in Texarkana. Electrotherapy equipment is provided for student use. Credit may be arranged for coursework previously completed.

#289 Eleanor Scott, R.M.T.
531 Londonderry Ln. #120
Denton, TX 76205
(817) 566-1880

HOURS OF TRAINING: 300

IN-CLASS HOURS: 250

DURATION OF COURSE: 3 months

COST: $1,700 plus cost of ABMP membership

FINANCIAL AID: payment plan

YEAR FOUNDED: 1994

MODALITIES AND SUBJECTS: hydrotherapy, joint range of motion, health and hygiene, business practices, clinical practice

UNIQUE ASPECTS OF SCHOOL OR CURRICULUM: Student/teacher ratio of not more than 6:1 allows for individual attention.

The following individuals are also certified as non-school instructors by the State of Texas. Contact them for program information:

Inga Alanne, 11301 Richmond Ave., Houston, TX 77082   (713) 293-9049

Steve Allen, 2405 Trafalgar, Austin, TX 78723   (512) 454-8631

Virginia Brown, 2413 Sierra Lane, Plano, TX 75075   (214) 867-7073

Virginia Brown, 1600 N. Central Expressway, Plano, TX 75074   (214) 578-8555

Virginia Brown, 1502 11th, Wichita Falls,
TX   (214) 766-6132

Michael Graves, 3930 Kirby Dr., ste. 205,
Houston, TX 77098   (713) 528-2097

Michael Heffernan, 620 E. Market, Rockport,
TX 78382   (512) 729-0817

Katherine Herbert, 1214 Moskowitz, Seabrook,
TX 77586   (713) 480-9161

Bruce Jones, 6065 Hillcroft #515, Houston,
TX 77081   (713) 783-6287

Brenda Kieser, 7011 Harwin #100, Houston,
TX 77036   (713) 783-9988

Harlin Magee, 1105 Tuffit Ln., Austin,
TX 78753   (512) 339-1305

Joe Santos, 907 N. Blvd., University City,
TX 78217   (512) 828-6661

Bettijane Schoeffler, 1117 Willknox, Galveston,
TX 77551   (409) 744-3022

Olivia Trevino, 1104 Gardenia (rear), McAllen,
TX 78501   (512) 783-5303

Dee Vetrone, 29526 Brookchase, Spring,
TX 77386   (713) 298-5166

Sundra Walker, 9002 Parkhill Forest, Houston,
TX 77088   (713) 820-4349

Wanona Wellspring, 6206 Shadow Bend, Austin,
TX 78745   (512) 443-2663

Lois Werner, 1899 Westlake Dr., Austin,
TX 78746   (512) 328-0098

Utah

State Licensing: 600 hours or 1,000-hour apprentice-ship

National Certification Exam not accepted

Schools:

#290 Myotherapy Institute of Utah
3350 South 2300 East
Salt Lake City, UT 84109
(801) 484-7624 or (800) HEAL-YOU

HOURS OF TRAINING: 600 (30 credits)

DURATION OF COURSE: minimum of two 10-week quarters

DAY/EVENING/WEEKEND: day and evening programs available

COST: Application fee $25, registration fee $100, tuition $150 per credit ($4,500 for 600 hours)

FINANCIAL AID: Contact the school for information about financial aid and payment plans.

YEAR FOUNDED: 1987

ACCREDITATIONS/APPROVALS: ACCSCT, IMF, Utah Department of Rehabilitation, Veterans' Administration

MODALITIES AND SUBJECTS: survey of bodywork modalities, acutherapy, polarity, shiatsu, Touch for Health, infant massage, executive mini-massage, cryotherapy, hydrotherapy, kinesiology, pathology, basic study skills, practice building and Utah law, psychology for the massage therapist, first aid/CPR, t'ai chi, plus six electives (choose from advanced shiatsu, advanced Touch for Health, sports massage, bookkeeping, marketing, nutrition and herbology, reflexology, spinal touch therapy, trigger point therapy)

UNIQUE ASPECTS OF SCHOOL OR CURRICULUM: The school's Center for Advanced Therapeutic Studies is conducting a continuing research project to quantify the effectiveness of various bodywork modalities. The school also offers a "distance" massage training consisting of videotapes, audio tapes and printed material for students who wish to learn massage therapy at home.

ADVANCED PROGRAMS: 600-hour advanced program includes clinical pathology, joint pathology, Oriental modalities, spinal touch, applied kinesiology, organo body balancing, cranial therapy, nutritional therapy, homeopathy, clinical practice lab, electives and research studies

#291 Utah College of Massage Therapy
25 South 300 East
Salt Lake City, UT 84111
(801) 521-3330

HOURS OF TRAINING: 712

DURATION OF COURSE: six months days, one year evenings

COST: $5,112 day program or $4,812 evening program including course manuals and clinic uniform

FINANCIAL AID: Pell grants, Federal Family Education Loan Program, Vocational Rehabilitation, Veterans' Benefits

YEAR FOUNDED: 1986

ACCREDITATIONS/APPROVALS: COMTAA, ACCET

MODALITIES AND SUBJECTS: Esalen, shiatsu, acupressure, Touch for Health, trigger point therapy, sports massage, Russian sports massage, injury massage, proprioceptive neuromuscular facilitation, craniosacral bodywork, on-site, infant massage, deep tissue bodywork, Feldenkrais, body mechanics, medical terminology, pathology, educational kinesiology, Russian classical massage, hydrotherapy, Qigong, t'ai chi, yoga, anatomical massage, body energy techniques, client prospecting, reflexology, first aid/CPR, AIDS awareness, professional development

Vermont

No State licensing

Schools:

#292 Body Music
41 Main St.
Burlington, VT 05401
(802) 860-2814

HOURS OF TRAINING: 400

IN-CLASS HOURS: 296

DURATION OF COURSE: six week-long modules over a two-year period

COST: $2,800

FINANCIAL AID: Vermont Student Assistance grants available to Vermont residents.

YEAR FOUNDED: 1989

GRADUATES PER YEAR (APPROX.): 12

MODALITIES AND SUBJECTS: inclusive attention, kinesiology, developmental patterns, language patterns, feet, backs, pelvis and shoulders, heads, brain massage, perception, dealing with emotions, vibrational physics, practicum

UNIQUE ASPECTS OF SCHOOL OR CURRICULUM: The program trains practitioners in Resonant Kinesiology, a style of bodywork based on the educational rather than medical model. It uses touch, sound and movement to evoke change, growth and healing.

#293 Vermont Institute of Massage Therapy
93 College St.
Burlington, VT 05401
(802) 862-1111

HOURS OF TRAINING: 234

DURATION OF COURSE: 9 months days, 12 months evenings

COST: $2,600

FINANCIAL AID: State aid through Vt. Student Asst. Corp.

YEAR FOUNDED: 1986

GRADUATES PER YEAR (APPROX.): 25 to 30

MODALITIES AND SUBJECTS: advanced massage, reflexology, pressure points, small business preparation, deep relaxation

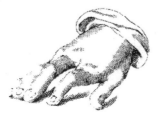

Virginia

No State licensing

Schools:

#294 Fuller School of Massage Therapy
3500 Virginia Beach Blvd., #100
Virginia Beach, VA 23452
(804) 340-7132

HOURS OF TRAINING: 200 to 500

DURATION OF COURSE: 5½ to 7 months, 2 mornings or 2 evenings per week

COST: 200 hours $1,650 including two required books;

FINANCIAL AID: approved for veterans' training, payment plans

YEAR FOUNDED: 1983

GRADUATES PER YEAR (APPROX.): 25

MODALITIES AND SUBJECTS: reflexology, hydrotherapy, myofascial and deep tissue techniques, Oriental massage, acupressure, sports massage, myotherapy and neuromuscular therapy, on-site, range of motion, therapeutic stretches, body mechanics, CPR/first aid, business management and professional ethics

UNIQUE ASPECTS OF SCHOOL OR CURRICULUM: class size is limited to 16, with 2 instructors, for very personalized attention.

ADVANCED PROGRAMS: Up to 300 hours of advanced training may be taken as individual courses — advanced anatomy and physiology, mind/body integrative therapy, marketing/business practice, hydrotherapy, advanced sports massage, injury assessment and therapy, myofascial release, Oriental massage, medicinal herbs/aromatherapy/nutrition, integration of clinical skills. 300-hour advanced certificate is awarded for completion of all advanced course work.

CONTINUING EDUCATION: Advanced programs may be taken individually as continuing education.

#295 The Reilly School of Massotherapy
P.O. Box 595
67th Street And Atlantic Ave.
Virginia Beach, VA 23451
(804) 428-0446

HOURS OF TRAINING: 225 or 600

DURATION OF COURSE: 225-hour program takes 7 to 8 months evenings and weekends; 600-hour course takes six months full-time, longer part-time.

COST: 225 hours $1,550; 600 hours $3,995

FINANCIAL AID: payment plans, tuition reduction, scholarship, work-study, veterans' benefits

YEAR FOUNDED: 1987

GRADUATES PER YEAR (APPROX.): 40

MODALITIES AND SUBJECTS: history of massage, sports massage, integrative massage, Jin Shin Do, foot reflexology, therapeutic touch, body/mind integration, hydrotherapy, professional ethics, Cayce home remedies, clinical experience/practicum, dreams and meditation, biofeedback and visualization, t'ai chi, yoga, introductions to Rolfing, osteopathy, acupuncture, kinesiology, polarity, and cranial-sacral therapy

UNIQUE ASPECTS OF SCHOOL OR CURRICULUM: Included in the 600-hour program is a holistic program based on the philosophy of healing found in the Edgar Cayce readings.

CONTINUING EDUCATION: Cayce/Reilly massage, Jin Shin Do, other programs as scheduled.

#296 Richmond Academy of Massage
2004 Bremo Rd., suite 102
Richmond, VA 23226
(804) 282-5003

HOURS OF TRAINING: 208 classroom hours plus approximately 300 hours outside class

DURATION OF COURSE: six months, two evenings per week and some Saturdays

COST: $2,000

FINANCIAL AID: payment plan

YEAR FOUNDED: 1987

ACCREDITATIONS/APPROVALS: approved for veterans' benefits

MODALITIES AND SUBJECTS: sports massage, geriatric massage, shiatsu, trigger point therapy, on-site

#297 Virginia School of Massage
P.O. Box 2187
Charlottesville, VA 22902
(804) 293-4031

HOURS OF TRAINING: 500

DURATION OF COURSE: 18 months or one year accelerated

DAY/EVENING/WEEKEND: day and evening programs available

COST: $3,750

FINANCIAL AID: some partial scholarships, payment plans

YEAR FOUNDED: 1989

GRADUATES PER YEAR (APPROX.): 40

MODALITIES AND SUBJECTS: deep tissue work, myofascial release bodywork, kinesiology, building communication skills, ethical and successful business practices

Washington

State Licensing: 500 hours

National Certification Exam accepted

Approved out-of-state schools:

American Institute of Massage, Costa Mesa CA
Atlanta School of Massage, Atlanta GA
Bancroft School of Massage, Worcester MA
Bonnie Prudden, Tucson AZ (see Trigger Point)
Boulder School of Massage, Boulder CO
Colorado Institute of Massage, Manitou Springs CO
Colorado School of Healing Arts, Evergreen CO
Connecticut Center for Massage, Newington CT
Desert Institute of Healing Arts, Tucson AZ
East-West College, Portland OR
The Feldenkrais Guild, P.O. Box 489, Albany OR
Health Enrichment Center, Lapeer MI
Heartwood Center, Garberville CA
International Professional School, San Diego CA
Mueller College, San Diego CA
Myotherapy Institute of Utah, Salt Lake City UT
New Mexico Academy, Santa Fe NM
New Mexico School, Albuquerque NM
New Perspectives Institute, Seattle WA
Oregon School of Massage, Portland OR
The Rolf Institute, Boulder CO
Dr. Jay Scherer's Academy, Santa Fe NM
Swedish Institute, New York NY

Schools:

#298 Alexandar School of Natural Therapeutics
4032 Pacific Ave.
Tacoma, WA 98408
(206) 473-1142

HOURS OF TRAINING: 600

DURATION OF COURSE: 6 months days, 10 months half-days or evenings (plus some weekend seminars)

COST: $5,800

FINANCIAL AID: payment plans, Department of Vocational Rehabilitation, Veterans Administration, Employment Security, Labor and Industries retraining programs

YEAR FOUNDED: 1982

MODALITIES AND SUBJECTS: shiatsu, on-site, somassage, sports massage, medical massage, deep tissue massage, joint mobilization, passive, active, active assistive and resistive exercises, kinesiology, Barnenieff Movement Fundamentalism, aromatherapy, hydrotherapy, nutrition, palpation skills, body psychology, student clinic, practice management and business practice

#299 Bellevue Massage School
15600 NE 8th, suite B1214
Bellevue, WA 98008
(206) 641-0848

HOURS OF TRAINING: 660

COST: $5,100

YEAR FOUNDED: 1977

UNIQUE ASPECTS OF SCHOOL OR CURRICULUM: Classes are kept to a maximum of 15 for personalized instruction. Introductory programs are offered, and cost is applied to full program tuition.

#300 The Bodymind Academy
12623 NE 110th St.
Kirkland, WA 98033
(206) 367-9060

HOURS OF TRAINING: 619

COST: $4,800

FINANCIAL AID: payment plans

MODALITIES AND SUBJECTS: sports massage, neuromuscular therapy, trigger point, medical treatment massage, injury treatment, shiatsu, deep tissue, myofascial, reciprocal inhibition, proprioceptive neuromuscular facilitation, learning processes, medical terminology, case study internship program, client assessment and charting, emotional release during massage, abuse and the body, kinesiology, palpation, self-care, AIDS trainings, first aid/CPR, laws, ethics, insurance billing, practice management and professionalism

UNIQUE ASPECTS OF SCHOOL OR CURRICULUM: The training incorporates emotional sensitivity, medical knowledge and bodywork modalities into a healing process that is grounded in experiencing touch as a catalyst for healing in your own body.

ADVANCED PROGRAMS: The school also offers certification programs in Shiatsu, Counseling Hypnotherapy, and Breathwork. Completion of all four core programs is the first step toward certification as a BodyMind Practitioner.

#301 The Brenneke School of Massage
160 Roy St.
Seattle, WA 98109
(206) 282-1233

HOURS OF TRAINING: 650

DURATION OF COURSE: one year

DAY/EVENING/WEEKEND: day and evening programs available

COST: $5,750

FINANCIAL AID: Pell grants, Stafford Loans, PLUS loans, DVR, Commission for the Blind, Veterans Administration, Employment security, Labor and Industries Retraining program, payment plans

YEAR FOUNDED: 1974

ACCREDITATIONS/APPROVALS: COMTAA, ACCET, Washington Workforce Training and Education Coordinating Board, approved for CEU's for Certified Athletic Trainers

PREPARATION FOR OUT-OF-STATE LICENSING EXAM: Ohio

MODALITIES AND SUBJECTS: on-site, hygiene, record keeping, ethics and professional development, kinesiology, pathology, sports massage, myofascial or trigger point work, AIDS education, student clinic, treatment clinic, case studies, business, hydrotherapy, plus electives.

Electives may include evaluation and treatment of thoracic outlet and carpal tunnel syndrome, naturopathic hydrotherapy, advanced business seminar, therapeutic touch, connective tissue massage, Hellerwork, polarity, manual lymphatic drainage, infant massage, Reiki, shiatsu, cranio-sacral, foot reflexology, common running injuries, Progoff Intensive Journal, somassage, lomi lomi and loku lomi, herbology, naturopathic medicine, cadaver anatomy, advanced sports massage.

ADVANCED PROGRAMS: 264-hour Clinical Intern program (hospital-based massage), connective tissue massage, manual lymphatic drainage, sports massage

CONTINUING EDUCATION: shiatsu, foot reflexology, herbology, pregnancy massage, lomi lomi, infant massage, connective tissue massage, running injuries, therapeutic touch, evaluation and treatment of common thoracic outlet and carpal tunnel syndromes — courses may vary; contact school for current listings.

#302 Brian Utting School of Massage
900 Thomas St.
Seattle, WA 98109
(206) 292-8055

HOURS OF TRAINING: 1,100 including 300 hours externship

IN-CLASS HOURS: 800

DURATION OF COURSE: 12 months

DAY/EVENING/WEEKEND: day and evening programs available

COST: $5,500

FINANCIAL AID: payment plan

YEAR FOUNDED: 1982

ACCREDITATIONS/APPROVALS: COMTAA, Veterans' Administration

PREPARATION FOR OUT-OF-STATE LICENSING EXAM: Oregon

GRADUATES PER YEAR (APPROX.): 125

MODALITIES AND SUBJECTS: deep tissue techniques, connective tissue massage, NMT, sports massage, circulatory massage, pregnancy massage, movement, hydrotherapy, pathology, cadaver anatomy, injury evaluation and treatment, professional ethics, communication skills, business skills and marketing, student clinic, community internship

CONTINUING EDUCATION: shiatsu, Thai massage, manual lymphatic drainage, deep tissue, onsen; contact school for current listings.

#303 Inland Massage Institute
W. 1717 Francis Ave., suite 103
Spokane, WA 99205
(509) 328-3116

HOURS OF TRAINING: 624

DURATION OF COURSE: one year

DAY/EVENING/WEEKEND: day and evening programs available

COST: $4.600

FINANCIAL AID: payment plans, Department of Labor and Industries, Division of Vocational Rehabilitation, Veterans' Administration, Commission for the Blind

YEAR FOUNDED: 1985

GRADUATES PER YEAR (APPROX.): 70

MODALITIES AND SUBJECTS: kinesiology, pathology, prenatal and infant massage, sports massage, acupressure, therapeutic touch, reflexology, on-site, clinical massage, hydrotherapy, business, ethics, psychology, nutrition, exercise, marketing, CPR/first aid

UNIQUE ASPECTS OF SCHOOL OR CURRICULUM: Credit may be awarded for prior massage education. Clinical massage and pathology are emphasized.

#304 New Perspectives Institute
Northwest Hellerwork
3418 Densmore Ave. North
Seattle, WA 98103
(206) 632-1160 or (800) 243-5194

HOURS OF TRAINING: 1,250

DURATION OF COURSE: 6 2-week intensives over a period of 18 months

COST: $12,850

YEAR FOUNDED: 1979

ACCREDITATIONS/APPROVALS: WA State Workforce Training, Ed. Coordinating Board

GRADUATES PER YEAR (APPROX.): 16 to 20 in each 18-months cycle

UNIQUE ASPECTS OF SCHOOL OR CURRICULUM: Hellerwork is a system of structural bodywork that integrates movement education, energetics and dialogue. It is based on the inseparability of body, mind and spirit, and it emphasizes self-awareness and balance. Graduates of this training are prepared for the Washington Massage Licensing Exam and are also certified Hellerwork Practitioners.

ADVANCED PROGRAMS: through Hellerwork, Inc. (see listing in Bodywork section)

CONTINUING EDUCATION: Somatics

#305 Seattle Massage School
7120 Woodlawn Ave. NE
Seattle, WA 98115
(206) 527-0807

5005 Pacific Highway E, suite 20
Fife, WA 98424
(206) 926-1435

2721 Wetmore Ave.
Everett, WA 98201
(206) 339-2678

HOURS OF TRAINING: day and evening program 891 (66 credits); optional evening program 628 (51 credits)

DURATION OF COURSE: 11 to 18 months

COST: 66-credit program $7,990, 51-credit program $6,790

FINANCIAL AID: federal Pell grants, Stafford loans, PLUS/SLS loans, veterans benefits

YEAR FOUNDED: 1974

ACCREDITATIONS/APPROVALS: COMTAA, ACCET

GRADUATES PER YEAR (APPROX.): 175 Seattle campus, 110 Everett campus, 150 Tacoma campus

MODALITIES AND SUBJECTS: pathology, professional development and business skills, first aid/CPR, AIDS training, treatments for specific injuries, hospital internship, chronic pain, clinical practice and treatment, hydrotherapy, Maniken anatomy, kinesiology, deep tissue, trigger point, postural balancing, polarity, sports massage, holistic healing principles, student clinic, communication and learning skills, teaching assistant program

UNIQUE ASPECTS OF SCHOOL OR CURRICULUM: Originally in Seattle, the school began adding branches in 1991 and anticipates additional locations in the future.

CONTINUING EDUCATION: contact school

**#306 Soma Institute of Neuromuscular
        Integration
        730 Klink Rd.
        Buckley, WA 98321
        (206) 829-1025**

HOURS OF TRAINING: 580

DURATION OF COURSE: 6 months

COST: $9,000 (2% discount for full payment)

FINANCIAL AID: payment plan

YEAR FOUNDED: 1978 (1986 current owner)

GRADUATES PER YEAR (APPROX.): 6 to 10

MODALITIES AND SUBJECTS: Massage program includes kinesiology, psychology for the bodyworker, remedial exercise, joint mobilization, pathology and clinical practice. Soma training includes myofascial anatomy and physiology, skeletal anatomy and structural integration

UNIQUE ASPECTS OF SCHOOL OR CURRICULUM: Soma neuromuscular integration is a system of 10-session bodywork which accomplishes structural and emotional changes through deep tissue manipulation of the fascial system of the body. Graduates are trained both as licensed massage therapists and as Soma practitioners.

CONTINUING EDUCATION: contact school

**#307 S.W. Washington Massage Therapy Center
        School and Clinic
        5601 N.E. St. Johns
        Vancouver, WA 98661
        (206) 969-2210**

HOURS OF TRAINING: 700

IN-CLASS HOURS: 550

DURATION OF COURSE: one year

DAY/EVENING/WEEKEND: day and evening programs available

COST: $4,750

FINANCIAL AID: payment plan

YEAR FOUNDED: 1984

ACCREDITATIONS/APPROVALS: private vocational school association

PREPARATION FOR OUT-OF-STATE LICENSING EXAM: Oregon

GRADUATES PER YEAR (APPROX.): 30

MODALITIES AND SUBJECTS: kinesiology, reflexology, infant massage, on-site, russian massage, connective tissue massage, Touch for Health, sports massage, deep tissue, body-mind (pain control and stress management) techniques, history of massage, hygiene,

communication skills, hydrotherapy, community involvement, clinic practice, pathology, internship, independent study

UNIQUE ASPECTS OF SCHOOL OR CURRICULUM: small class size for individual attention; emphasis on medical massage

**#308 Spectrum Center School of Massage
        1001 N. Russell Rd.
        Snohomish, WA 98290
        (206) 334-5409 or (800) 801-9451**

HOURS OF TRAINING: 534 plus 100 hours outside class

DURATION OF COURSE: 10 months

DAY/EVENING/WEEKEND: day and evening programs available

COST: $4,350

FINANCIAL AID: payment plans

YEAR FOUNDED: 1981

ACCREDITATIONS/APPROVALS: vocational rehabilitation

GRADUATES PER YEAR (APPROX.): 36

MODALITIES AND SUBJECTS: pathology, kinesiology, lymphatic drainage, medical terminology, on-site, study skills, human behavior, hydrotherapy, business practices, clinical treatments, deep tissue, trigger point, Cyriax, muscle energy, polarity, pregnancy massage, sports massage, AIDS

UNIQUE ASPECTS OF SCHOOL OR CURRICULUM: All teachers have at least 7 years teaching experience. Small class size and use of teaching assistants allows for individualized instruction.

CONTINUING EDUCATION: contact school

**#309 Tri-City School of Massage
        26 E. Third Ave
        Kennewick, WA 99336
        (509) 586-6434
        (school located in Southeast Washington)**

HOURS OF TRAINING: 850

IN-CLASS HOURS: 576

DURATION OF COURSE: approx. six months, coursework two evenings per week

COST: $3,800 includes books

YEAR FOUNDED: 1968

ACCREDITATIONS/APPROVALS: COMTAA

GRADUATES PER YEAR (APPROX.): 14

MODALITIES AND SUBJECTS: connective tissue, positional release, reflexology, sports massage, acupressure, magnetic therapy, massage in pregnancy, infant massage, iridology, on-site, health and hygiene, pathology, hydrotherapy, first aid/CPR, AIDS awareness, thesis, clinical application, business and professional ethics, applied anatomy and kinesiology, medical gymnastics, body mechanics

Wisconsin

No State licensing

Schools:

#310 Aesthetics University
2457 N. Mayfair Rd., suite 204
Wauwatosa, WI 53226
(414) 259-5115 or (800) 377-5115

Contact the school for program information.

#311 Balanced Touch Institute of Massage
N-7576 Timber Dr.,
Rib Lake, WI 54470
(715) 427-3369

No catalogue

HOURS OF TRAINING: 500

DURATION OF COURSE: 2 years, one evening per week

YEAR FOUNDED: 1988

GRADUATES PER YEAR (APPROX.): 12

MODALITIES AND SUBJECTS: therapeutic touch, craniosacral massage, shiatsu, stress reduction techniques, business

UNIQUE ASPECTS OF SCHOOL OR CURRICULUM: Two-year, once-a-week format helps students integrate massage practice into their lives prior to graduation.

#312 Blue Sky Educational Foundation
4811 W. Bradley Road
Milwaukee, WI 53223
(414) 354-5321

HOURS OF TRAINING: 500

DURATION OF COURSE: one day per week and some weekends for nine months

DAY/EVENING/WEEKEND: day and evening programs available

COST: $4,535

FINANCIAL AID: payment plan

YEAR FOUNDED: 1985

ACCREDITATIONS/APPROVALS: IMF, City of Milwaukee

MODALITIES AND SUBJECTS: learning strategies, mind-body and self care, relaxation techniques,

anatomy of a muscle spasm, ayurvedic facial massage, hatha for health professionals, clinical preceptorship, student massage journal, homeopathy, juicing for health, food as medicine and nourishment, ayurvedic cooking, medical terminology, postural analysis, techniques for low back pain, lymphatic massage, reflexology, techniques for cervical spine and upper limbs, herbal massage, sports massage, vegetarian cooking, somatic education (movement and repatterning), facial massage, treating common problems, introduction to the business world, nutrition and hyperactivity

UNIQUE ASPECTS OF SCHOOL OR CURRICULUM: Blue Sky is a non-profit organization committed to a sustainable future and to emotional, physical and spiritual well-being.

CONTINUING EDUCATION: Ohashiatsu, meditation, Reiki, on-site, sports massage level two, somatics level two, t'ai chi

#313 Capri College
6414 Odana Road
Madison, WI 53719
(608) 274-5390 or (800) 747-8953

See listing for Capri College, Iowa

#314 Lakeside School of Natural Therapeutics
1726 N. 1st St.
Milwaukee, WI 53212
(414) 372-4345

HOURS OF TRAINING: 500

DURATION OF COURSE: 6 months days, 10½ months evenings & Saturdays

COST: $4,700

FINANCIAL AID: payment plans

YEAR FOUNDED: 1985

ACCREDITATIONS/APPROVALS: COMTAA

MODALITIES AND SUBJECTS: history of massage, clinical considerations, ethics, business practices, reflexology, sports massage, trigger point therapy, shiatsu, energy work, CPR/first aid, hydrotherapy and heliotherapy, sensitivity and professional practice issues, arthritis intervention, skin care and oils, corrective exercises

#315 Lives Unlimited School of Healing Arts
401 Wisconsin Ave.
Madison, WI 53703
(608) 256-3733

Contact the school for program information.

#316 Madison School of Massage Therapy
       6273 University Ave.
       Middleton, WI 53562
       (608) 238-7277

No Catalogue

HOURS OF TRAINING: 650

IN-CLASS HOURS: 582

DURATION OF COURSE: six months

COST: $4,175

FINANCIAL AID: payment plans, limited work-study

YEAR FOUNDED: 1993

GRADUATES PER YEAR (APPROX.): 40

MODALITIES AND SUBJECTS: pathology, kinesiology, sports massage, deep connective tissue therapy, polarity, hydrotherapy, introduction to manual lymph drainage, Reiki and myofascial release, business practices, law, ethics, self-massage, movement, CPR

ADVANCED PROGRAMS: teacher training

CONTINUING EDUCATION: contact school

Index

You can write to the author c/o

Enterprise Publishing
P.O. Box 179
Carmel, NY 10512

For your school or business to be included in subsequent editions, please send your address and phone number to Enterprise Publishing at the above address.

You can order individual copies of this book for $23.95 postpaid from Enterprise Publishing at the above address (New York State residents please add Sales Tax). Allow three to four weeks for delivery.

Discounts are available for quantity purchases. Massage and bodywork schools, massage and bodywork retail outlets and other interested institutions please write to Enterprise Publishing for wholesale discounts.

Distribution to bookstores and the book trade is by Independent Publishers Group, 814 N. Franklin St., Chicago, IL 60610 and major industry wholesalers.

The information in this book was accurate, to the best of the author's and publisher's knowledge, as of January 1, 1995. Please consult with the organization or company directly before relying on the accuracy of any information.